Nutrition and its Disorders

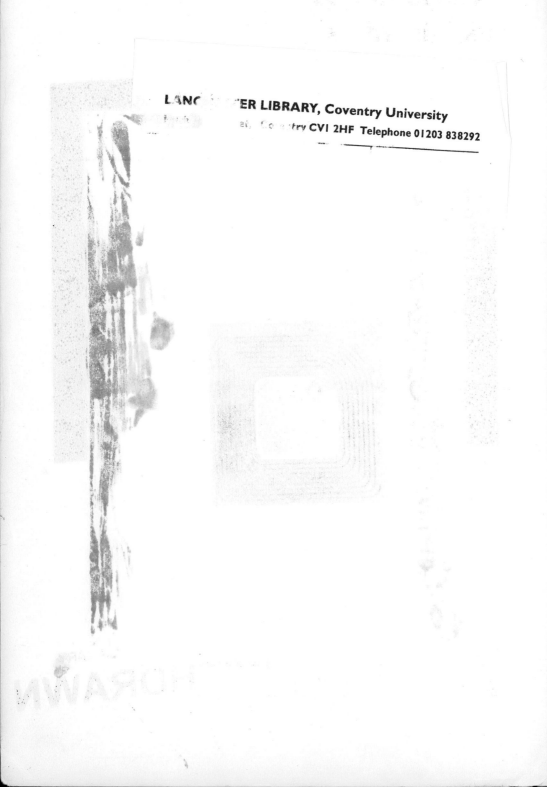

Nutrition and its Disorders

Donald S. McLaren

MD (Edin) PhD (Lond) FRCP (Edin) DTM & H (Eng)
Reader in Clinical Nutrition, Department of Medicine, Royal Infirmary, Edinburgh, UK;
Formerly Professor of Clinical Nutrition, and Director, Nutrition Research Program,
School of Medicine, and Associate in the School of Public Health,
American University of Beirut, Lebanon

Michael M. Meguid

MB (Lond) PhD (MIT) FRACS FACS
Professor of Surgery and Director, Surgical Nutrition Service, University Hospital, State
University of New York, Syracuse, USA

FOURTH EDITION

CHURCHILL LIVINGSTONE
EDINBURGH LONDON MELBOURNE AND NEW YORK 1988

CHURCHILL LIVINGSTONE
Medical Division of Longman Group UK Limited

Distributed in the United States of America by
Churchill Livingstone Inc., 1560 Broadway, New York,
N.Y. 10036, and by associated companies, branches
and representatives throughout the world.

First Edition 1972
Second Edition 1976
Third Edition 1981
Fourth Edition 1988

ISBN 0-443-03782-5

British Library Cataloguing in Publication Data
McLaren, Donald S.
Nutrition and its disorders.—4th ed.
1. Nutrition
I. Title II. Meguid, Michael M.
613.2   TX353

Library of Congress Cataloging-in-Publication Data
McLaren, Donald Stewart.
 Nutrition and its disorders.

Includes bibliographies and index.
1. Nutrition disorders. 2. Nutrition.
I. Meguid Michael M. II. Title. [DNLM: 1 Nutrition Disorders.
WD 100M161n]
RC620.M25 1988   616.3'9   877.18186

Produced by Longman Singapore Publishers Pte Ltd
Printed in Singapore.

Preface to the Fourth Edition

Interest in and knowledge of nutrition as it relates to health and disease have grown at such a pace since the appearance of the third edition in 1981 that it seemed only right that two heads would prove to be better than one for the task. Moreover, there is now a balance struck between medical and surgical aspects, problems of the third world and western industrialized societies, and between age with its experience and youth with its enthusiasm!

Every part has been thoroughly read and corrected or revised where indicated. Many sections have been completely rewritten. The book is considerably larger but the style remains highly condensed so that the amount of information provided is really surprising. Many new tables and figures appear.

The book was originally written, and has been repeatedly revised and updated, out of the experience of teaching nutrition to medical students at all levels, but it has appealed to a much wider readership both within and without the health professions. Interestingly, surveys in the UK show that it is very popular for borrowing from public libraries! It should continue to prove to be an invaluable and inexpensive textbook for undergraduate students of medicine and also during their early postgraduate training.

Those who teach nutrition to medical students and to young doctors invariably have their primary specialty training in other related fields such as internal medicine, surgery, gastroenterology, paediatrics, community medicine, biochemistry, etc. and are unlikely to be fully conversant with all the latest aspects of medical nutrition. This book seeks to meet their needs and they should find the book of great assistance in planning and delivering their courses and lectures.

With these needs in mind the selection of books and articles for further reading has been enlarged as well as updated and an entirely novel feature has been included: a selection of multiple choice questions and answers.

Edinburgh   DSM
Syracuse   MMM
1988

Preface to the First Edition

Nutrition impinges on almost every aspect of medicine to a greater or lesser degree. It should form an integral part of the curriculum in physiology and biochemistry (normal nutrition), pathology, paediatrics, internal medicine and other clinical studies (primary nutritional disorders and secondary nutritional disorders) and in community medicine (nutrition in the community). This is the plan followed here and the four sections of this book bear the titles given above in brackets. The wide scope of nutrition frequently results in its being neglected or even omitted altogether from the curriculum offered to the student.

It is unrealistic to expect that departments or chairs of nutrition will be established in medical schools save in exceptional circumstances. Much of the teaching of nutrition to the medical profession goes on in the schools of hygiene or public health where contact with the mainstream of medicine in the medical school is minimal at best. However, none would deny that the education of every doctor is deficient without a good grounding in the subject and it is certainly expected of him by his patients and the public. Perforce the responsibility in this matter lies largely with the teachers in the disciplines mentioned above and it is with their needs and interests in mind that the present text has been written to provide a progressive approach to the integrated teaching of the subject.

Although this book has been written out of the experience gained during ten years of teaching in a medical school many others concerned with human health and welfare will find nutritional aspects of their disciplines covered here.

1972   DSM

Contents

I

Normal nutrition

'*Der Mensch ist was er isst*'—Man is what he eats
LUDWIG FEUERBACH (1804–1872)

1. INTRODUCTION

The dictum quoted above makes a very good starting point in our consideration of nutrition. Coming from one of the nineteenth century philosophers of materialism, who aroused the enthusiasm of Marx and Engels, it was of course meant in a philosophical sense originally. It is nevertheless true that all the elements of which the body is composed derive from the food eaten, together with the air breathed.

One of the most remarkable things about nutrition, so common-place that it is hardly given a thought, is the fact that there is no such thing as an ideal diet. Any of the almost infinite variety of diets composed of foodstuffs cultivated locally and consumed in amounts to satisfy hunger throughout the entire history of mankind and all over the world, has proved capable of meeting all of the complex nutritional requirements of man for normal growth, healthy life under widely varying conditions and successful continuity of the species. It almost seems that under these circumstances knowledge of nutrition is superfluous. Man eats for only three reasons: to satisfy hunger, from custom and for pleasure. None of these relates to the nutrient content of the food. However, few live throughout their lives in such an idyllic state, and nutrition is of all-pervasive importance throughout the lifespan of man, as we shall see.

In the strictest sense nutrition is a process and may be defined as *the process by which the organism utilizes the nutrients in food*. *Nutriture*, or more commonly *nutritional status*, is the state of the body produced by the process and results from the balance between the supply of nutrients on the one hand and the expenditure by the organism on the other.

The process of nutrition is a complicated one involving digestion, absorption, transport, storage, metabolism and elimination of the many constituents that make up the very varied diets which we call our food. All of this has as its purpose the *maintenance of life, growth, reproduction, normal functioning of organs* and *production of energy*. Through the complex interrelationships of man with his food, human nutrition cannot be considered in isolation, but must be related to the growing, processing, marketing and consumption of food, as well as to economics, sociology, demography and even politics!

Conceptually it is helpful to consider nutrition in the context of an Agent-Host-Environment interaction system. This concept is visualized in Figure 1 and applied to the interacting elements involved in nutrition. The *human body* is the Host; that part of the environment we normally consume is *food*. The Agent in nutrition is that part of food which nourishes and the term *Nutriment* is applied to this. Food and nutriment are not synonymous; not everything in food nourishes the body, for example fibre (p. 32), additives (p. 20) and toxins (p. 23).

Nutriment may be divided into *macro-* and *micronutrients* (Fig. 2) according to the amounts consumed. Macronutrients comprise the bulk of any diet and consist of carbohydrates (p. 31), fats (p. 33) and proteins (p. 34). They are sources of energy, comprise most of the body structure and none is essential for the body in itself but only for what it yields on digestion (i.e. glucose and other monosaccharides, fatty acids and glycerol, and amino acids respectively).

Vitamins are non-energy producing organic compounds occurring naturally in food and necessary for health. *Fat-soluble vitamins* (A, D, E and K) are stored by the body. *Water-soluble vitamins* (thiamin, riboflavin, niacin, pyridoxine, folic acid and vitamin B_{12} of the B group and vitamin C), with the exception of vitamin B_{12}, are little stored and most function as coenzymes.

Of the 92 natural chemical elements, more than 50 are found in human body tissue and fluids. Four of these, oxygen, hydrogen, carbon and nitrogen, make up 96 per cent of the body weight. More than half of this is oxygen and, together with hydrogen as water, accounts for three-fourths of body weight.

The remaining 4 per cent of body weight is composed of essential elements, most of which are minerals, and also traces of mineral contaminants from the environment. These elements can be divided into four groups, according to whether or not they are known to have a function and, if so, the amount required by the body.

1. *Essential macroelements* (required in amounts of 100 mg/day or more): calcium, phosphorus, sodium, potassium, chlorine, magnesium, sulphur.

2. *Essential micro- or trace elements* (required in amounts of no more than a few mg/day and sometimes only a few μg): iron, copper, cobalt, zinc, manganese, iodine, molybdenum, selenium, fluorine, chromium.

3. *Essential microelements necessary for animals but not proved for man:* tin, nickel, silicon, vanadium and most recently arsenic and possibly cadmium and lead.

4. *Trace contaminants with no known function:* mercury, barium, strontium, boron, aluminium, lithium, beryllium, rubidium, gold, silver and others.

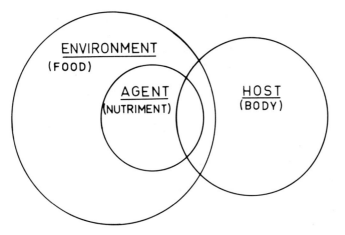

Fig. 1 Agent–Host–Environment concept applied to nutrition

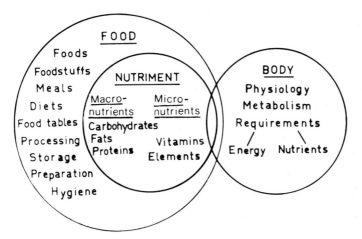

Fig. 2 Interrelationships of food, nutriment and the body in more detail

2. THE BODY

Chemical composition

Protein (16 per cent), fat (18 per cent), carbohydrate (0·7 per cent), water (60 per cent), minerals (5·2 per cent) and traces of vitamins make up the average adult body. Most fat is stored and in obesity it may be 70 per cent of the body weight. The percentage as fat is almost twice in females what it is in males (see p. 8).

Body carbohydrate is mainly glycogen, mostly in skeletal muscle (about 300 g), but in higher concentration in the liver (about 90 g). Glucose in the circulation is the labile form of carbohydrate. Carbohydrate stores are consumed within the first day or so of starvation.

Almost 10 per cent of the water can be lost but in starvation and other states of malnutrition total body water, expressed as a percentage of body weight, usually increases (see p. 99).

There is a considerable reserve of labile protein, amounting to several kilograms, in skeletal muscle available for gluconeogenesis in exercise and starvation (p. 72). The body protein varies considerably in composition in different organs although metabolically it is all in dynamic equilibrium.

About 90 per cent of body lipid is in adipose tissue, almost entirely as triglycerides. The rest is structural phospholipid in cell membranes, mitochondria and organelles; cholesterol and prostaglandins.

The adult body contains about 3·5 kg mineral, just under half of which is calcium, almost all of which is in the skeleton, and about one-quarter is phosphorus. Iodine is in high concentration in the thyroid gland and fluorine is found mostly in bones and teeth. Iron is mainly in the form of haemoglobin and also stored in the bone marrow. Most trace elements are concentrated in the liver.

The liver is the main storage site of vitamins A and B_{12}. Vitamins D and E are mainly in the fat depots.

Body compartments

On the basis of the different ways in which chemical compounds diffuse throughout the body and become diluted in the body fluids it is possible to conceive of the body as consisting of several compartments. Two main divisions are (1) adipose tissue (fat + fat cells) and (2) lean body mass (soft isssue + dense connective tissue + bone + essential lipids). About 60 per cent of the body weight is water (total body water TBW) composed of intracellular water (ICW) 35 per cent and extracellular water (ECW) 25 per cent. The latter is all the water outside the cell (plasma water 5 per cent; intersitial water and lymph 18 per cent; and transcellular water 2 per cent). The distribution of electrolytes in the major fluid compartments (Fig. 3) is of great importance in water and electrolyte physiology (p. 78) and it disorders (p. 136 and 158).

Total body water

Several substances freely diffuse throughout the body water, e.g. urea, antipyrine, tritium and deuterium. After sufficient time has been allowed for the substance to distribute itself evenly through the water of the body the concentration in the blood is determined and on the basis of the dose given and concentration in the sample the volume of the diluent (body water) can be calculated.

Extracellular water

Inulin, sucrose, sodium thiosulphate, sodium thiocyanate and bromide

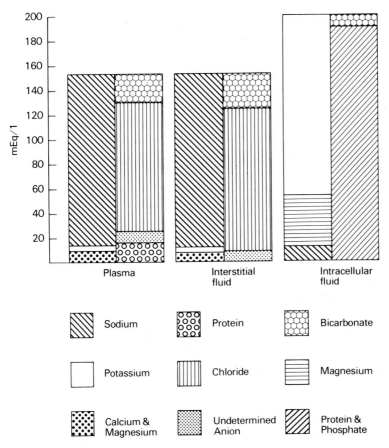

Fig. 3 Electrolyte composition of the major body fluid compartments. (Fig. 11.2 from Haycock G B 1976 In: McLaren D S, Burman D (eds) Textbook of Paediatric Nutrition. Churchill Livingstone, Edinburgh.)

(labelled isotopically), appear to occupy a 'space' which is thought to be coextensive with the extracellular space. The dilution principle is used. This space is about 18 to 24 per cent of the total body weight in health.

Cell water and cell mass

This is estimated indirectly by subtracting extracellular from total body water. On average, cells are 70 per cent water and therefore in a man of 65 kg body weight, total body water of 40l and extracellular water of 15l,

$$\text{cell water} = 25l \text{ and cell mass} = 25l \times \frac{100}{70} = 35\cdot7 \text{ kg}$$

or about 55 per cent of body weight.

Direct estimates for research purposes of cell (lean body, fat-free) mass can be made by measuring ^{40}K in a whole body counter, or N by prompt γ analysis or neutron activation; both of which elements are rather uniformly distributed in cells.

Fat

This compartment is the most variable, not only in disease, as in starvation or obesity, but also in health. It was first estimated by applying Archimedes' principle to show that draftees into the US Navy who had been professional footballers in civilian life had been wrongly registered as unfit by a medical board on the grounds that their weight was excessive for their height! It was shown that they were exceptionally muscular and had very little fat. In this method, as originally for the crown of the king of Greece, the body is weighed first in air and then under water. The ρ (density) $= m$(mass)/V (volume). V is obtained by displacement, the difference between the body weight in air and in water is the mass (m) of the water displaced. Human fat is known to have a density of 0.90 and lean body mass approximates a density of 1.10. These figures can be substituted in the formula used by Archimedes to give:

$$\frac{100}{\rho(\text{body})} = \frac{100-x}{1 \cdot 10} + \frac{x}{0 \cdot 90}$$

where x is the percentage of fat

$$x = \frac{495}{\rho(\text{body})} - 450$$

Measurement of subcutaneous fat with skinfold calipers is much more simple and can be used in the field. Standardization of the technique is difficult. By correlation of the results obtained in groups of healthy subjects using values obtained at four sites (triceps, biceps, subscapular and suprailiac) with densitometry results, formulae have been developed for estimation of toal body fat. For example, if the sum of these four skinfolds on one side of the body (the left is routinely used) is 50 mm in a subject aged 17–29 years, this denotes body fat of 19·0 per cent in the male and 26·5 per cent in the female. Standards for all age groups and both sexes have been published. There appear to be ethnic differences.

Recently it has become evident that the distribution of body fat is much more important in relation to predisposition to disease than its total amount (p. 152).

The skeleton

Skeletal mass is greater in men than women and there are racial differences.

Large frame is usually associated with large muscle mass and these together have an important influence on body composition. Simple methods for assessment of frame size have been developed and more attention is now being paid to it in relation to weight-for-height standards (p. 147).

Growth and body composition

Major changes occur in man, as in other mammals, during growth and development.

Water

Water constitutes 82 per cent of the fat-free weight at term and 72 per cent in the adult. The total body water as a percentage of body weight reaches the adult level by about 6 months of age when it is about 65 per cent.

At birth the extracellular fluid accounts for about 45 per cent of body weight. The proportion falls steeply in the first two months as the intracellular fraction rises. Although the total water reaches the adult level in a few months the proportion of extracellular water slowly falls until puberty.

Protein

Until recently it was held that growth occurred in three phases: (1) early fetal life — rapid hyperplasia (increase in cell number), (2) late fetal and early post-natal life — hyperplasia and hypertrophy (increase in cell size), and (3) later postnatal, hypertrophy and protein synthesis. Some evidence also suggested that in phase (2) undernutrition could cause permanent retardation of cell number (e.g. in the c.n.s., p. 108) or overfeeding of energy could cause permanent increase in cell number (e.g. in adipose tissue, i.e. obesity, p. 150). More strictly controlled experiments have failed to demonstrate such clear-cut phasing of growth and have cast doubt on the hypothesis implicating disordered nutrition affecting cell number.

During infancy, with the decrease in the percentage of body weight due to water, protein content of the major tissues increases from 12 per cent at birth to about 24 per cent by maturity.

Fat

The proportion of body weight due to fat increases from about 5 per cent at birth to 10 per cent or more by about 3 months of age with the decrease in body water. In the second 6 months of life the child becomes thinner and more muscular.

Minerals

During fetal life and early childhood a process of chemical maturation takes place. The total amounts of minerals in the body show a steady increase with age. Body growth accounts for most of the increase in electrolytes, iron, copper and zinc. The amount of chloride per kilogram body weight falls. For calcium more than half, for phosphorus about half, and for magnesium less than half the increment is used for increasing the concentration of these minerals in bone.

Pregnancy

Desirable weight gain during pregnancy is about 11 kg. This increase is made up of fetus (3·5 kg), placenta (0·65 kg), intersitial fluid (1·2 kg) and maternal blood (1·8 kg). The 1·6 kg unaccounted for is mostly protein and fat (see p. 84).

Old age

Body water decreases as a result of shrinkage of cells and contraction of the extracellular fluid. Bone rarefaction appears to occur universally (p. 217).

Sex

Body composition differences between the sexes are mainly due to the greater adiposity of the female (25 versus 14 per cent). The female skeleton and the musculature are also relatively lighter. Storage iron is much less in the female (p. 62).

3. FOOD

FOOD AND CULTURE

In all probability man first fed himself by gathering leaves, fruits, berries, roots, nuts and bark. Hunting developed later, for animal skins for covering as well as for food, and crop cultivation probably began in parts of the Middle East about 9000 BC.

Most men, like many animals, are omnivorous but large sections of mankind are virtually vegetarian through necessity and many individuals so from choice. For a strictly vegetarian diet to be nutritionally adequate the sources of food must be varied. Some vegetarian groups, such as Seventh Day Adventists, have enhanced longevity but this must be, at least in part, attributed to abstinence from alcohol and tobacco and healthy activities. *Veganism* is an extreme form of vegetarianism in which all animal flesh and animal products (e.g. milk, milk products and eggs) are excluded. Such a diet is deficient in vitamin B_{12}. In affluent societies, in the third world, as well as in technologically developed countries, *food fadism* has gained tremendous popularity in recent years. Much of the advice as to what is supposed to be a healthy diet on radio, television and in magazines is given by those who have no training in or understanding of the science of nutrition. In this, as in other areas the public is very gullible, usually prepared to spend large sums or go to extremes of inconvenience in the hope of achieving a long and healthy life with some oversimplified, often dangerous, 'magic bullet' type of solution of their problems. Fads about food range all the way from life-threatening, grossly deficient regimes like the systems of macrobiosis, Zen Buddhism or some liquid formulae, to the purchase of food almost exclusively from 'health food' stores to avoid all contact with chemical fertilizers, pesticides, etc. Unfortunately the standards of hygiene under these circumstances are often deficient and levels of natural contaminants can be high. The upsurge of interest and concern of the public over healthy eating is greatly to be welcomed and the medical and other concerned professionals should be sufficiently well informed and morally responsible to ensure that advice given is based on current scientific knowledge (p. 281).

No person or group of persons eats all the edible material available to them. The classification of edible matter into food and non-food has arisen as a result of many complex social, religious and economic factors. Such classification comprises a deep-seated facet of every cultural pattern, is learned by imitation in early childhood and is extremely resistant to change.

This division bears no relationship to nutritive value. The connection between nutritional deficiency disease and over-reliance on a non-nutritious food is not recognized by most people. Unfortunately improvements in diet usually take a long while before their effects are evident. It is extremely difficult to alter harmful food habits by educational means. The following is a classification of foods:

Cultural super-foods. All cultures have one or more of these. They are usually the staple and main source of energy. If it is a grain it is usually over-milled and white (wheat or maize flour, rice). Super foods have special emotional value with often semidivine status. The children of those peoples with a cutural superfood that is relatively rich in protein (wheat, millet) will have more protection against kwashiorkor (but not marasmus) than those whose super-food has a low protein content (plantian, cassava) (see p. 102).

Prestige foods. These are reserved for feasts and ceremonies and are expensive, being rich in protein. Examples include the camel hump among Bedouin Arabs, and the pig in New Guinea. In American culture the T-bone steak may be considered to be a prestige food.

Body image foods. In certain systems of thought in India, the Near East and Latin American, the body physiology is classified into 'humours', especially 'hot' and 'cold'. Foods and illnesses are similarly classified. For example diarrhoea in India is a 'hot' illness. Milk is also a 'hot' food there and consequently to the mother is a dangerous food to feed to her child with diarrhoea or during recovery. She will, however, readily use home-made acidified milk because it is categorized as 'cold'.

Sympathetic magic foods. With these foods it is believed that the magical function of appearance may affect the eater. Examples are the walnut as a brain food in Gujerat because of its convoluted appearance, and underdone steak still fed to many athletes, symbolizing energy and muscularity.

Physiological group foods. Foods may be reserved for certain groups (usually male elders) but more commonly groups are restricted with regard to eating certain foods (especially women when pregnant and lactating, and very young children). In general the restricted foodstuffs are nutritious, e.g. fish, eggs and meat, and these practices are clearly harmful nutritionally.

FOODSTUFFS

The term foodstuffs includes any article which nourishes the body (Table 1).

Table 1

A. Foodstuffs of vegetable origin

1. *Cereals.* The seeds of family Gramineae
   Examples: rice, wheat and millets
2. *Pulses* (legumes). The dry seeds of family Leguminosae
   The peas and beans (edible leguminous green pods are not pulses and will be placed under vegetable fruits)
3. *Vegetables.* These are subdivided into:
   (a) *Roots.* These come from many different families
       Examples: yams, onions, carrot
   (b) *Leaves and shoots*
   (c) *Gourds*, including pumpkin and squashes (family Cucurbitaceae)
   (d) *Vegetable fruits.* A group for vegetables not included under the above headings, they come from many families.
       Examples: tomato, ladies' fingers, fresh pods, bread fruit
4. *Nuts and seeds*, including all seeds other than cereals, pulses and condiments
   Examples: coconut, sesame seeds and buckwheat
5. *Fresh dessert fruits.*
   Examples: oranges and bananas
6. *Dried fruits.*
   Examples: dates and prunes
7. *Condiments and spices*

B. Foodstuffs of animal origin

1. Meat, birds, fish, shell-fish and eggs
2. Milk and milk products

C. Miscellaneous foodstuffs

Examples: vegetable oils, honey, sugar, yeasts, jams, mushrooms, oils, feculas, insects, and beverages

---

The staple foodstuff constitutes the main food of a community, usually one of the cereals — wheat, rice, maize and, to a lesser extent, barley, rye, oats and millets. For about 200 million people, roots such as yam, sweet potato and cassava form the staple. Smaller groups subsist on other foodstuffs. Examples include fish for Eskimos, fermented milk for some nomadic tribes and the plantain for some tribes of Africa.

No single foodstuff can provide a complete diet. Not only is it inadequate nutritionally but its low palatibility renders it inedible over any length of time. Nevertheless hundreds of millions of people, especially in south and east Asia, subsist on little else than their main staple, rice, which provides as much as 95 per cent of the total energy intake.

Cereals

Wheat (Triticum vulgare) and its preparations

Wheat is the most extensively cultivated cereal and is nearly all consumed in the form of preparations of flour, mainly breads. The protein complex gluten (a mixture of gliadin and glutelin) is present only in sufficient amount in wheat and rye to make the dough viscid, and causes it to rise when gas is liberated in the baking process, whether from natural yeast fermentation or the addition of artifical baking powder. Most bread is of this kind: unleavened breads are less common and the loaves are flat.

White bread is produced by low extraction of the flour and in Britain thiamin, iron and calcium are added although this is no longer mandatory. Much of the iron is not absorbed (p. 43). *Brown bread* is a mixture of whole wheat and white flour. *Wholemeal bread* consists only of whole wheat flour; bleaching and improving agents (p. 21) are not permitted. These three breads constitute respectively about 78, 12 and 10 per cent of the market, with white bread falling and wholemeal rising. The latter contains about three times the fibre in white bread; but even if it were to replace white bread completely the daily intake of crude fibre would only rise by about 3 g or less than 10 per cent of the total. Vegetables and fruits provide more fibre than cereals.

In many countries biscuits, cakes and confectionery, breakfast cereals and toast are other important wheat products; as are macaroni, spaghetti and vermicelli in Mediterranean countries and other parts, and chapattis in Indian communities.

Rice (Oryza sativa)

South-east Asia is the great rice producing and consuming area of the world. Rice normally eaten after husking and boiling needs to have grains of such a quality that they do not adhere into a soggy mass. Varieties are chosen that ripen early so that the sticky sugar and dextrin of the unripe grain have been converted fully into starch. Highly milled raw rice loses much of its content of the B group vitamins in the process. Light milling is preferable from the nutritional point of view and parboiling (boiling before milling of the grain) will disperse the vitamins throughout the endosperm. A policy of enrichment or reinforcement of rice with nutrients has to face many difficulties in practice and, in general, health policy should rather be one of conservation of naturally occurring nutrients. Rice is devoid of carotene and, as consumed, very low in thiamin unless parboiled.

Maize (Indian corn) (Zea mays)

This is the only cereal originating in the New World. It often grows in places unsuitable for other cereals. It may be eaten as a kind of porridge, as in parts of Africa, or as a gruel for young children. In Central America it forms pancakes or tortillas.

The main protein of maize, zein, is devoid of tryptophan and the nicotinic acid present is largely unavailable except when lime treated as in the making of tortillas. (p. 39).

Millets

These are the seeds of Graminae which are smaller than wheat or rice, and therefore difficult to prepare as food, and are usually accepted by man only where the other cereals are unobtainable. Sorghum is the largest and most often used, and in India and Africa is eaten as cakes or porridge. It is the chief cereal in Upper Egypt and Sudan where it is mixed with wheat, barley, fenegreek or beans to make a kind of bread. The protein content and nutritional quality are good.

Legumes (pulses)

Legumes tend to complement cereals nutritionally, especially with regard to essential amino acids, and the combination makes a sound basic diet. Beans or peas are the seeds of Leguminosae and are called pulses when dried. Split peas are called *dhals* in India and smaller dried peas are *grams*. Although their nutritional value is high (between 20 and 35 per cent protein) they are much more indigestible than cereal and can be consumed only in quite small quantities. Most contain substances that impair digestion, e.g. the antitrypsin of the soya bean. Soya bean and groundnut have a high fat content, and both are widely cultivated for their oils which are rich in linoleic acid. Soya bean emulsion or 'milk' has long been used in the Far East as a substitute for cow's milk.

Roots and tubers

Among those containing more than 20 per cent starch are the Irish potato, sweet potato, yams, taro and manioc (cassava). In some parts of the world these are the main article of diet although they contain only 2 per cent or even less of protein, and this often of poor amino acid quality.

The ordinary or Irish potato is a cheap crop and yields more energy/ hectare than any cereal. Protein is only about 2 per cent but of high biological value. Minerals and B vitamins and vitamin C are in small amounts but the potato is an important source as it is consumed in large amounts. The yellow forms of sweet potato contain carotene. The tubers of wild species of yam contain toxic substances but selective cultivation has produced varieties that are free of these. Certain varieties of taro keep for months and made possible the populating of Pacific Islands by long sea voyages. Some varieties are grown mainly for their leaves. Manioc grows on poor soil and is the most prolific tropical root crop and requires little cultivation. The outer coat of the root is rich in a glycoside, *linamarin*, which reacts with an enzyme, *linamarase*, to form cyanide (p. 25). The roots must be peeled and washed before cooking. Tapioca is prepared from cassava roots. The tender leaves are eaten as a vegetable in some places. They are rich in carotene.

Roots with less starch include carrot (rich in vitamin A precursors), onion, radish and turnip.

Leaves, fruits and nuts

Many leaves are good sources of vitamin C and leaves contain carotene in proportion to the depth of their green colour due to chlorophyll — both substances are involved in photosynthesis. Some attempts have been made to promote the utilization of their far from negligible protein content to combat what has been seen as a global protein shortage, but this is now generally recognized to be a misconception of the nature of the problem (p. 276).

Gourds and pumpkins contain 90 per cent or more of water and thus have little nutritional value although they have a demulcent effect with hot curries and make a pleasant salad. They are easy to grow and keep well.

Starchy fruits, such as plantain and banana, are of low protein content but as a flour may form the staple food. Nuts are seeds larger than cereal grains and with a hard shell. They are relatively indigestible and are eaten in small quantities. Nuts and seeds are much cultivated for their oils. Major sources are cottonseed, groundnut, rapeseed, sesame, sunflower and maize. Most of these are rich in polyunsaturated fatty acids and are being increasingly used for cooking in Europe and America because of the known blood cholesterol lowering effect of these acids (p. 204).

Oil is also obtained from palm nuts for cooking, notably coconut oil which has mainly saturated fatty acids and red palm oil which is rich in β-carotene. The latter is the main cooking oil in much of West Africa but is also exported from there and Indonesia for soap manufacture. Tragically, the latter country uses mainly coconut oil which is devoid of carotene, and suffers from a severe vitamin A deficiency problem (p. 109).

Fruits abound in warm climates and are usually sweet because the starch has been changed to sugar with ripening. Most are rich in ascorbic acid and carotene but provide little else of nutritional value.

Condiments, spices and beverages

The first two assist the appetite through their stimulating effect on taste and smell. The common beverages coffee, tea and cocoa contain the xanthines caffeine, tannin or theobromine, which are mildly stimulant and diuretic. A cup of coffee contains about the same amount of caffeine as, and a little less tannin than, a cup of tea. Long-term consumption has not been proved harmful and reports that coronary disease or some cancers are associated with high consumption are conflicting. Alcoholic beverages are of five kinds: beers, spirits, wines, fortified wines and strong liquors. They are nutritionally important because of their contribution to energy intake (7 kcal or 29.3 kJ/g) and because of the harmful effects of abuse (see p. 240).

Miscellaneous foodstuffs

Many other items which do not fall into any of these categories are consumed as food, often by small groups and in small amounts. Some of these are being investigated at the present time as possible sources of edible protein; among these may be mentioned algae, single cell protein and yeast.

Food of animal origin

Butcher's meat

Joints and cutlets consist of a variable amount of muscle, gristle (collagen) and fat, depending on the part of the carcass, and the age and condition of the animal. Pork, because of deposition of fat between muscle fibres, tends to be less digestible than beef or mutton. Moderate cooking improves digestibility by allowing penetration of digestive juices and making it softer to chew. Overcooking, however, coagulates protein and impairs digestibility. The fat of these meats is highly saturated.

In response to growing consumer pressure for reduction of saturated fat, farmers and the meat industry are growing animals and producing meat cuts and products that are leaner. In the West most of the poultry, much of the pork and more of the beef is produced by factory farming which converts protein mainly unacceptable to man to an acceptable form. No lessening of nutritive value has been shown.

Important taboos apply to the consumption of cetain meats, including pork by Moslems and Jews, any meat by high caste Hindus, and the slaughtering of the cow by any of the Hindu faith. In some parts other animals are eaten including the dog, the rat and the monkey.

Mammalian organs

Those commonly consumed are liver, kidney, heart, sweetbreads (thymus of young animals and pancreas), brain and tripe (stomach and intestines). The liver is espcially rich in vitamins and nucleoproteins. Sweetbreads and tripe are well digested. Brain is poorly digested and mainly valuable for its highly unsaturated fatty acids.

Milk and milk products

Everywhere these items tend to be expensive, and in most developing countries cattle do not thrive and milk is of poor yield. Transportation raises further problems. Buffaloes give a richer milk than cows and thrive on wet lowlands. Milk, preferably breast, is the ideal food for young children and has the important advantage of being liked by them and fully acceptable to their mothers. There is a high incidence of lactose intolerance among adults of some ethnic groups (p. 185).

Milk alone will support growth and development for the first 3–4 months of life. Thereafter it cannot readily be consumed in sufficient quantities to meet energy requirements and the diet must be supplemented. Both human and artificial milks are deficient in iron and vitamin D, adequate in vitamin A and rich in calcium (see p. 81).

Processed milks. These are of many kinds including unsweetened condensed (evaporated) milk, sweetened condensed, skimmed, whole milk powders, skimmed milk powders, milk powders with added sugar etc. and modified milks in which the fat is replaced by vegetable oils. All of these milks can be readily distributed and are generally safer and more convenient for household use than ordinary milk. Skimmed milk contains no vitamins A and D but is now fortified by all major agencies supplying developing countries. After the Second World War it formed a major approach adapted to the combat of childhood malnutrition and was part of the misconception underlying the 'protein fiasco' (p. 109). Fermented milks keep well in hot climates.

Butter, ghee and cheese. Butter is produced by the churning of cream and the tang is partly due to bacterial action on the protein during the process. It easily becomes rancid in warm climates.

Ghee often replaces butter in the tropics. Milk is boiled and the fats are skimmed off and again heated to remove the protein and most of the water.

Cheese consists of the proteins and fats of milk. Milk is clotted by rennet or curdled by vinegar or bacterial action. The whey is removed from the casein and fat under varying degrees of pressure, this, together with the species of bacterium used during the ripening process in a cool place, determining the type and flavour of the cheese.

Fowl

Birds like chicken and turkey that spend most of their time on the ground have tender breasts and tough legs. The reverse is true of migratory birds like snipe and woodcock. Duck, goose and other water birds have a high fat content and are less digestible. The 'white' meat of fowl has a lower saturated fat content than 'red' butcher's meat.

Eggs

Egg is a highly nutritious food. Whole egg protein has an amino acid pattern closest to the ideal for man. It is often used as reference protein and its bio-logical value (BV) is 100 (p. 37). Eggs contain no carbohydrate and are poor in niacin. Other vitamins and most minerals are in rich supply. One egg contains about 250 mg of cholesterol. Some believe that eggs should therefore be limited or even excluded in the treatment and prevention of atherosclero-sis (p. 204).

Fish

Those of cold climates contain more fat then the tropical varieties. Liver and body oils are rich in vitamins A and D. Dried fish contain 1.5 to 5 per cent of salt and 1·5 to 3 times the amount of protein present before drying. Fish flour is fat-free, odourless and almost tasteless and has been used in several countries to reinforce bread in school feeding programmes.

Fatty fish, such as mackerel, marine oils and whale and seal meat contain high levels of n-3 class polyunsaturated fatty acids that may alter blood coagulability and reduce the tendency to thrombus formation (p. 205).

Shell fish

Oysters, mussels, clams and other molluscs have little nutritional value except for their iron and iodine content. Crustaceans, e.g. lobsters, prawns and crabs, are about 18 per cent protein and make a valuable contribution to diets in the East. Some are poisonous due to infection by salmonellae and other bacteria after death, or due to poisons that accumulate during life, such as arsenic, and allergic reactions can occur.

MEALS AND DIETS

As meals follow a recurring pattern they constitute the diet and it is this that largely determines the nutritional status of individuals and communities (p. 258).

The pattern of meals varies considerably. Some groups eat virtually only once or twice a day. It is especially difficult for young children to have their needs met under these circumstances unless meals are specially prepared for them. Families usually eat at least the main meal together. When the special nutritional requirements of children are not appreciated, the older male members often eat first and alone and the women and children receive what is left. In a large family the toddler may be especially vulnerable if he is not the youngest child who will be taken care of by the mother while the older children get in first. A young child will fare badly in a situation where hands are dipped into a common dish for the main staple and a spoon will be needed to obtain the protein-rich relish. Some tribal peoples still practise prechewing of the food by the mother before giving it to the baby. Others hand feed young babies by what amounts to forced feeding and aspiration pneumonia may result.

A daily pattern of few (e.g. two) large meals common in an affluent society predisposes to excessive weight, together with hypercholesterolaemia, impaired glucose tolerance and ischaemic heart disease, perhaps through hyperlipogenesis. From the point of view of introducing change it should be realized that innovations that are likely to be acceptable will need to be time-saving. This is just what many of the newer processed foods are, but unfortunately, while they tend to add variety to the diet, they are not all of high nutritional value. When artificial milks and other commercial infant foods are available they end to oust breast-feeding and when hygiene is poor and there is ignorance of infant formulation they act as a precipitating factor in PEM (see p. 102). In affluent societies infantile obesity from overconcentrated formulae, introduction of semisolids before the 4th month, or the practice of giving a feed instead of water when the baby is thirsty (p. 150), prevalent about a decade ago, has been largely overcome by effective nutrition education of mothers.

FOOD TABLES

The physician may find them of value in both clinical and community medicine practice and in research. Thus if a patient presents with signs and symptoms suggestive of deficiency disease it is of importance to check the recent dietary history against the nutritive value of the foods being consumed. The dietary intake of communities, whether 'free living' or as 'confined groups' such as armed services, schools, orphanages, prisons, can also be studied by noting the amount of food consumed and the nutritive value of the foods and by making comparison with the usual recommended allowances. Finally, the devising of experimental and therapeutic diets neccessitates reference to food tables for the broad formulation of such diets. Chemical analysis of the diet itself will have to be carried out for precise work.

The limitations of food tables should be realized. The figures given are average values for a limited number of analyses. The range of 'normal' values may be considerable in a single place and even greater for the same item grown in different places. Water is the most variable constituent. Proximate principles—protein, fat, carbohydrate—do not vary greatly, with the exception of the fat content of meat. The energy value can usually be measured with considerable accuracy.

The vitamin and mineral contents of foods vary much more than do those of the proximate principles. Broad statements can usually be made, however, as to whether or not a diet is deficient in a certain vitamin. Minerals pose the special problems of great variability of content and the poor availability of the material in the food item; especially important in relation to iron (p. 61) and calcium (p. 60).

FOOD TECHNOLOGY

The massive food industry has developed in response to the need to feed vast numbers of town and city dwellers all over the world. Food technology has as its aim the provision of attractive and nutritious food for the consumer and the prevention of its adulteration. Quality control by analytical procedures and legislation and implementation of the necessary measures are vital steps in the process of ensuring the safety and quality of food consumed. Recently manufacturers have been quick to respond to public demand for informative labelling of foods (p. 27).

Processing

In industrialized countries about 80 per cent of all food is processed and the very lives of most of us are dependent upon this vast commercial enterprise. With proper manufacturing practice processed food can be, and almost always is, just as nutritious as the fresh variety. Appearance and taste usually are less pleasing. It is appropriate to touch on only a few aspects of this subject that relate to human nutrition, and attention will be focussed on the major cereals, wheat and rice, and some consideration given to the situation in the third world.

The grains of both these cereals have essentially the same structure. The husk or hull surrounds the grain and consists of inedible woody cellulose. It is readily removed by threshing from wheat but is fairly adherent in paddy or unhusked rice. The germ is the richest in nutrients, but vitamins are also found in the aleurone layer and to a lesser extent in the pericarp. The bran which results from milling contains varying amounts of all the structures, even including the endosperm.

Primitive methods

Crushing or grinding between stones or pounding with some form of pestle in a mortar is still used in homes by millions of people in the rural tropics. This is heavy work, often done by women, and as only the husk, the more fibrous outer coats, and plumule and radicle are removed the grain usually retains much of its nutritional value.

Flour milling

Many types of mills have been designed to produce flours or meals from wheat, rice, maize and other cereals. Stone mills have been driven by hand, cattle, wind, water and engine. Percussion and hammer mills produce a finer flour. Today most flour is produced by roller mills which are more efficient: efficient, that is, in achieving the miller's primary object of isolating and grinding the endosperm in as free a state as possible. 'Contamination' by bran spoils the colour, and bran and germ impair the baking quality. The final product is attractive but has lost much of its nutritional value.

Rice milling

This may be carried out on paddy without heat treatment to produce *white* or *raw rice*, or after the paddy has been soaked in water and steamed, when *parboiled rice* results.

In general, parboiled rice has a higher thiamin content then milled raw rice. The many varieties of rice behave differently in the milling process with greater loss of the thiamin-rich parts in some then in others, for example depending upon the thickness of the pericarp, shape of grain, moisture content. Milling beyond the removal of about 8 per cent of bran results in a sharp fall in the thiamin content of their rice.

Parboiling toughens the grain, makes the scutellum and aleurone layer more adherent and carries some of the water-soluble vitamins into the interior. There is, however, a 30 per cent loss of thiamin due to oxidation, and fermentation in prolonged soaking may increase this greatly. Washing of dirty rice has this adverse effect on vitamin content. Cooking should be done in a limited amount of water

Preservation and storage

Spoilage may be biological, by rodents, birds or insects; micro-biological from yeast, moulds and bacteria; or biochemical by enzyme action within the foodstuff. All of these processes can be retarded by manipulating the temperature, moisture, air content, etc. Precooking of meat and fish and scalding of vegetables prolong storage life. Recent developments include freeze-drying, where water is removed from a frozen product, aseptic canning of foods that have been sterilized by a high temperature, short-time process, refrigeration in transport and ionized radiation exposure of foodstuffs.

Grains should be dry and in good condition. Flours are more susceptible to bacterial and insect spoilage than the whole grains. Wholemeal flours with their richer content of nutrients store less well than white flours. Removal of fat in high milling also assists storage.

Stores must be damp-proof and, so far as possible, free from rats and insects. Humid climates increase the problems. Roots store well in sand, earth or straw.

Cold storage is of various forms. Meat and fish lose virtually none of their nutritive value. Fruits and vegetables lose only a little ascorbic acid.

Canning and bottling are generally carried out with the necessary precautions to minimize losses of vitamins from heat, oxidation and alkalinity, and the nutritive value of foodstuffs so preserved is not seriously diminished.

Drying by exposure to the sun is used extensively for the preservation of fish, meat and fruits in the tropics. Sunlight has a destructive effect on riboflavin. On the commercial scale three methods are used: (1) contact with a heated surface as roller drying of milk, (2) contact with dry heat and air, and (3) dehydration by vacuum oil technique. The latter method is superior in its preservation of vitamins in vegetables and meat and the foodstuffs are readily reconstituted with good retention of flavour and colour.

FOOD ADDITIVES

Chemicals are added to food by industry for a variety of reasons, the main examples of which are discussed below. Many countries have strict regulations as to what substances may be added to food and in many instances limits are set on maximum concentrations. In recent years governments have had to respond to pressure groups arousing alarm, largely unwarranted, in the public mind concerning the safety of food containing additives. Laboratory testing has been intensified and controls generally tightened. It may be said that, while it is virtually impossible to state categoricaly that any given additive is entirely harmless, additives at present in use have not been shown to have adverse effects in the amounts used.

Preservatives

Sulphur dioxide, sulphite and benzoic acid are now commonly used but it is not known with certainty that they are entirely innocuous. Physical, rather than chemical, methods are probably best, e.g. freezing, dehydration, sterilization by heat and, increasingly in the future, irradiation. Many countries, including the UK and USA, permit the preservation of certain foods by low level irradiation.

Colouring agents

The largest review of food colours has recently been completed in the UK and, for the first time, limits have been set for all permitted colours. The principle has been followed to restrict their use as far as possible. Another sound principle is to concentrate on preserving any natural colouring, as in such items as parsley, tomatoes, peas and beans, rather than covering up inadequacies by artificial additions.

Sweetening agents

The sweetest of the sugars found in food items is cane sugar. Saccharin is 400 times sweeter and for those who need to limit their energy intake has the advantage that it provides no energy, but as it is destroyed by heat is not used extensively by the food industry. There is inconclusive evidence that it may cause some forms of cancer; rather similar evidence years ago led to the banning of cyclamate, but there are moves being made for its return to use. Aspartame and several other intense sweeteners have been permitted in recent years.

Flavouring agents

This is the least well-defined category of additives, containing thousands of substances, natural and synthetic, many of whose chemical composition is either unknown or unstandardized. The only control at present on their use is 'good manufacturing practice'. One of these, monosodium glutamate (MSG), the salt of one of the non-essential amino acids, has a meaty flavour and has been added to stews, soups and sauces. Glutamic acid has been used for centuries to enhance flavour, especially in Chinese food. It is present in fermented soya bean curd and several plant and animal proteins are rich in it.

The so-called 'Chinese restaurant syndrome' consists of a burning sensation in the back of the neck spreading to the forearms and to the anterior thorax, accompanied by raised intraobital pressure, tightness and substernal discomfort.

Relatively low oral doses of glutamate have caused hypothalamic damage in infant mice. Baby foods are rich in natural glutamate and manufacturers have now ceased to add MSG for flavouring.

Flour improvers

These are used to 'strengthen' wheat flour and produce in baking a large or what is called 'bold' loaf. 'Agene' or nitrogen trichloride was used for many years for this purpose until it was shown that bread treated in this way produced hysterical symptoms in dogs. In the process methionine is converted into methionine sulphoximine and this appears to be the toxic substance.

Fat extenders

These are used in the manufacture of ice-cream, cakes and salad dressings, the best known being glycerol monostearate. They enable a more economical use of the fat by allowing more water to be incorporated and by stabilizing the emulsion.

Antioxidants

Natural oils and fats contain antioxidants, such as the tocopherols, that prevent the oxidative changes causing rancidity. They are often removed or destroyed in the manufacturing process. Gallic esters may be added to replace them in biscuit and cake manufacture.

Nitrates and nitrites

These compounds are widely distributed in soil, water and plants. Nitrates are converted to nitrites by bacterial action in the body. High levels of nitrite cause acute toxicity from the conversion of haemoglobin to methaemoglobin, especially in infants, with cyanosis, resulting in respiratory and circulatory failure and possible death. Nitrites are known to give rise in the body to *nitrosamines*, a group of compounds that has been shown to be carcinogenic in animals. The most important nitrosamine in food is thought to be n-nitrosopyrrolidine. Sodium nitrite is used to cure meat and poultry, processed fish and some cheeses. It gives cured meats their characteristic colour and flavour and, more importantly, inhibits the growth of *Clostridium botulinum* and prevents botulism (p. 29). Recent evidence, not accepted by some, that nitrite itself is carcinogenic in animals, thus poses an as yet unresolved dilemma for legislators and food industry alike. Even so only about 20 per cent of nitrite intake comes from cured meats and proposed legislation would not affect the other 80 per cent.

CHEMICALS USED IN AGRICULTURE

Weeds, insects, rodents and animal parasites require control if farm yields are to be high. Improper use of chemicals can result in contamination of food destined for man. There is a growing lobby for chemical-free farming.

Pesticides and weed killers

The use of these chemicals is mainly hazardous to farmers and food industry workers. Scores of such compounds are in use, prominent among them being DDT (dichlorodiphenyl trichlorethane), BHC (benzene hexachloride) and dieldrin, all organochloride insecticides.

After 25 years of incalculable service to man, DDT has been banned or restricted in its use. The molecule is very stable and its rate of biodegradation is slow in warm-blooded animals, and it appears to be hardly metabolized at all in cold-blooded creatures. It thus tends to pass up a food chain, eventually to man. Alternative insecticides are clearly desirable but none is as cheap and few as safe to use. Millions of lives have been saved annually by its use in controlling the vectors of such diseases as malaria, typhus, plague and trypanosomiasis. Not a single death has been attributed to DDT poisoning nor has a clinical syndrome of chronic DDT poisoning been recognized even among some workers heavily exposed to it for 20 years.

Parathion on barley and mercury (p. 26) dusted on wheat for planting to prevent fungal disease have caused fatal toxicity.

Antibiotics.

In addition to being used to treat infectious diseases in farm animals, they have been incorporated into feed to promote rapid growth in a way that is ill-understood. Direct harmful effects to man are not known, but indirectly this has resulted in the development of bacterial resistance, e.g. of strains of *Salmonella typhimurium* and *Escherichia coli* that are human pathogens, and clinical cases of infection, especially among immunocompromised patients and the elderly have been rising alarmingly in recent years.

Hormones

Anabolic steroids — androgens, oestrogens, and progestogens — both natural and synthetic increase muscle mass in animals, as they do in athletes. Controlled use probably causes no harm to the human consumer, but there is much abuse currently and it is difficult to justify their use when meat production is grossly surplus to need. The EEC has proposed a ban on hormone implants effective from January 1988.

DIETARY TOXINS

Goitrogens

Many dietary factors have been experimentally shown to cause enlargement of the thyroid, but none has been proved to be responsible for goitre in man. Most important among these are probably cyanoglycosides, the thiocyanates, and derivatives of 2-thiooxazolidone. The two last are involved in the goitrogenic activity of Brassicae and other members of the family Cruciferae. The most potent of all naturally occurring goitrogens is probably *goitrin*, found in seeds of many Brassicae and edible portions of turnip as a precursor, *progoitrin*. Much of the goitrogenic activity that may pass into milk from animal feed is destroyed by scalding and freezing.

Seafood toxins

About 100 fish families have been reported to be toxic. It has been estimated that 60 to 70 per cent of all poisoning by seafood takes place in Japan, where marine organisms contribute as much as 10 per cent of the total food supply. Numerically, four types of poisoning are the most important: ciguatera, moray eel, scombroid, and puffer fish.

Favism

Ingestion of fresh or uncooked broad or fava bean, *Vicia faba*, may cause this dramatic syndrome with haemolytic anaemia. The responsible principle has not been identified.

This agent acts as an oxidant in individuals with deficiency of the enzyme glucose-6-phosphate dehydrogenase (G6PD) in red cells. This enzyme plays a critical role in the oxidative pathways of glucose metabolism, from which the erythrocyte obtains much of its energy. In these individuals there is consequent impairment of reduction of NADP to NADPH resulting in a low level of reduced glutathione which normally prevents denaturation of haemoglobin and fragility of the red cell. These individuals are haematologically normal until exposed to the oxidant. G6PD deficiency is transmitted as a sex-linked trait and occurs in about 10 per cent of North American black males who have enzyme levels 7 to 15 per cent of normal. It may also occur in populations in the Far and Middle East, Sicily and Sardinia, and in Sephardic Jews. The degree of deficiency tends to be more severe than in blacks, and these groups commonly react to fava bean while blacks rarely do so.

Younger red cells are apparently more resistant to haemolysis, as patients uaually recover once the intitial attack of acute haemolysis is over.

Mycotoxins

Ergotism. Claviceps purpurea is a fungus that commonly infects rye, and less often other cereals such as wheat, barley and oats. The mature sclerotium of the fungus is the source of ergot. In man two distinct forms of ergotism are seen, the gangrenous and convulsive, depending upon the combination of active *laevo* ergotamine compounds. Vast epidemics of 'Saint Anthony's fire' from consuming contaminated crops in time of food shortage occurred in the past, and small outbreaks still happen from time to time.

Aflatoxins are produced by species of *Aspergillus*, which often contaminate peanuts and other protein-rich foods consumed by man. *Aspergillus flavus* produces at least four aflatoxins (B_1, B_2, G_1, G_2, denoting the blue and greenish colours emitted by them under ultraviolet light). Liver cancer results in duck, trout, guinea-pigs, rats and rhesus monkeys when the feed contains only a few parts per million. The evidence for liver damage in man from consumption of contaminated groundnut is equivocal. Contamination of glutinous rice in northern Thailand is associated with epidemics of Reye's syndrome, a highly fatal disease in young children with liver necrosis and encephalopathy. An epidemic of acute hepatitis in western India was associated with consumption of contaminated maize. A recent report that aflatoxin contamination was associated with kwashiorkor but not with marasmus in Sudan is more likely to be casual than causal.

Oxalates

Despite numerous case reports in the literature attributing poisoning to oxalic acid in plants the evidence available is not convincing. It is improbable that chronic toxic effects would occur without a very high intake of oxalate-containing foods and a very low intake of calcium and vitamin D over a long period. For oxalate and bladder stone see page 211.

Halogenated hydrocarbons

Complex aromatic substances are more dangerous than short-chain aliphatic halogenated compounds, because they tend to persist in the environment and accumulate in the body. Most concern centres around the presence of polychlorinated biphenyl (PCB) compounds in human milk. They are currently permitted in closed systems in the electrical industry but may occur as a contaminant in recycled paper.

Gossypol

This is a pigment obtained from cottonseed which has been shown to have numerous toxic effects in animals. Cottonseed flour intended for human consumption should not contain more than 0.045 per cent by weight.

Radioactivity

When a nuclear explosion occurs, something like 200 different radioactive substances are found. Most of the radionuclides have short half-lives and rapidly decay. In practice, attention may be focused on four radionuclides: strontium-90, iodine-131, caesium-137 and carbon-14. The main portal of entry of fallout into the body is by ingestion. After the scare at Three Mile Island, USA, and the disaster in Chernobyl, USSR, public apprehension and protest have become focused on the real danger associated with human error.

Lathyrism

This disease is characterized by spastic paralysis, especially involving the legs. It occurs mainly in parts of India. Epidemiologically the disease is associated with the consumption of large amounts of the peas, *Lathyrus sativus*, *L. ciceva* or *L. clymenum*. They survive drought well and consequently are turned to for human food in times of famine. There is evidence to suggest that the toxic factor in *L. sativus* is L-oxalyl-amino-alanine. It has been found that the toxic factor(s) can be removed either by cooking the seeds in an excess of water or by steeping them in hot water.

Cyanide

Smoking increases the concentration in plasma of cyanide and thiocyanate and the excretion of the latter in urine. In experimental animals cyanide in quite small doses causes demyelination. In man heavy pipe smoking is associated with impairment of vision and visual field defects (p. 218).

Tropical ataxic neuropathy and endemic goitre (p. 23) in parts of Africa may be related to the consumption of cassava (p. 12). The thiocyanate that results is known to inhibit uptake of iodine by the thyroid (p. 23). The high incidence of a neurological disorder, resembling amyotrophic lateral sclerosis, in Guam and other Pacific islands has been attributed to intoxication with *cycasin*, a cyanogenic glycoside present in food prepared from the cycad nut, but proof is lacking.

Senecio poisoning

Herbs of this genus contain an alkaloid which produces lesions in the liver of experimental animals, and naturally in horses and cattle, that closely resemble those of *veno-occlusive disease* in man. It is thought that malnutrition may sensitize some children to develop liver damage (p. 180).

Akee poisoning (see p. 184)

Mercury

Concern has been expressed recently about the possibility of mercury poisoning from eating swordfish and tuna-fish. Serious mercury poisoning was reported from Japan in the 1950s from the eating of mercury-contaminated fish caught in polluted water. Levels of contamination seem to be much lower in other parts of the world and people eating considerable amounts of tuna-fish have been shown to have quite low levels of mercury in blood and hair. In methylated form mercury tends to accumulate and because of its lipid solubility cross the placenta and may damage the fetus.

Lead

This is especially dangerous to the infant brain. The main source is lead used in soldering in can construction for milk products. Recent work suggests that lead may play a part in motor neurone disease, as well as being a well-known cause of anaemia, peripheral neuropathy and encephalopathy.

Arsenic

It tends to be concentrated in such marine animals as grey sole and shrimps. Most is rapidly excreted in urine.

FOOD CONTROL

The setting up of food standards in order to try to ensure the health of the consuming public is of concern to both national governments and international agencies. A joint expert committee of Food and Agriculture Organization (FAO) and World Health Organization (WHO) has the subject of food additives under regular review and these bodies have set up a commission which works on a *Codex Alimentarius* with the objective of preparing international food standards and regulating food trade and technology throughout the world. Food control should preferably be done by governmental bodies with the powers to implement the decisions taken, but with the major technical representation from independent scientists. In the United Kingdom the Ministry of Agriculture, Fisheries and Food has a Food Advisory Committee that operates on these lines.

Labelling

In the United States, the United Kingdom and some other countries, orders have been introduced regulating the labelling of commercial foods. These orders were originally designed to govern the definition, formulation and promotion of such products with regard to their nutrient content, in order to protect the public from false or misleading claims by the manufacturers. They are now seen by some as a means of encouraging consumers to learn healthy eating, but it is doubtful whether this can ever be proved.

DOMESTIC AND INSTITUTIONAL FOOD PREPARATION

Cooking

Cooking has an important effect on the digestibility of certain foods. Cereals, roots and pulses cannot be readily digested by man otherwise, and only in this way is the tough cellulose wall surrounding the cells disrupted and the digestive enzymes allowed to penetrate.

The starch is swollen by the heat and assists in the rupture of the cell walls. Meat is made easier to chew by cooking as the tough collagen fibres are converted by heat to gelatin and digestive juices are allowed more ready access.

The heating of fats to high temperature (over 250°C) has rendered them toxic to animals. This is probably more drastic treatment than fats receive in most kitchens and restaurants, but overheating and prolonged heating should be avoided.

Cooking does cause certain nutrient losses and such practices as cooking for a long period, recooking, and keeping food warm for long periods are not recommended. Losses mainly concern ascorbic acid and thiamin, which are both water soluble, and ascorbic acid is subject to oxidation by exposure to air and enzymic action. Prolonged soaking in water permits the leaching out of these vitamins. Oxidation can be reduced by salt which inactivates enzymes. Acidity protects while alkalinity is destructive.

Wastage

This may arise in a variety of ways. Spoilage occurs when storage is poor, e.g. souring of milk and rancidity of fat in hot weather, contamination with cockroaches, with associated hygiene hazards. Food originally destined for man but fed to domestic pets is one form of waste. Plate waste is perhaps the most difficult to estimate and to control. It is greater in the homes of the affluent than the poor. The total waste may be as much as 500 kcal (2.1 MJ)/head/day. An allowance of about 10 per cent above physiological needs when estimating the retail supply or rations for group feeding is customary. Wastage presents serious economic and nutritional problems especially in long-stay institutions for the mentally and physically handicapped and the aged.

FOOD HYGIENE

Foods as a source of infection

Milk

Heavy bacterial growth can occur in this almost ideal culture medium. Contamination may occur during milking from the udders, the hands or droplet infection from milkers, from pails, churns or from bottles and when milk is pooled infection may spread to the whole supply. Besides the common organisms of food poisoning (salmonellae and staphylococci) milk may also be the vehicle of tuberculosis, streptococcal sore throat, scarlatina, diphtheria and brucellosis. Milk handled in bulk shuld be pasteurized immediately before boiling or drying. Inoculation with *Lactobacillus acidophilus* in the preparation of sour milk (yoghurt) prevents overgrowth of pathogens and gives a safe product especially useful in hot climates and where hygiene standards are low.

Meat

Made up dishes with meat, such as pies, mince and sausages are a common cause of food poisoning. Improperly stored carcasses may harbour salmonella and *Clostridium perfringens*. Encysted forms of worms (trichiniasis, taenia) may be present in beef and taenia in pork.

Fruit and vegetables

These provide a medium for the growth of bacteria and infection is usually light and contracted from the unwashed surface. In the tropics fruits that can be peeled before eating are preferable and salads should be avoided in hotels and restaurants. Fruit and vegetables that cannot be peeled should be soaked in detergent and then rinsed thoroughly. If this is not feasible, as for strawberries for example, they should be avoided.

Types of food infections

Food poisoning

This is an acute illness, usually including one or more gastrointestinal symptoms, caused by the recent consumption of food or drink. Most cases are due to organisms — by direct invasion of the intestinal wall, for example salmonella, or by production of an enterotoxin, eg. *Clostridium perfringens and botulinum Staphyloccus aureus.* Both within the family and outside, salmonella is the most common cause. Especially outside the family *C. perfringens, S. aureus* and *Bacillus cereus/sp.* account for a fair number of outbreaks; V. *parahaemolyticus* is a rare cause.

For a final diagnosis, laboratory tests are necessary but helpful clues are given by the duration of the incubation period, which may be short (2–6 hours), medium (8–24 hours), or long (1½–7 days). Most chemical poisoning and infection with *S. aureus* and *B. cereus* (emetic type) are short; salmonellas, clostridia and *B. cereus* (diarrhoeal type) are medium; and viral, *E. coli* and *G. lamblia* are long.

Other pathogens in food

The enteric fevers (typhoid and paratyphoid) are caused by salmonella organisms. Carriers are a common source and all food handlers should be checked regularly to exclude this state. Water, milk and various foods, such as shellfish and watercress can be the vehicle.

Bacillary dysentery (*Shigellae*), cholera (*Vibrio cholerae*), Weil's disease (*Leptospira icterohaemorrhagiae*) are other bacterial diseases spread through food or drinking water.

The protozoon *Entamoeba histolytica* causes amoebic dysentery and is transmitted by water or foods such as raw vegetables contaminated with human faeces. The flagellate *Giardia lamblia* is often commensal, but giardiasis is a common cause of diarrhoea, steatorrhoea and malabsorption in children and travellers. A number of worms are spread through food. Muscles of the pig may contain cysts of *Taenia solium*, the pig tapeworm, or trichinella. The infected meat of cattle transmit *Taenia saginata* and sea fish *Diphylobothrium latum.* The cystic stage of the dog tapeworm may produce hydatid disease (echinococcosis) in man. Ascaris (roundworm) and threadworms are also transmitted by faecal contamination of food or water by the ova.

It seems that to a considerable extent people develop immunity to their own local gut pathogens. However, travellers and tourists often fall prey to unfamiliar organisms away from home. 'Traveller's diarrhoea' or *tourista* is commonly caused by local strains of enterobacteria or by *Giardia lamblia.*

Treatment

Acute gastritis and diarrhoea are treated by rest in bed, withdrawal of solid food for 24 to 48 hours, water and electrolyte replacement, and antibiotics are only indicated if there are extragastrointestinal symptoms (see p. 176).

Prevention

A number of more or less commonsense rules, if followed, can help to keep outbreaks to a minimum, especially in hot climates and in crowded cities where the opportunities for contamination of food and water are great and sanitation is primitive. Water for consumption, however, can be boiled if the supply is suspect and a chlorinator can be added when water has to be carried for drinking. Food grown at home is safer than bought food and fruits and vegetables should be carefully washed after purchase. Those not capable of proper cleansing, e.g. strawberries, are best avoided. Storage of food should be in the coolest place, preferably in a refrigerator, and away from flies and vermin.

Strict and constant vigilance is necessary in restaurants and institutions where food is handled in bulk. Food should be inspected on receipt for freshness. Fruit and vegetables should be water sprayed immediately on receipt, before being taken into the kitchen area proper. Low temperature refrigeration is needed for safe storage of food cooked in bulk and often stored for some time before being eaten. Frozen poultry should be well thawed, properly cooked and stored in the cold if not to be eaten at once after cooking. Before being hired, kitchen staff should be screened for the typhoid carrier state, intestinal ova, skin infections and tuberculosis. Personal hygiene must be taught and adequate toilet facilities provided for them and for those they serve.

4. NATURE AND SOURCES OF NUTRIENTS

A sound diet is one that meets the nutrient, energy and aesthetic requirements of the individual, and contains nothing, either naturally or added, that is harmful to the body.

Here we shall consider something of the chemistry and dietary sources of nutriment.

ENERGY

Living creatures obey the first law of thermodynamics which states the principle of conservation of energy. They cannot create or destroy energy; they can only transform it. While green plants can utilize solar energy by photosynthesis, animals get their energy directly or indirectly from plants in the form of carbohydrates, protein or fat.

The various forms of energy in the body (chemical, mechanical, thermal, electrical) are interchangeable. Interconversion is never an efficient process: at best about 25 per cent from food, and most of the energy cannot be utilized for other purposes and is lost as heat.

The energy required for the activity of the organs has to come from chemical energy from oxidative processes. These activities include transport of electrolytes between intra- and extracellular spaces as well as heart action and the like.

The unit of energy in SI units is the joule (J) defined as $m^2 \, kg^2 \, s^{-2}$. It is related to the previous unit, the calorie, as follows: 1 kcal equals 4·1868 or approximately 4·19 J.

Bomb calorimetry is used to measure the energy content of food and other material. The 'bomb' is the central chamber in which the sample is placed and exposed to a high pressure of oxygen. In the presence of platinum as catalyst combustion of the material is initiated by an electric current. Complete combustion occurs and the heat liberated raises the temperature of the surrounding water.

Table 2 The heat of combustion and the available energy in the three proximate principles in a mixed diet

	Heat of combustion kcal(kJ)/g	Available energy kcal(kJ)/g
Carbohydrate	4.1 (17.18)	4.0 (16.76)
Protein	5.65 (23.67)	4.0 (16.76)
Fat	9.4 (39.39)	9.0 (37.71)

In a mixed diet energy is derived from carbohydrate, protein and fat. The heats of combustion of various proteins and fats differ only slightly but carbohydrates show greater differences (least for glucose and greatest for starch). The body is able to oxidize carbohydrate and fat completely to carbon dioxide and water, but protein oxidation is incomplete and the energy value of nitrogenous excretion products in urine has to be taken into account.

The efficiency of absorption has also to be allowed for. This is approximately 92 per cent for protein, 95 per cent for fat, and 97 per cent for carbohydrate. Table 2 shows the heat of combustion and available energy of the three proximate principles in the diet, the latter being known as the 'Atwater factors'.

For ordinary clinical and group-feeding practice the energy value of diets may be calculated from tables of food analyses using the Atwater factors. The research worker until recently had to carry out bomb calorimetry on food, stools and urine, but now a double labelled water method is being used (p. 45).

CARBOHYDRATES

These compounds are composed of carbon, hydrogen and oxygen, usually with the last two elements in the proportion in water, H_2O. Many are digested by man but not cellulose which forms the roughage of the diet.

Monosaccharides are simple sugars with up to six carbon atoms to each molecule (trioses, tetroses, pentoses and hexoses). The hexoses, glucose, fructose, galactose and mannose, are of major importance.

Glucose is present in only trace amounts in foods, except for some fruits, but starch is composed of glucose and it is part of the molecule of the common disaccharides sucrose, lactose and maltose. The body must have glucose for energy. It obtains it in different ways under different circumstances (p. 50). Fructose has the same empirical formula as glucose but differs structurally. It comes mainly from sucrose but is present in honey and some fruits. It is metabolized differently from glucose (p. 49).

Galactose is a hexose. Some hexose derivatives, such as sorbitol, mannitol and dulcitol, are incorporated industrially into some foods.

Disaccharides. Sucrose, from cane and beet, is the sugar in common domestic use and provides one molecule each of glucose and fructose.

Lactose is milk sugar and yields glucose and galactose on hydrolysis.

Polysaccharides. The three main polysaccharides in the human diet are all polymers of hundreds of glucose molecules.

Starch. There are two polysaccharides in starch: amylose and amylopectin. In this form the carbohydrate that can be utilized by man is stored in granules in roots and seeds of many plants. Moist heat, as in cooking, causes the starch to swell and become more soluble.

Glycogen. This is the animal equivalent of starch and is especially found in liver and muscle. It readily dissolves in water.

Dietary fibre

Dietary fibre is not an inert, unpalatable substance. Fibre has physical and chemical properties which significantly alter gastrointestinal function and human metabolism. Dietary fibre is that portion of plant cell wall or structural material ingested which is resistant to digestion by secretions of the human gastrointestinal tract. It consists of the carbohydrates cellulose, hemicellulose A, hemicellulose B, pectin and the non-carbohydrate lignin. Hemicellulose A is a polymer consisting of xylose, galactose, glucose, mannose and arabinose units. Hemicellulose B contains these sugars plus uronic acid derivatives. Lignin consists of phenylpropane units.

Crude fibre is the foodstuff residue left after treatment with boiling sulphuric acid, sodium hydroxide, water, alcohol and ether, and consists mainly of cellulose and lignin. Twenty to 50 per cent of total dietary fibre is crude fibre. Crude fibre chemical analysis underestimates the contribution of dietary fibre from all foods but especially from refined cereals. Wheat bran, for instance, is 35 to 40 per cent dietary fibre but is only 8 to 10 per cent crude fibre. Crude fibre excludes about 80 per cent of the hemicellulose, 50 to 90 per cent of lignin and about 50 per cent cellulose.

The major food sources are cereals, vegetables, fruits and nuts. In the average Western diet, cereals provide about one-third to one-half of the total (about 20 g/day) with most of the rest coming from vegetables. The intake is about five times higher in the diets of developing countries.

Dietary sources

The usual diets of man contain 300 to 500 g of carbohydrate providing 50 to 95 per cent of the total energy. In rural communities most of this is in the form of starch from cereal grains but in industrial societies a high proportion is from sucrose, about 40 per cent of absorbable carbohydrate compared with 25 per cent in 1900. This replacement of starch by sucrose is the biggest change that has taken place over the last century in Western diets. It may have played some part in the increased incidence of atherosclerosis and its complications (p. 201) and diabetes mellitus (p. 183) and has a role in dental caries (p. 219).

FATS

Fats are a concentrated source of energy. The fats of everyday life are mainly triglycerides, phospholipids and sterols and are included in the general term lipid. Lipids are water insoluble, organic solvent soluble, esters of fatty acids (actual or potential) and capable of utilization by living organisms.

Triglycerides. Lipids in plant foodstuffs or the fat depots of animals are mainly in the form of triglycerides. These are esters of glycerol and fatty acids with even numbers of carbon atoms. About 40 different fatty acids occur in nature. Fats are mixtures of a number of different triglycerides. Medium chain triglycerides (MCT) have a role in the dietary management of disorders of lipid metabolism (p. 187).

Fatty acids. These are classified according to their degree of unsaturation, i.e. number of double bonds. Saturated fatty acids have no double bonds and have the general formula $CH_3 (CH_2)_n COOH$ with n any even number from 2 to 24. Commonly occurring examples are lauric acid ($n = 10$), myristic acid ($n = 12$), palmitic acid ($n = 14$) and stearic acid ($n = 16$).

Of unsaturated fatty acids with one double bond (monoethanoid fatty acids) oleic acid is the most widely distributed in nature.

Fatty acids with two or more double bonds (diethenoid and polyethenoid acids) include three that are referred to as 'essential fatty acids' (EFA). They are linoleic acid, linolenic acid and arachidonic acid (see below).

Certain other unsaturated fatty acids, notably eicosapentaenoic acid (20:5 ω 3), in which the liver and tissue oils of fish such as mackerel, herring and cod are rich, have antithrombotic effects on platelets and may be important in preventing thrombosis in the coronary arteries (p. 205).

Trans fatty acids result from partial hydrogenation of cis isomers of unsaturated fatty acids, as by commercial processing of vegetable oil. In western countries they comprise about 15 per cent of total dietary fatty acids. They may have a role in aterogenesis (p. 201).

The physical state of fat is determined by its fatty acid composition. Fats solid at room temperature consist mainly of saturated fatty acids. Those that have a high proportion of unsaturated acids, for example olive oil and cod liver oil, are liquid. These latter can be turned into solid fats by hydrogenation in which saturation is produced. Vegetable oils are thus converted into margarine and other artificial butters.

Phospholipids. After the triglycerides these are the next most common kind of lipid, and a great variety exist in the body. Many have an important structural role as part of cell membranes. They include lecithin, sphingolipids and sphingomyelin.

Sterols. These are important solid alcohols. Cholesterol is a sterol present in all animal tissues but eggs are the only common food especially rich in it. It is synthesized by mammals. Other sterols with a metabolic function are ergosterol and 7-dehydrocholesterol, precursors of vitamin D (see p. 76). Closely related compounds called steroids include sex hormones, adreno-cortical hormones, steroidal alkaloids, cardiac glycosides and some carcino-genic hydrocarbons.

Essential fatty acids

Rigid exclusion of fat from an otherwise adequate diet results in a deficiency syndrome due to lack of certain polyunsaturated fatty acids. The two major essential fatty acids (EFA) are linoleic acid (18:2 ω 6) and arachidonic acid (20:4 ω 6) made from the former in the liver. The formulae indicate the number of carbon atoms and the number of double bonds, with the position of the double bond nearest to the methyl terminus, counting from the same, indicated by the symbol ω.

Most common vegetable oils contain linoleic or linolenic acid. Corn oil (34 to 42 per cent), cottonseed oil (40 to 48 per cent) and soya bean oil (50 to 60 per cent) are especially rich in linoleic acid. Arachidonate is found as a minor constituent only in common animal fats.

Dietary sources

Diets low in fat are often insipid and unpalatable. Fat may supply between about 10 per cent and 40 per cent of the total energy. The higher figure is usually due mainly to saturated fat of animal origin and may be associated with a high incidence of atherosclerosis (p. 201). In the early 1900s total fat was 25 per cent less and animal sources, such as butter and lard, were much higher. Diets low in fat are nearly always also low in protein and other nutrients. High fat diets do not necessarily predispose to obesity (p. 147). Those who are very active need a high-fat diet in order to be able to meet their high energy requirements.

PROTEINS

Proteins have molecular weights ranging between about 5000 and 500 000. Besides carbon, hydrogen and oxygen, they also contain nitrogen, sulphur, phosphorus and other elements. Amino acids, of which 20 plus are commonly found in nature, are the basic building blocks of protein and, conversely, result from hydrolysis of protein. In proteins amino acids are joined together in peptide linkage, the amino group of one being linked to the carboxyl group of the next with the elimination of water. The infinite variety of possible linkages of hundreds of amino acids in proteins gives the latter not only their infinity of number but also of structural formation. Not only are proteins, together with water, the basis of body and tissue structure but they are enzymes, hormones and play a role in transport and many other processes.

Animals are incapable of synthesizing the amino group and therefore must eat plants or other animals. The animal body is limited in its ability to convert one amino acid to another. The liver is the site of this conversion, in part by transamination through the enzyme transaminase, the coenzyme of which is pyridoxal phosphate (p. 74). Those amino acids that cannot be converted, or not at a sufficient rate to meet the body's needs, must be in the diet and are the essential amino acids for the species.

There are now considered to be 10 for man. Histidine is probably essential for adults as well as infants and recent reassessment of the evidence on arginine includes it. The others are lysine, methionine (giving rise to cystine), valine, leucine, isoleucine, tryptophan, phenylalanine (giving rise to tyrosine) and threonine.

Both essential and non-essential amino acids are necessary for protein synthesis. In the absence of any one essential amino acid protein synthesis ceases. In addition to this general role most of the amino acids have special parts to play in metabolism.

Glycine is the simplest amino acid. All others have an asymmetrical carbon atom and can exist in L-(natural) and D-forms. Glycine is used by the liver for detoxication of phenols. It is a precursor in such compounds as purines, porphyrins, conjugated bile acids and creatine.

Glutamic acid. The amino group is readily lost to keto acids and in this way glutamic acid is a major source of other amino acids (p. 72). It has a meaty flavour and is much used in the food industry (p. 21). In the brain, glutamic acid, together with γ-amino butyric acid (GABA) which it gives rise to by decarboxylation, are believed to have facilitatory and inhibitory actions, respectively, on brain function (p. 121). Glutamine is converted by kidney tubules to ammonia which combines with some of the sulphuric acid produced from protein for excretion as ammonium sulphate. Evidence has recently been provided for a key role for glutamate in the control of whole-body amino acid metabolism.

Arginine is required for urea formation in the ornithine-arginine cycle (p. 72).

Lysine like threonine does not exchange its amino group with other acids. Cereals tend to be deficient in lysine but diets as eaten are more often limiting in the sulphur amino acids (p. 277).

Valine, leucine, iso-leucine. These branched chain acids are metabolized mainly in skeletal muscle. Their level in plasma, particularly that of valine, falls rapidly in protein deprivation and rises rapidly when protein is fed (p. 106).

Methionine, cysteine, cystine. Cysteine can be made from methionine except perhaps by the newborn. These amino acids are the main source of sulphur in the diet. Methionine has a special role in transmethylation.

Histidine. Deficiency causes a dermatosis. It is the precursor of histamine.

Tryptophan gives rise to serotonin (5-hydroxytryptamine) and to some of the nicotinic acid in the body (p. 56). It has the lowest concentration of all amino acids in dietary and tissue proteins and amino acid pools. Its tissue content is carefully regulated and it probably has a unique role in protein synthesis.

Alanine has been shown to be the main contributor to gluconeogenesis from amino acids (p. 72).

Hydroxyproline is excreted in urine, mainly in peptide form, in proportion to the turnover of collagen. This provides a useful index for assessing skeletal growth (p. 106).

Dietary sources

Unlike carbohydrate and fat, protein intake varies little with income in realtion to total energy intake. Most people obtain about 11 per cent of their energy intake from protein. The source of protein, however, differs greatly, with most of the total being from animal sources in affluent communities and the reverse being the case among the poor. Overreliance on any single protein source results in inadequate intake of certain essential amino acids. While proteins of animal origin have a higher BV than vegetable, mixtures of the latter, especially a cereal with a legume, have a complementary effect and can meet all protein requirements.

Protein value of foods

This depends on both the quantity and quality of protein, as well as other factors such as energy intake and times of meals.

The quantity of protein is calculated by determining the nitrogen content, usually by the method of Kjeldahl, and multiplying by a factor of 6·25. This figure approximates to the average nitrogen content of many proteins. When applied to food analysis it also includes the nitrogen of non-protein compounds such as vitamins, purines.

Dietary proteins differ widely in their content of the amino acids that are essential to man. Very few are like zein of maize in being totally devoid of some essential amino acids. An ideal *reference protein* would contain all the essential amino acids in optimum amounts for human use and be completely digestible and utilizable. For infants the proteins of human milk appear to fulfil these theoretical criteria. The proteins of whole egg are the most conveniently available and are widely used as a reference standard. In order to make an evaluation of the quality of the dietary proteins various tests have been devised in which the results obtained with reference protein, taken to be 100 by definition, are compared with those obtained with the protein under test in identical conditions. Tests on human subjects are more difficult to carry out than those on animals, and the rat, which has amino acid requirements not very different from those of man, is often used.

The following are some of the tests most commonly in use.

PER (protein efficiency ratio)

Rats are fed the test diet containing 10 per cent protein for 4 weeks. The weight gain in grammes per gramme protein consumed constitutes the PER. This is a simple test and the results correlate quite well with those of more elaborate methods.

BV (biological value)

Nitrogen balance is the sum of the gains and losses of all tissue proteins of the body. The fraction of absorbed nitrogen retained in the body is defined as the BV. Then

$$BV = \frac{I - (U + F)}{I - F}$$

where I = intake, U = urinary nitrogen, F = faecal nitrogen

The subject consumes a diet containing no (or very little) protein and the output of nitrogen in urine and faeces falls to what is termed the 'endogenous nitrogen output'. If reference protein is then fed it will be fully utilized and none will be excreted as extra nitrogen in the urine. If the test protein is of poorer quality than reference protein, some will be excreted. Comparison with reference protein as 100 gives the BV of the test protein.

NPU (net protein utilization)

Of more practical value than the BV is the NPU in which the digestibility of the protein is also taken into account. NPU is retained/intake. Nitrogen balance studies are carried out on a nitrogen free diet and on the test diet. In a more rapid method nitrogen balance is estimated directly by carcass analysis of animals.

NDpV and NDpCal (J) per cent. (Net dietary protein value and Net dietary protein calories (joules) per cent.)

NDpV is the product of protein concentration and NPU (operative), i.e.

measured on the diet fed without standardization of conditions. This represents the utilizable protein in the mixture and is a function of both quality and quantity. On the basis that people eat to satisfy energy needs the expression of NDpV in terms of calories (joules) from protein calculated as a percentage of the total metabolizable energy in the diet gives NDpCal (J) per cent.

Chemical score

Several schemes have been prosposed in which the adequacy of the amino acid composition of the test protein is compared with that of reference protein. This may be confined to the essential amino acid in greatest deficit, i.e. the limiting amino acid, or may include all of the essential amino acids, making the procedure very cumbersome. A compromise is sometimes reached by using those amino acids that tend to be deficient in diets; lysine and the sulphur amino acids.

VITAMINS

Vitamin A (retinol)

Retinol is a colourless, fat-soluble alcohol ($C_{20}H_{30}O$) corresponding to half of a molecule of an unsaturated hydrocarbon, β-carotene consisting of two β-ionone rings joined by a long central chain. The biodegradation of β-carotene to retinol takes place via retinal (vitamin A aldehyde) in the small intestine.

Plants are ultimately the source of all vitamin A-active substances. Of the nearly 500 naturally occurring carotenoids known, less than 10 can be converted by the animal organism to vitamin A. Dark green leafy vegetables (such as spinach, turnip tops and parsley), and carrots, are good sources of vitamin A as are yellow fruits (e.g. papaya and mango). Pale leaved vegetables and cereals are low in provitamin A. Red palm oil, extracted from the fruit coat of *Elaeis guineensis*, the traditional cooking oil in much of West and Central Africa, contains as much as about 100 000 i.u. (33 000 μg) of provitamin A activity per 100 g oil. Recently HPLC (high performance liquid chromatography) has provided an accurate and rapid method for estimating individual carotenoids.

Preformed vitamin A is concentrated mainly in the liver, but also occurs to some extent in milk, plasma and kidney. Fish liver oils are especially rich in the vitamin. Butter, cheese, cream, whole milk and egg yolk are good sources.

In developing countries almost all of the vitamin A intake may be provided by vegetable sources. In Europe and North America about two thirds comes from animal and one third from vegetable sources.

Thiamin (vitamin B$_1$, aneurin)

This water-soluble vitamin of the B complex, made up of pyrimidine and thiazole moieties, is rather unstable to heat. At pH 5 or higher it is destroyed by autoclaving and at pH 7 or more by boiling or even storage at room temperature.

In the average European diet cereal products provide about one-third; meat, fish and poultry almost one-fourth and dairy products one-eight of the necessary thiamin. Whole grain cereals contain the greater part of their thiamin in the germ, pericarp and endosperm most of which is removed by milling but remains after home pounding. Parboiling disperses this and other water-soluble vitamins throughout the grain, thereby preserving a high proportion (p. 19). Enriched or whole wheat bread is a significant source of the vitamin when consumed in large amounts, as in low-income families.

Thiamin may be lost in cooking by leaching, destruction by heat and oxidation. Loss is greatest in the presence of alkali.

Riboflavin (vitamin B$_2$)

Riboflavin is 6, 7-dimethyl-9 (*d*-ribityl)-isoalloxazine. It is widely distributed in both animal and vegetable foods. One quart (1·14l) of milk provides all the recommended intake, provided precautions are taken to minimize exposure to sunlight. Cereals are quite low except after germination, when fermented products taken in the form of snacks as in the Far East, may make a considerable contribution towards satisfaction of the requirement.

Niacin (nicotinic acid)

Niacin is very stable in solution as well as in the dry state. It was originally isolated as an oxidation product of nicotine and later from nicotinamide adenine dinucleotide (NAD, coenzyme I) and nicotinamide adenine dinucleotide phosphate (NADP, coenzyme II).

Major sources are yeast, liver, meat, poultry, and legumes. Although milk and eggs are low in preformed niacin they are high in tryptophan content and so have a high niacin equivalent. Much of the niacin in cereals such as maize and rice, is present in bound forms (e.g. niacytin) and is separated only with difficulty unless the food is prepared with alkali, as in *tortilla*. Niacytin appears to be unavailable to man. Most of the niacin in cereals is in the husk and is removed by milling.

Vitamin B$_6$ (pyridoxine, pyridoxal, pyridoxamine)

All three substances are equally effective as vitamin B$_6$ in animal nutrition.

Vitamin B$_6$ is widely distributed and few foods can be considered as poor sources. Among the richest are meats, liver, vegetables, whole grain cereals and egg yolk.

Pantothenic acid

Several independent lines of investigation finally converged in the isolation from various sources of this further member of the heat-stable fraction of water-soluble vitamin B.

All food groups make significant contributions to the dietary intake. Organ meats and whole grain cereals are the richest sources, but processing in dry heat causes considerable destruction of the vitamin.

Biotin (vitamin H, anti-egg white injury factor)

Rats fed a well-balanced ration but with egg white as the sole source of protein develop severe skin lesions and die. A yeast factor, biotin, was found to cure the condition. Heat treatment deprives egg white of its toxic properties by freeing biotin from avidin.

Most biotin in food occurs bound to protein. Liver, kidney, egg yolk and yeast are the richest sources. Cauliflower, nuts and legumes are good plant food sources.

Folic acid (folacin, pteroylglutamic acid (PGA), vitamin M, vitamin B_c, L. casei factor)

Folic acid is a yellow crystalline compound, a member of a family of closely related substances containing three moieties: pterin, p-aminobenzoic acid and glutamic acid. It occurs in many plant and animal tissues in the unstable forms of reduced methyl or formyl polyglutamates.

Liver, kidney, yeast and mushrooms rate among the best sources of folic acid but it is found in most natural foods. Significant losses occur in cooking, canning and on exposure to light.

Vitamin B_{12} (cobalamin)

This is the food factor curative in pernicious anaemia. The molecule consists of a modified metalloporphyrin with cobalt in the centre, linked to a nucleotide. Several cobalamins occur in food bound to protein by peptide bonds which are dissociated by cooking or digestion.

Vitamin B_{12} is unique among the vitamins in being synthesized almost exclusively by micro-organisms. Many sources contain the vitamin in its coenzyme form linked to it specific protein. Good sources are liver, kidney, meat and fish.

Vitamin C (ascorbic acid)

By precipitation with basic lead acetate, a nitrogen-free unstable substance with antiscorbutic activity was isolated from lemon juice. This activity appeared to be related to the reducing power of the substance and yet freshly oxidized solutions retain this property. Investigation of redox systems in plants and animals led to the isolation of an identical crystalline, optically active substance with the formula $C_6H_8O_6$ designated hexuronic (later ascorbic) acid.

Apart from a few animal products such as kidney, liver, roe and milk, only fruits and vegetables contribute natural vitamin C to the diet. Citrus fruits, guavas, turnip and broccoli greens and Brussels sprouts are especially rich in the vitamin.

Vitamin C is especially susceptible to food processing procedures because of its high solubility in water and the ease with which it is oxidized chemically or enzymatically. Significant losses do not occur with the usual household methods of cooking but are considerable in large scale preparation of food. In controlled modern commercial methods of blanching, dehydration, canning and bottling there is relatively little destruction.

Vitamin D (calciferol)

About 10 compounds are known to have vitamin D activity but only 2 are of practical importance. Ergocalciferol (vitamin D_2) is manufactured by exposing ergosterol, a sterol in fungi and yeasts, to ultraviolet light. Cholecalciferol (vitamin D_3) is the form produced by ultraviolet radiation of 7-dehydrocholesterol in the skin. By its structure, formation in the body and function calciferol is more like a hormone than a vitamin (p. 76).

Relatively few foods provide the vitamin. Really rich sources are fish liver oils (several thousand $\mu g/100g$; 1 μg equals 40 i.u.). Unfortified cow and human milk are poor sources; containing no more than $0.03\ \mu g/dl$.

Vitamin E (tocopherol)

Eight tocopherols and tocotrienols have been identified with vitamin E activity, the most potent being a tocopherol. Vitamin E occurs in greatest concentration in vegetable oils, the proportion of the different tocopherols varying considerably. The amount of vitamin E is related, in general, to the amount of polyunsaturated fatty acids. Freezer storage of foods fried in oil causes about 70 per cent decrease of tocopherol content. Heating of cooking oils destroys almost all the tocopherol present, although esters are little affected. Very little is lost in normal cooking procedures.

Vitamin K

Vitamin K exists in nature in at least two forms, K_1(phytonadione) and K_2, both derivatives of 2-methyl, 1,4-naphthoquinone (menadione).

Good food sources of vitamin K, are dark green leafy vegetables and some fruits, tubers and seeds. Vitamin K can be synthesized by many bacteria, including those normally present in the human intestine, which usually provide an adequate supply in man.

WATER

Water comprises anywhere from 50 to over 90 per cent of all living matter. In addition to that obtained from food and drink metabolic water is available from the oxidation of carbohydrate, fat and protein. Water intake in health is usually determined by habit and custom; less often is it a response to actual sensation of thirst.

ELEMENTS

The minerals and other elements required by the body can be classified according to the way the body handles them.

1. *Readily absorbed and excreted.* After digestion most food is easily absorbed as simple compounds of hydrogen, oxygen, carbon, nitrogen, sodium, potassium and chlorine. These elements are also freely excreted in the urine, and as carbon dioxide, in the breath.

2. *Imperfectly absorbed and readily excreted.* Calcium, magnesium and phosphorus in food are in part combined as indigestible and insoluble compounds; consequently chemical analysis of the diet does not reflect their availability to the body. After absorption they are freely excreted.

3. *Poorly absorbed and poorly excreted.* Included are iron, copper, cobalt, zinc and manganese but excessive accumulation is known to occur with only the first two.

Sodium

It is widely distributed in relatively small amounts in foods and is often added during processing. A separate supply in addition to that present in foods is not necessary. Intakes vary enormously between populations and relative to the prevalence of hypertension (p. 206) and stroke (p. 201). The daily range is 50 to 400 mmol in western societies, but as low as 2 to 10 mol in some hunter-gatherers.

Chlorine

In the diet and in the body it is closely associated with sodium as chloride.

Potassium

The usual daily intake is 50 to 150 mEq obtained from a wide variety of foodstuffs. Different samples of the same food vary greatly in potassium content.

Calcium

In the typical western diet about 75 per cent comes from milk and milk products, and the rest about equally from meat, fish, and eggs, cereal products, beans, fruits and vegetables. The daily per capita intake is about 1·0 g. The calcium in milk is in complexes from which it is readily released whereas binding to oxalate in vegetables and phytate in cereals may render much of the calcium present unavailable. Other significant sources of calcium may be in water if it is hard (up to 50 mg or more per litre), and lime added in making tortillas and fish pastes.

Phosphorus

Animal foods are rich in phosphorus but it is widely distributed in nature and dietary deficiency does not occur. It is a component of phytic acid in whole grain cereals which binds with calcium and impairs absorption.

Magnesium

It is widespread in animal and vegetable foodstuffs and deficiency is of endogenous origin.

Iron

No single food group is responsible for a major portion of the iron intake. Milk and milk products are especially low in iron, although it is well utilized. Loss may be considerable by solution into cooking water which is discarded.

Iron is one of those elements that is poorly absorbed and poorly excreted. The terrestrial environment is rich in iron and the body is thus normally protected against the dangers of overload. The major source in most diets, and exclusively for vegetarians, is non-haem iron of which 10 per cent or less is absorbed. Haem iron from meat is much more readily absorbed.

Iodine

The iodine content of fresh water is small and very variable, about 1 to 50 µg/l. Its importance lies rather in the indication it can give of the likely iodine content of cereals and vegetables grown in soil which water irrigates. Sea water is a poor source but sea food of all kinds is the richest source. Most soils are poor in iodine and consequently most foodstuffs are poor sources.

Zinc

Most diets provide 10 to 15 mg per day. Those high in protein and wholegrain products are richer but much of the zinc in vegetable sources is not absorbed.

Fluorine

Almost all soils, water supplies, plants and animals contain small but widely varying amounts of fluorine. It is therefore a normal constituent of all diets. Tea (0·475 mg/100 g) and coffee (0·25 mg/100 g) are rich sources.

Copper

Copper is widely distributed in foods, the average adult ingesting 25 to 50 mg per day. Rich sources (> 8 p.p.m.) include organ meat, oysters, nuts, dried legumes and whole grain cereals. Milk is a poor source.

Selenium

Intake depends largely on the soil content where food is grown and varies widely. It is closely associated with protein, the dietary intake of which has an influence.

Chromium

It occurs in two dietary forms: as Cr^{3+} and in a biologically active molecule that appears to be dinicatinatochromium^{3+} complexed with amino acids.

Manganese

Whole cereals, nuts, legumes and green leafty vegetables are rich sources and dietary deficiency is not known.

Molybdenum

This element is derived mainly from vegetables, the content being related to that in soil.

Cobalt

Cobalt can only be utilized in vitamin B_{12} as far as is known and, consequently, rich dietary sources of the vitamin also provide cobalt.

5. PHYSIOLOGY OF NUTRIENTS

In this chapter we shall see what happens to the nutrients in the diet once they are eaten. This will cause us successively to consider the processes of eating, digestion, absorption, transport, storage and excretion.

Physiology and energy

The energy expenditure of the body when at rest and in other states may be measured either by *direct* or *indirect calorimetry*. By *direct calorimetry* the subject enters a specially constructed chamber in which all the heat produced is measured. In this way it has been shown that the body obeys the first law of thermodynamics, in that the total energy expended by heat produced and mechanical work done is equal to the net energy from the food consumed, caculated by deducting the energy content of the faeces and urine from the total energy content of the food. It was also found that total energy expenditure is quantitatively related to oxygen consumption (approx. 5 kcal or 20·95 kJ/litre). On this basis it is possible to carry out the much simpler procedure of *indirect* calorimetry in which oxygen consumption is measured.

Several types of apparatus have been used for measuring oxygen consumption: respiratory chambers of elaborate construction, the Benedict Roth spirometer used in hospitals for measuring basal metabolism, the Douglas bag designed to collect expired air for the measurement of its O_2 and CO_2 content, and the readily portable Max Planck respirometer.

When pure protein is being oxidized about 4·5 kcal (18·86 kJ) are made available when 1 litre of oxygen is used up. Corresponding figures for fat and carbohydrate are 4·7 and 5·0 kcal (19·70 and 20·95 kJ)/l respectively. The usual mixture of these oxidized by a healthy adult yields about 4·8 kcal (20·06 kJ)/l. If the oxygen consumption over a given period is known, the metabolic rate can be calculated using this figure. Thus if 20 l of oxygen are consumed in 1 hour, the metabolic rate is about $20 \times 4·8 = 96$ kcal (402·2 kJ)/hour.

If the metabolic mixture differs considerably from the usual, then errors up to about 4 per cent could be introduced by using the compromise figure of 4·8 kcal (20·1 kJ)/l. An estimate can be made of the types of material that are being oxidized by obtaining the respiratory quotient (RQ). This is defined as the ratio of carbon dioxide produced to the oxygen used up per unit time. When carbohydrates are oxidized, one molecule of carbon dioxide is given off for every molecule of oxygen used up and the RQ is 1. For fats the RQ is about 0·7 and for protein about 0·8. On a natural diet the RQ is about 0·8.

Recently, a doubly labelled water method, using $H_2^{18}O$ and ^2H_2O, has come into use for estimating rate of CO_2 production and water output. With the RQ known energy expenditure can be calculated. The method is specially useful in studies of lactation.

Basal metabolic rate

Energy expenditure varies in relation to muscular work. Contrary to popular belief, it is not increased by mental activity. When the subject is completely at rest and no physical work is being done, energy is still required to maintain body temperature and for the activity of the organs for what is termed the resting or basal metabolism. The basal metabolic rate (BMR) is measured in the investigation of some diseases, notably in hypo- and hyperthyroidism, when it is, respectively reduced and increased. The test is done at least 12 hours after the last meal with the subject lying down at complete rest in a comfortable warm room. Results are conventionally expressed in kcal (or kJ)/m²/hour. It has been shown that basal metabolism of many different species is remarkably similar if expressed in this way, although differing widely if related to body weight. For comparisons of individuals of the same species, however, this is not the best standard, because the surface area does not reflect the body shape or body composition. As might be expected, the BMR is closely related to the lean body mass (p. 5) and when so related, differences between the sexes, found when surface area is used, disappear. In adults the variations in body shape and composition are almost entirely due to differences in adipose tissue. Tables are available of the resting rate of energy expenditure of adults of different body type.

The BMR is high during the early years of life. It is about 10 per cent below the standards for those adapted to life in the tropics. Sitting or standing increases the metabolism by 20 or 30 per cent.

Thermogenic effect of food

The taking of food increases the metabolism on the average by about 10 per cent. It has usually been claimed that protein has a greater effect than carbohydrate or fat but recent work has failed to demonstrate any difference. The thermogenic effect is apparent earlier with carbohydrate than after protein or fat and this makes comparison difficult. It appears to reflect protein synthesis rather than catabolism. This is consistent with the finding of an increased thermogenic effect after a meal when a malnourished subject is recovering and when protein synthesis is greatest.

Of considerable importance to the maintenance of a stable weight is the finding that exercise after a meal approximately doubles the thermogenic response to the meal.

Energy expenditure and activity

Rates of energy expenditure have been measured for many activities using indirect calorimetry. The types of activity have been graded and the expenditure may be anywhere between about 2·5 kcal (10·48 kJ)/min for light work to over 10 kcal (41·9 kJ)/min for heavy work (p. 95, Durnin and Passmore).

Energy for hard work is derived from muscle glycogen and when this is consumed the rate of exercise has to be reduced to that for which oxidation of free fatty acids can yield the necessary energy. The greatest glycogen stores can be obtained by emptying them by undertaking prolonged exercise, keeping them low for three days on a low carbohydrate diet and then repleting them by a few days on a high carbohydrate diet. This has been shown to be a valuable training regime for athletes requiring short, severe bursts of activity.

Eating

The regulation of food intake is a highly complex process. Psychological and cultural influences play upon the basic physiological mechanisms.

Hunger is the complex of sensations evoked by changes in the physiological state of the body that in man and the higher animals compels to ingestion of food. *Fullness* is the feeling when hunger is abolished and is associated with the alimentary tract.

Appetite is the desire for food and is an affective state, and *satiety* is the corresponding affective state in repletion, signifying a desire not to eat.

Early investigations suggested that contractions of the stomach were responsible for producing the sensation of hunger. Later experiments, in which the stomach was denervated, provided contrary evidence. Attention was later shifted to the role of the hypothalamus. Patients with obesity with lesions confined to the hypothalamus provide clinical support and conclusive evidence has come from discrete lesions of this region induced in experimental animals.

Bilateral destruction of ventromedial parts of the hypothalamus produces obesity as a result of an insatiable appetite. These areas constitute the 'satiety centre'. Contrariwise, destruction of the extreme lateral parts of the hypothalamus causes aphagia, and the animal dies of starvation unless force-fed. These form the 'feeding centre'. The interaction of these ill-defined 'centres' and the integrative action of other parts of the central nervous system control the food intake.

It would appear that the regulation of food intake is primarily concerned with the intake of energy, which is adjusted to balance the energy requirement. The short-term adjustment mechanism is not clear. We do not know exactly why we stop eating when we do. When activity is changed abruptly there is no immediate corresponding change in the food intake, but on a week-to-week basis appetite does appear to regulate food intake and help to maintain body weight constant.

The nature of the stimuli acting on the hypothalamic centres has been the subject of much research and there are three major hypotheses. It is generally believed that stimuli act mainly on the satiety centre and indicate the need to stop eating.

The glucostatic hypothesis

Cells in the satiety centre act as chemoreceptors sensitive to their own rate of utilization of glucose. With high blood glucose the gluco-receptors are stimulated and they signal the feeding centre that food intake should decrease. The reverse happens when the glucose level is low. There is considerable supporting experimental evidence for this mechanism which would also act in such a way as to protect the glucose supply of the brain. There are also some objections, including the fact that when human subjects are given a high fat, low carbohydrate diet they may show no fluctuations in blood glucose but still experience typical cycles of hunger and satiety.

The lipostatic hypothesis

This suggests that coincident with the release of free fatty acids, unknown metabolites are released from the fat depots into the blood, and act on the hypothalamic centres. In this way the centre might be kept informed of the state of the fat depots. This theory is better suited to explain long-term adjustment of energy intake than short-term regulation.

The thermostatic hypothesis

Appetite is decreased in warm and increased in cold surroundings. While the increased heat production associated with the metabolism of foods after their absorption may have some effect on the amount of food eaten it is probably of minor importance in actual regulation.

Cultural and psychological factors

Man usually eats not when he is hungry but according to schedules dictated by custom and convenience. Affluent societies may hardly ever experience real hunger while underprivileged communities may rarely know what satiety is. Nevertheless, the long-term regulation of food intake seems to be remarkably efficient in most, and body weight is maintained almost constant.

Sometimes psychological factors override all others. Compulsive eating may represent compensation for anxiety or boredom (p. 149) or equally powerful drives may lead to semistarvation (p. 149).

Control of energy balance

Exactly how energy balance is maintained is not understood. Three factors promote stability: (a) hunger and satiety are imprecise but keep intake within a fairly narrow range; (b) fat storage involves energy expenditure and overfeeding results in thermogenesis; (c) large changes in body weight are associated with changes in metabolic rate; a long-term version of (b). Even in obesity the degree of control over energy balance is remarkable (p. 148).

CARBOHYDRATES

Digestion and absorption

Saliva contains ptyalin, an enzyme that splits starch. It is inactivated by acid when the food reaches the stomach. Most of the digestion of carbohydrates goes on in the small intestine where amylase (diastase) secreted by the pancreas works optimally in the slightly alkaline medium there to break down starch and glycogen to disaccharides. These and the disaccharides of the diet are absorbed into the mucosa of the small intestine and within the epithelial cells are acted upon by various disaccharidases, lactase, sucrase and maltase, to form the monosaccharides which are taken up into the portal blood. These enzymes are sometimes deficient (see pp. 108 and 185).

Glucose and other hexoses are absorbed by the small intestine through an active transport mechanism.

Transport and storage

Glucose is continuously being utilized by all body tissues, necessitating its delivery by the circulation. An early morning fasting blood sample contains 3·3 to 5·5 mmol/l (60–100 mg/100 ml) glucose. This level remains relatively constant as a result of homoeostatic regulation.

Some tissues are more sensitive than others to a fall in blood glucose. The brain is probably most dependent, as glucose is the major energy source that crosses the blood-brain barrier, although in prolonged starvation ketone bodies ae utilized. Muscle and some other tissues can derive part of their energy needs from other sources, such as ketone bodies. Heart muscle can utilize fatty acids and lactic acid.

Blood glucose is derived partly from the portal absorption of products of carbohydrate digestion. This contribution varies greatly between individuals, and from day to day, and ceases at night. Glucose in blood also comes from the hydrolysis of glucose-6-phosphate in liver, kidney and intestine. This comes ultimately from glycogen (glycogenolysis) or from all other precursors (glucogenesis) which also includes gluconeogenesis indicating new glucose formation from non-carbohydrate sources.

It was long ago demonstrated, although largely forgotten, that the metabolism of glucose and that of fructose are different, as evidenced by respiratory quotients of $<1·0$ and $>1·0$ respectively. Diets rich in sucrose, and consequently fructose, produce hyperlipidaemia and that fat synthesis occurs is suggested by rise in blood pyruvate indicating glycolysis in the Embden-Meyerhof pathway. Pyruvic acid can be converted to acetyl CoA which gives rise to fatty acids. (see pp. 65 and 68).

Normally no more than a trace of glucose is lost in the urine. From the blood, glucose diffuses into cells where it is phosphorylated (see p. 64).

Factors influencing blood glucose concentration

As indicated in Figure 4 the sum of the 'fates' of glucose must equal the sum of the sources. The rate of glucose utilization is determined partly by the concentration in the blood and other parts of the extracellular space. Sustaining blood glucose at hyperglycaemic levels favours the formation of products derived from glucose, especially liver glycogen and fatty acids. Insulin lowers the blood sugar by facilitating the passage of glucose into cells where synthesis of glycogen by muscle, and of fatty acids by liver and adipose tissue, is increased. In diabetes mellitus, conversely, there is evidence of glucose underutilization. Many of the consequences of diabetes resemble the effects of starvation, except for the hyperglycaemia.

Glucose tolerance

The capacity to dispose of glucose may be tested by oral or intravenous dosing. For routine use the oral test using 1 g glucose/kg body weight is satisfactory. A fasting level of 4·95 mmol/1 (90 mg/100 ml) will usually rise to a maximum of about 7·7 mmol/1 (140 mg/100 ml) in about 1 hour. By the end of 2 hours the level should be back to normal. The initial hyperglycaemia increases the rate of glucose utilization by cells and causes the pancreas to discharge insulin at an increased rate.

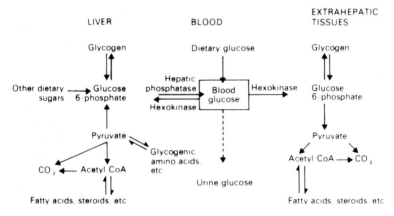

Fig. 4 Sources and fates of blood glucose. (From White, Handler and Page, 1973, *Principles of Biochemistry*, 5th edn McGraw-Hill, New York.)

In the diabetic the fasting blood glucose is elevated. After glucose administration it rises higher, often exceeding the renal threshold and causing glycosuria. Insulin response is impaired and the decline in blood glucose is slow.

Dietary fibre

This is a complex mixture of unabsorbed compounds, varying in composition and physiological action (p. 33). Bile salts may be bound and their reabsorption prevented. Lack of dietary fibre has been attributed to an increased incidence of diverticular disease, appendicitis, hiatal hernia, colon cancer, gallstones, constipation, haemorrhoids, varicose veins, atherosclerosis, diabetes mellitus, obesity and dental caries.

A low residue diet leads to a decrease in faecal mass and a prolongation of transit time, altering bile acid metabolism in the the colon. Normally the conjugated bile salts are transported to the ileum, reabsorbed, and recycled to the liver. A small fraction is not absorbed and moves to the colon, where the anaerobic microflora dehydroxylate cholate and form deoxycholate, which is an effective chemical carcinogen.

Colonic disease, particularly carcinoma of the colon, has been linked with fibre depletion and faecal stasis. Prolonged dietary fibre supplementation normalizes abnormal human transit time, produces an increase in the major ions of normal faeces, i.e. volatile short-chain fatty acids, and increases faecal wet weight by 50 per cent.

Generally there is an increase in faecal output with an increasing excretion of faecal energy from fat and nitrogen sources. A decrease in transit time has also been observed. Certain fibres (pectin) significantly delay gastric empty-ing. In addition, bran inhibits the action of bacteria on bile salts and thus may prevent the formation of carcinogens. The increase in faecal bulk may be the result of the increased production of volatile fatty acids (acetic, butyric, propionic) by bacterial action on dietary fibre. These fatty acids may act as cathartics. Fibre may absorb water and function as a bulking agent and promote peristalsis. Bran inhibits this bacterial degradation of bile salts and also diminishes the time of contact of the carcinogen with the mucosa by de-creasing the transit time.

Fibre, particularly apple pectin, delays gastric emptying. This fibre has been used in certain clinical conditions associated with rapid emptying of gastric contents into the intestine seen after partial surgical resection of the stomach (postgastrectomy syndrome). Fibre may also improve glucose tolerance by delaying gastric emptying, particularly in patients with diabetes mellitus.

A more rapid transit time may have a positive effect in removing cholesterol from the system. Dietary fibre has physical properties that have a potential for binding fats, cholesterol and minerals, such as zinc, copper, iron and perhaps magnesium. A fibre intake in excess of 30 to 40 g/day can mean the loss of important nutrients.

FATS

Digestion and absorption

Fat in food delays the emptying of the stomach, possibly due to the liberation of an unidentified hormone, when fat enters the duodenum causing inhibition of gastric movements.

Emulsification is necessary for the digestion of fat and this begins in the duodenum below the point where the bile and pancreatic juice enter. The for-mation of droplets less than 0.5 μm in diameter is necessary for absorption and these are produced in the presence of bile salts, fatty acids and monoglycerides liberated by pancreatic digestion.

Bile salts have lipophobic groups at one end of the molecule and lipophilic groups at the other. They combine with fatty acids and monoglycerides and form *micelles* which, by the presence of lipophobic groups inside and lipophilic outside the molecule, allows solubility in water.

Pancreatic and intestinal juices contain lipases which split triglycerides into fatty acids, diglycerides and monoglycerides and glycerol. Hydrolysis often stops at the stage of monoglyceride. Some resynthesis of triglyceride may take place.

The microvilli of the intestinal mucosa receive a microemulsion of lipid which passes within the cells. Here the triglycerides formed are more characteristic of the host than of the food. Probably about 40 per cent of ingested triglycerides is hydrolysed completely to fatty acids and glycerol, about 10 per cent is absorbed unchanged and the rest as mono- or diglyceride. Most fat absorbed enters the circulation through the thoracic duct but medium and short chain fatty acids enter via the portal tract (p. 187).

Transport and storage

The insolubility of lipids in water creates a problem regarding their transport in the watery plasma. They are carried as chylomicrons, secondary particles, low and high density lipoproteins and free fatty acids, all of which are bound to protein.

In the postabsorptive state, plasma contains about 500 mg of total lipid per 100 ml (about 25 per cent triglyceride, 40 per cent cholesterol — two thirds esterified, one-third free, 35 per cent phosphatides — more lecithin than cephalins).

Shortly after the ingestion of a fatty meal the lymphatic channels become distended with milky chyle rich in triglycerides. Most of this fat is present as chylomicrons. Discharge of this chyle into the venous circulation produces an *absorptive lipaemia*. Chylomicrons are removed from blood in a matter of minutes, brought about by plasma lipoprotein lipase (clearing factor). It appears in the plasma during lipaemia and its activity is enhanced by heparin. The fatty acids liberated are picked up by serum albumin.

Lipids circulate in plasma attached to specific proteins, forming lipo-proteins of which there are four classes. Two of these, chylomicrons and VLDL (very-low-density lipoproteins) are composed predominantly of triglyceride and are respectively the transport form of dietary and endogenous lipid. LDL (low-density lipoprotein) contains most of the plasma cholesterol. HDL (high-density lipoprotein) is 50 per cent protein and 25 per cent phospholipid and may be protective against coronary heart disease (p. 203).

Disorders involving hyperlipaemic states (p. 190) and their implications in atherosclerosis (p. 201) are dealt with later. Lipids, mostly as triglyceride, are formed in all organs but may be regarded as being stored mainly in the fat depots.

Adipose tissue is a reservoir of energy of considerable size in health, that very readily yields energy in highly concentrated form in times of restricted nutrition. Located largely subcutaneously, it provides protection for the more thermosensitive tissues against excessive heat loss to the environment. The subcutaneous fat depots also protect against mechanical trauma. Recent work suggests that brown fat, located mainly in the neck and shoulder regions, may play a part in adult thermogenesis as well as in the 'non-shivering thermogenesis' of infants (p. 151).

In life lipid in the depot is in the liquid state and appears to be as saturated as it can be in relation to the ambient temperature. Thus deeper depots with a higher ambient temperature have a more highly saturated composition. Energy yield from oxidation is proportional to degree of saturation. The effect of diet reflects in depots the origin of the depot fatty acids. Thus in prolonged feeding with corn oil the adipose tissue resembles the composition of corn oil more than it does normal adipose tissue.

Under normal circumstances linoleic acid (18:2 ω 6) and its metabolic products 20:3 ω 6 and arachidonic acid (20:4 ω 6) are present in detectable quantities in plasma lecithin. The pattern is disturbed in deficiency (p. 136). Pyridoxine is required for the conversion of linoleic acid to its 20 carbon metabolite.

PROTEINS

Digestion and absorption

Proteolytic enzymes hydrolyse protein to amino acids and some small peptides which are then absorbed.

The peptic cells of the stomach secrete pepsin which acts well in the acid medium of that organ. Polypeptides are formed. Rennin in the stomach of new-born mammals causes clotting of caseinogen, a protein of milk.

Pancreatic juice contains the main proteolytic enzyme, trypsin, which converts proteins into polypeptides and about half of these are further broken down to amino acids. Undigested meat fibres and an increase in faecal nitrogen are evidence of pancreatic dysfunction.

Animal protein is more rapidly and more efficiently absorbed than protein of vegetable origin. Faecal nitrogen comes only partly from the diet (exogenous nitrogen). The endogenous nitrogen consists of nitrogen entering the alimentary canal from the circulation, as amino acids, and of nitrogen in intestinal secretions and shed epithelial cells.

Individual amino acids are absorbed at slightly different rates but the postabsorptive curve of amino nitrogen is smooth, being markedly elevated within half an hour of protein ingestion and remaining so for several hours.

Transport, storage and excretion

Almost all of the amino acids absorbed from the intestine enter the circulation by the portal blood, where they are in free solution. Small amounts of low molecular weight peptides and, especially in the young, molecules of some proteins, including immunoglobulins from breast milk, do appear to penetrate the mucosa. Foreign proteins may cause immunological sensitization and be the basis for idiosyncrasies towards food proteins such as milk protein and egg white (p. 227).

In contrast to carbohydrates (glycogen) and fats (triglycerides) there is no equivalent storage of protein or amino acids, although the considerable total turnover of protein in the large mass of skeletal muscle provides a labile reserve of energy by gluconeogenesis that may be drawn upon when intake is reduced, and during exercise. Amino acids are quickly removed from the circulation and appear in all tissues and organs of the body. The plasma aminogram is constant in health. It is subject to considerable fluctuations in relation to dietary, circadian and other influences. It is distorted charcteristi-cally in protein deprivation and kwashiokor (see p. 106).

From the circulation amino acids may be taken up into one of many pathways. These include (1) incorporation into protein, (2) incorporation into a small peptide, (3) utilization of the nitrogen and/or carbon for synthesis of another amino acid, (4) or of some other nitrogenous compound, (5) removal of the a-amino group and formation of urea and oxidation of the resultant a-keto acid.

If amino acids are ingested in amounts in excess of requirements they may be excreted as such to a small extent or, more economically, their nitrogen is removed and excreted and the corresponding a-keto acids oxidized for their energy value or converted to glycogen or fatty acids for storage. Furthermore there is a constant need for the degradation of amino acids to go on for the biosynthesis of many nitrogenous compounds such as purines, pyrimidines, porphyrins, adrenaline, thyroxine, nicotinic acid.

The body is able to utilize nitrogen and carbon skeletons from a variety of sources. A synthetic diet that provides nitrogen only in the form of essential amino acids, plus the small amount in vitamins, can support maximal growth. When the intake of protein nitrogen is inadequate, synthesis of nitrogenous compounds continues at a reduced level but incomplete or imperfect proteins cannot be made.

The proteins in plasma play an active part in the transport process itself as well as having several other functions.

Albumin normally ranges from 35 to 56 g/l and, because of its small size (molecular weight 69 000) and its abundance, has an important role in exerting most of the plasma oncotic pressure that retains fluid within the circulation. Albumin also serves to transport sparingly soluble metabolic products and many other substances, including fatty acid ions, bilirubin, sulphonamides, hormones and vitamins. Plasma albumin level is depressed late in protein deficiency. Retinol-binding protein, prealbumin and transfer-rin fall earlier on (p. 106). Transport proteins are synthesized in the liver.

y-Globulins occur in plasma in concentrations normally from 6·0 to 12·0 g/100 ml. Antibodies found in blood are mainly assoicated with y-globulins. These proteins are synthesized in the reticulo-endothelial cells. Their level in plasma reflects past experience in relation to infectious diseases. Their formation is not affected by protein deficiency.

Nitrogenous compounds of the urine

A normal adult excretes daily an amount of nitrogen (about 12 g) roughly equivalent to that ingested in the same period and is said to be in nitrogen balance. A small fraction of the total urinary nitrogen is made up of a variety of compounds including creatinine and uric acid, the concentration of which is virtually constant. NH_3 excretion is a function of acid-base relationships and arises in the kidney mainly from glutamine. Urea forms normally 80 to 90 per cent of urinary nitrogen. Inadequate protein intake and low status result in diminished production of urea by the liver and lessened excretion. Abnormally high intake leads to excessive urinary loss as urea.

VITAMINS

Vitamin A

In the lumen of the small intestine micelle formation takes place and dietary vitamin A esters are largely hydrolysed. Bile salts assist in this process, and tocopherol prevents destruction by oxidation. Within the mucosal cell carotene is coverted via retinal into retinol and, together with preformed vitamin A in whatever form it was ingested, is esterified, mainly as palmitate.

In the mucosal cell most of the retinyl palmitate is incorporated into chylomicrons and in this form passes via the thoracic duct into the systemic circulation and thence to the liver for storage. Here nearly all the vitamin A is present as ester, mostly as palmitate. About 90 per cent of the postabsorptive circulating vitamin A is retinol coupled to retinol-binding protein (RBP) and a prealbumin. The normal concentration of vitamin A in postabsorptive blood is 20 to 50 μg/100 ml. Most of the carotenoids are concentrated in the β-lipoprotein fraction and the normal range is 80 to 120 μg/100 ml.

Retinol is oxidized to retinal (vitamin A_1 aldehyde, retinene) for utilization by the retina. It is one of the stereoisomers of retinal, the neo-b (11 cis) isomer, that takes part in the visual system.

Thiamin

Thiamin is readily absorbed in the small intestine but is not stored to any extent in the body. Any excess over requirement is excreted in the urine and reflects status. Biochemical test are more sensitive (p. 116).

Riboflavin

Riboflavin is not stored to any extent in the body, although the liver with 16 μg/g and the kidney with 25 μg/g usually contain higher concentrations than other tissues, e.g. muscle (2 or 3 μg/g). Urinary excretion, as in the case of thiamin, is used to measure the body status regarding the vitamin, but biochemical tests are more sensitive (p. 110).

Niacin

The body obtains niacin not only directly from the diet but indirectly about half from the conversion of tryptophan and possibly also from that synthesized by intestinal micro-organisms. The pathways of tryptophan metabolism in man are shown in Figure 5. Three vitamins are involved — thiamin, riboflavin and vitamin B_6. There are six possible points where pyridoxine-dependent enzymes may act. Measurement of urinary excretory products after a tryptophan load forms the basis of one method of detecting pyridoxine deficiency (see vitamin B_6).

Several metabolic products are excreted in the urine, of which N^1-methylnicotinamide and its pyridones are the most important. The ratio of pyridone to N^1-methylnicotinamide per gram of creatinine in urine has been used as a criterion of niacin nutritional status. A ratio of less than 1:1 is considered indicative of pellagra and a ratio between 1:1 and 1–3:1 as borderline.

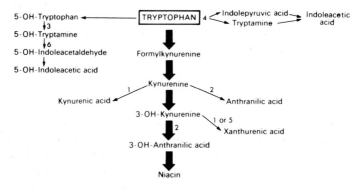

Fig. 5 Metabolic pathways for tryptophan in man with major pathways designated by heavy arrows. Pyridoxine-dependent enzymes are indicated by numbers on arrows. Key: 1, kynurenine transaminase; 2, kynureninase; 3, aromatic L-amino acid decarboxylase; 4, trytophanase; 5, hydroxy-kynurenine transaminase; 6, monoamine oxidase.

Vitamin B_6

Pyridoxal, pyridoxamine and pyridoxine are found mainly in the extracellular fluid, from which they may be readily transported intracellularly. The most important intracellular forms are pyridoxal-5^1-phosphate and pyridoxamine-5^1-phosphate. All the free forms are interchangeable and each can be phosphorylated. The latter forms are interchangeable. Pyridoxal-5^1-phosphate is degraded in the liver to 4-pyridoxic acid, which is then excreted in the urine.

There is virtually no storage of pyridoxine in the body; any excess is oxidized to pyridoxic acid, which is metabolically inert. About 0·4 mg is normally excreted in the urine daily.

Pantothenic acid

Human blood normally contains 18 to 35 μg pantothenic acid per 100 ml, mostly present in the cells as CoA. About 3 mg are excreted daily in the urine.

Biotin

Biotin is so readily made by intestinal bacteria that deficiency is most unlikely to arise except when all intestinal bacterial growth is suppressed or when diets are excessive in egg white (p. 129).

Folic acid

Folate is absorbed rapidly, primarily from the proximal small intestine, by a mechanism resembling that for iron and vitamin B_{12} through an active, energy-dependent process for small quantities but by diffusion in unphysiological amounts. Polyglutamates from food are broken down and reduced to dihydro- and tetrahydrofolates (THF), the latter being the active or co-enzyme form, present in serum, liver and other tissues as 5 N-methyl THF. Ascorbic acid helps to maintain folic acid co-enzymes in a reduced or active form.

Vitamin B_{12}

With a molecular weight of about 1500, vitamin B_{12} is probably the largest and most complicated vitamin. In physiological concentrations it can diffuse across the plasma membrane of the intestinal cell only after combination with intrinsic factor, a glycoprotein secreted by the parietal cells of the gastric mucosa. The site of absorption is limited to the terminal part of the ileum. Vitamin B_{12} circulates in three forms bound to specific proteins (transcorrin I and II), namely methyl-cobalamin, 5^1deoxyadenosylcobalamin, and hydroxo-cobalamin. Only the first two are active coenzyme forms. The normal serum level is 140 to 750 picograms per ml. Several milligrams are normally stored in the liver.

Vitamin C

The largest concentration of vitamin C is found in the adrenal gland, with high levels also present in liver, spleen and brain. Blood ascorbic acid consists of two fractions: one in the plasma and the other in the 'buffy coat', i.e. leucocytes and platelets. The renal threshold value in human plasma is about 1·4 mg/100 ml, whereas buffy coat and liver values range from 25 to 32 mg/100 g.

Vitamin D

Vitamin D from the skin (D_3), the major source, and the diet (D_2) is hydroxylated in the liver to 25-hydroyxvitamin D_2 and D_3 (25-OH-D_2 and D_3), the main forms in the circulation. Further hydroxylation takes place in the kidney to the steroid hormone 1,25-$(OH)_2D_3$ or to 24, 25$(OH)_2$-D_3 depending upon calcium and phosphorus status. Parathyroid hormone and calcitonin, secreted by the thyroid gland are also involved in calcium homeostasis (p. 76).

Vitamin E

The tocopherol content of human tissues, including plasma, has been found to vary widely among individuals, with highest concentrations in the pituitary, testes and adrenals. The usual concentration in plasma in adults is between 0·8 and 1·4 mg/100 ml. Much lower levels (0·05 to 0·40) are common in infancy: these are lower still in premature infants.

Vitamin K

Vitamin K is readily synthesized by bacteria of the type normally found in the human intestinal tract. Deficiency is therefore clinically rare unless absorption is interfered with, but during the newborn period, because of the sterility of the intestinal tract, deficiency is not uncommon.

WATER

It so happens that the volume of water and other fluids drunk is normally equal to the urine output. This fact is used in the simple 'fluid balance' sheet kept by the nursing staff in most hospitals to assist in the prevention of dehydration.

A complete water balance study, however, involves in addition to measurement of water in the diet solids, the metabolic water (usually a small contribution), the faecal water, and the evaporative water from the skin and lungs.

Water regulation. The kidney plays the major part, with thirst in a secondary role. Urine volume is very variable and usually reflects the fluid intake. Normally the kidneys can concentrate urine to 1200 mmol (sp. gr. 1·030) with a minimum daily volume of about 830 ml. If the load of urinary solutes, especially protein and salts, is reduced to 300 mmol or less the daily volume may be only 500 ml. This is of importance in case of shipwreck and other emergencies where water is short.

The urine volume is normally regulated by osmoreceptor cells in the hypothalamus that are sensitive to changes in plasma solute concentration. Dilution of the plasma is sensed by these cells which by nerve impulses to the posterior pituitary cause the inhibition of the secretion of the antidiuretic hormone (ADH) and diuresis starts. The reverse occurs in dehydration. Damage to the hypothalamus or posterior pituitary results in uncontrolled diuresis (p. 000). Kidney function is immature for several days after birth and the fluid intake is greater than the output. The balance is lost by evaporation. The large volumes of fluid lost readily in febrile illnesses and diarrhoea and vomitting by infants make dehydration a common danger.

Thirst

Osmoreceptors in the hypothalamus sample the osmotic pressure of the blood and control nerve impulses from the supraoptic nucleus to the posterior pituitary gland. When the osmolarity is reduced antidiuretic hormone (ADH) is released to increase reabsorption of water by the kidney tubules. The reverse occurs when osmolarity rises.

ELEMENTS

Sodium

The dietary intake is largely reflected in the urinary output. There is usually a diurnal variation, with maximum excretion at midday. Sodium conservation occurs by tubular reabsorption under control of adrenal cortical hormones. There is no mechanism comparable to thirst to warn the body of impending salt depletion such as occurs in excess losses in sweat. Heavy manual labour or high fever may cause salt depletion without thirst.

Loss of sodium through the gastrointestinal tract is usually small. The high concentrations in the digestive juices are reabsorbed.

Very little sodium is excreted through the skin in the absence of active sweating. When sweating does occur the loss may be considerable, even amounting to more than the urinary output. Acclimatization to heat usually results in a more dilute sweat.

Chloride

It is involved in water balance, osmotic pressure regulation and acid-base balance. As hydrochloric acid in gastric juice it initiates digestion of protein.

Potassium

Urinary loss largely reflects dietary intake. Increased losses occur when tissue breakdown is going on, where 1 g nitrogen is associated with 2·7 mEq of potassium. Potassium output through the gastrointestinal tract resembles that of sodium described above. Sweat losses are usually negligible. A vegetable diet gives rise to an alkaline urine because in these foodstuffs the cations, Na and K, are associated with weak organic acids. Flesh foods produce a slight excess of anions, PO_4 and SO_4, and in meat eaters the urine is strongly acid. Omnivorous man usually has a slightly acid urine but the healthy kidney can easily make adjustments by secreting alkali or acid.

Calcium

Only about 20 to 30 per cent of dietary calcium is normally absorbed. This is an active process involving oxygen and glucose or some other sources of energy. Vitamin D has a key role to play in this process. It has been shown to regulate the synthesis of a protein involved in the transport of calcium across the intestinal wall (p. 76).

Equally important are those factors that interfere with the absorption of calcium. Phytic acid (inositol phosphoric acid), present in larger amounts in whole wheat and oatmeal than in white bread, impairs calcium absorption. Calcium is usually added to wheat flour, except wholemeal (p. 11). Many cereals contain phytase, which leads to considerable destruction of phytic acid during the leavening process. Phytate phosphorus may also be largely liberated by the digestive juices and cause no impairment of calcium absorption. Considerable adaptation to diets high in cereal and phytic acid content and poor in calcium is known to take place.

Oxalates present in fruits and vegetables are seldom consumed in sufficient quantities for the insoluble calcium oxalate formed to create a problem.

Calcium balance. In health this can be maintained on very dissimilar dietary intakes. A high intake leads to poor absorption and increased urinary excretion. When the intake is low the efficiency of absorption is increased and excretion is diminished. Adaptation to low intakes has occurred in population groups over long periods of time and has been induced experimentally in subjects for a year or longer. There is, however, some evidence for the occasional occurence of pure calcium deficiency rickets (p. 132).

In hypocalcaemia parathyroid hormone acts with $1,25(OH)_2D_3$ to raise blood calcium and prevent a rise in phosphorus by impairing tubular reabsorption. In hypophosphataemia parathyroid hormone is not secreted and $1,25(OH)_2D_3$ raises the level to normal. Calcitonin causes a lowering of an artificially raised blood level of calcium by a direct effect on bone.

Calcium in the serum is in three forms, ionized (65 per cent), proteinbound (30 per cent) and diffusable unionized (5 per cent). The ionized fraction is controlled by parathyroid hormone and it is the concentration of this fraction that is altered in pathological states.

Phosphorus

It constitutes about 1 per cent of the body weight; 80 per cent being bound to calcium in bones and teeth. It is involved in many cellular reactions (p. 79).

Magnesium

It is present in all soft tissues and 70 per cent is in bone from which, like calcium and phosphorus, it may be mobilized when the need arises.

Iron

Man in more limited than other mammals both in his ability to absorb and to excrete iron. Iron in vegetables is absorbed not more than 2 to 10 per cent and from animal sources (haem compounds) 10 to 30 per cent. Animal protein improves iron absorption from other sources, as does vitamin C but phytates decrease it.

Most of the functional iron is in the red cells, about 800 to 900 mg in adult man. The metabolism of iron is described in the caption to Figure 6.

The minute amount of ferritin in serum (normal male 94, female 34 ng/ml), has recently been shown to be a sensitive measure of iron status. The level is low in childhood and gradually increases to adult life in the male, but not in the adult female.

Iodine

Absorption takes place in all parts of the gastrointestinal tract in the form of iodide. Part is taken up and stored in the thyroid gland and released as thyroid hormones, the rest circulates as part of the 'iodide pool'. Most iodide is excreted by the kidney.

Blood normally contains about 8 to 12 μg/100 ml iodine. About one-fifth is as iodide which freely enters red cells and does not vary significantly in different thyroid states. The rest, organic iodine, is detected as protein-bound iodine (PBI) in serum. In the thyroid gland the thyroid hormones that are synthesized there are held in combination with a high molecular weight protein, thyroglobulin, and they are economically released to the circulation after enzymic proteolysis of thyroglobulin.

Iodine plays its role in metabolism through the action of the thyroid hormones which have a fundamental effect on cellular oxidation.

Zinc

Little (<10 per cent) of dietary zinc is normally absorbed. The form in which the zinc is present has a considerable influence on its absorption, and phytic acid and fibre bind it. In blood, zinc is found in plasma (12–17 μmol/l) attached loosely to albumin and about twice as much firmly bound to globulins. Plasma levels relate rather closely to dietary intake. Most zinc is lost via the faeces, that which has been absorbed is re-excreted mainly through the pancreatic juice. Only a small amount appears in the urine.

Fluorine

Almost complete elimination occurs at low levels of intake. Very high levels indeed have to be reached for harmful retention to occur. Fluoride is treated similarly to chloride and is widely distributed throughout the extracellular

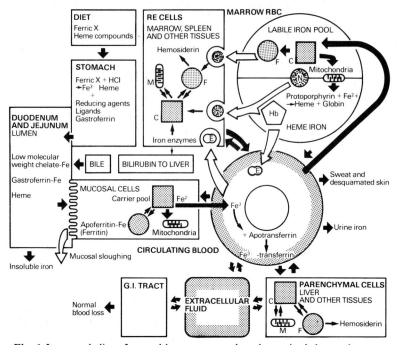

Fig. 6 Iron metabolism. Ingested haem compounds and organic chelates, when subjected to the action of hydrochloric acid (low pH) in the stomach, are broken down to form haem molecules and ferric ions. The ferric ions react with reducing agents, ligands and gastroferrin. Only iron kept soluble, either as haem molecules or by binding to low-molecular-weight chelates or gastroferrin, can undergo absorption, which occurs chiefly in the duodenum and proximal jejunum. Luminal iron incorporated into the mucosal blood cell enters the carrier pool (C). Most of this iron is deposited as ferritin (F) or utilized by mitochondria (M) for enzyme synthesis and then is lost by sloughing. The remainder is absorbed by being transferred from the carrier pool to the plasma, where it is bound tightly in the ferric state to the β_1-globulin transferrin. Iron leaves the plasma primarily by entering the labile iron pool of the erythroid series, from which there is considerable feedback of iron into the plasma, mainly via reticulo-endothelial (RE) cells. Within the developing erythroid cells of the bone marrow, ferrous ions combine with protoporphyrin to form the porphyrin haem, which in turn combines with globin to form haemoglobin. Haemoglobin is released into the circulation within circulating red cells (E) that have an average life span of 117 days. At the time of their disintegration, these cells are removed from the circulation by the spleen and other reticuloendothelial tissues with excretion of the split porphyrin as bilirubin in the bile and conservation of almost all the iron, which re-enters the plasma and is bound once more to transferrin. These phagocytic RE cells normally are the chief source of iron entering the plasma. Approximately two-thirds of normal total body iron loss (1.0 mg/day) occurs as the result of the gastrointestinal blood loss of 1.2 ml/day (0.6 mg Fe per day). Approximately 18 per cent of the iron leaving and entering the plasma does so in equilibration with extracellular fluid transferrin; the formation and breakdown of myoglobin and the haem enzymes; iron absorption; and iron storage. Arrows are not quantitative. (Fig. 49.4 from Stanbury, Wyngaarden, Fredrickson 1978 Metabolic basis of inherited disease, 4th edn. McGraw Hill, New York.)

space. Most of a large dose is deposited in the bones. Levels in blood and other tissues are very low.

Copper

The main site of absorption is the upper small intestine. Only 5 to 10 per cent of ingested copper is normally absorbed. In plasma about 80 per cent of copper is firmly bound as the enzyme caeruloplasmin. Very little of this copper is exchanged daily. The remaining copper is loosely bound to albumin and is believed to constitute true transport copper. Most excretion occurs in urine, the extent varying considerably and bearing no relation to intake.

Chromium

Inorganic Cr is only about 1 per cent absorbed; against 20 per cent of the complexed form. In plasma it binds to transferrin and is probably stored with ferric iron.

Manganese

The mechanism of absorption is not known, but excretion is in bile. It is involved in mucopolysaccharide metabolism.

Molybdenum

Its absorption is inhibited by copper and sulphate. It is part of the enzymes xanthine oxidase, aldehyde oxidase and sulphite oxidase.

6. METABOLISM OF NUTRIENTS

CELLULAR ENERGETICS

Within a system, if a reaction involves a fall in free energy, it will proceed without the need for energy from an external source. If the reaction necessitates a rise in free energy, energy must be supplied from outside. There is also a half-way stage between the two in which the reactions have to be brought into an active state. Many of the reactions in cells which involve a fall in energy do not take place unless the reactants are brought together under the right circumstances. Large and complex molecules generally have more free energy than small and simple ones. The increase in free energy necessary for the building up and maintaining of the complex structure of the human body has to be provided by the energy contained in the food.

The sum total of the biochemical processes of the body is the *metabolism*. The breakdown of complex into simple molecules is *catabolism* and synthesis of complex molecules is *anabolism*. Catabolic reactions release free energy while those that are anabolic require energy from outside. Thus the energy derived from the breakdown of complex substances in the food is used for such processes as the synthesis of complex molecules by the body, maintenance of body temperature, and muscular contraction. The carbohydrates, fats and proteins of foodstuffs are gradually broken down into three simple acids, acetic, oxaloacetic and *a*-ketoglutaric. Little free energy is released until the three lines of catabolism converge on what is the key point in catabolism: the *citric acid cycle*. In this cycle complete oxidation occurs to carbon dioxide and water and in the process coenzymes are reduced which are then themselves oxidized through the cytochrome system. As a result much free energy is liberated and this is stored for used in energy-requiring processes in the form of ATP (adenosine triphosphate).

Two of the three phosphate groups of ATP can be easily removed and for each there is a fall in free energy of about 8 kcal (33.5 kJ)/mol ATP used. These are the high energy phosphate bonds. The third phosphate group is difficult to remove and the yield is only about 2 kcal (8.4 kJ)/ mol.

If a reaction involves a fall in free energy it will not necessarily take place. The reactant must be in an active state. There may also be several possible different products of reaction. It is the function of the special class of proteins known as enzymes to direct reactions in a manner appropriate for the organism. The processes that give rise to ATP in the body are outlined on page 66.

CARBOHYDRATE METABOLISM

Glucose may undergo one of three changes after it leaves the circulation, two of which are of little importance. These latter are (1) oxidation to glucuronic acid which can be phosphorylated and enter the alternative pathway of glucose oxidation and (2) reduction to sorbitol which may then be oxidized to fructose.

The overwhelmingly important reaction is conversion to glucose-6-phosphate. Besides glucose, most of the galactose and fructose absorbed passes through glucose-6-phosphate before further metabolism. There are four possible pathways for the further metabolism of glucose-6-phosphate.

1. Hydrolysis to glucose and inorganic phosphate. ATP is not formed. It takes place only in liver, kidney and intestine and appears to be necessary for glucose to be released from the cells for transport to other organs.

2. Conversion to glucose-1-phosphate for the synthesis of polysaccharides.

3. Oxidation to 6-phosphogluconic acid, the start of the alternative pathway of glucose oxidation.

4. Isomerization to fructose-6-phosphate which is the main pathway of glucose oxidation via glycolysis and the citric acid cycle.

The main pathway

The first section of the pathway involves the conversion of glucose to pyruvic acid and is known as *glycolysis* or the *Embden-Meyerhof pathway*. The *citric acid* (*tricarboxylic acid* or *Krebs*) *cycle* takes pyruvic acid on ultimately to carbon dioxide and water. For a lucid outline of these reactions the account given by Horrobin can be thoroughly recommended.

Glycolysis

In glycolysis ATP is required for phosphorylation at two points and is formed at two points. There is , however, a net gain of two units of ATP, because the two steps requiring ATP occur before the splitting of the hexose chain while the two steps generating ATP occur after each hexose chain has been split into two three-carbon units. Hydrogen is generated and is removed by the co-enzyme NAD^+ forming NADH. If oxygen is available the most important product of glycolysis results: ATP (see later). NAD^+ cannot be formed from NADH if oxygen is not available. Then it is produced from NADH by the removal of H necessary for a reaction whereby pyruvic acid is reduced to lactic acid. Many of the enzymes involved require magnesium ions for their activity, probably for the binding of the substance to the enzyme.

Citric acid cycle

Pyruvic acid has to be converted to acetyl-coenzyme A before it can enter the cycle. This reaction is a complex one involving four vitamins. The oxidative decarboxylation of pyruvic acid is carried out by cocarboxylase which is thiamin pyrophosphate. Lipoic acid is a vitamin with two sulphur atoms, pantothenic acid is part of the molecule of CoA, and nicotinic acid is essential for the synthesis of NAD^+. The net result is the using up of one molecule each of pyruvic acid, CoA and NAD^+; and the generation of one molecule each of acetyl-CoA and NADH.

Acetyl-CoA enters the cycle by combining with oxalo-acetic acid to form citric acid. One turn of the cycle results in the complete oxidation of the acetyl group and the regeneration of oxaloacetic acid. Acetyl-CoA is also the major product of the oxidation of fatty acids (see p.68) and so fats may yield up their energy through the citric acid cycle.

Proteins can also be oxidized in the same way. In alanine, aspartic acid and glutamic acid, the replacement of ammonia by oxygen yields, respectively, pyruvic acid, oxaloacetic acid and a-ketoglutaric acid, which can all enter the cycle. Other amino acids can also be oxidized in this way although the preliminary steps are more complex. Pyruvic, oxaloacetic and a-ketoglutaric acids can also be built up into the corresponding amino acids. This poses a threat to the operation of the cycle if large amounts of oxaloacetic or a-ketoglutaric acids were lost. Oxaloacetic acid is the more important as it is by reaction with it that acetyl-CoA enters the cycle. If there is lack of oxaloacetic acid, acetyl-CoA and pyruvic acid accumulate and the latter is converted to oxaloacetic acid. The vitamin, biotin, is part of the enzyme responsible, which appears to be incapable of combining with pyruvate in the absence of acetyl-CoA. Thus the build up of acetyl-CoA facilitates the production of oxaloacetic acid needed for its metabolism.

Carbohydrate oxidation cannot be simply reversed. Some of the reverse steps in glycolysis are different. Glucose can be resynthesized from pyruvate but not from acetyl-CoA; once it has reversed the cycle it cannot be regenerated.

The alternative pathway

The alternative pathway is also called the hexose monophosphate shunt and direct oxidative pathway. In contrast to the main pathway, the coenzyme used for dehydrogenation is $NADP^+$ (not NAD^+). The reduced form of $NADP^+$, NADPH, is necessary for the synthesis of fatty acids and therefore this pathway might be expected to operate where fatty acids are being synthesized.

The synthesis of ATP

The main alternative pathways of glucose oxidation produce large amounts of the reduced coenzymes NADH, NADPH and $FADH_2$. Most of the ATP formed arises from the oxidation of these compounds.

The enzymes concerned with the oxidation of the reduced coenzymes mentioned above are found in the mitochondria and it is here that most of the ATP is generated. This occurs by what is known as the *electron transport chain*. Many links in the chain are still unknown but the compounds which constitute it include NADH dehydrogenase, succinic dehydrogenase, iron-containing cytochromes and ubiquinones. Electrons resulting from the oxidation of food materials pass along this chain until they eventually combine with oxygen to form water. In the process ATP is generated by what is known as *oxidative phosphorylation*.

The glucose–fatty acid cycle

Observations showing the antagonistic effect ketone bodies and fatty acids have on insulin and the known effect of glucose and insulin on the storage of fatty acids as triglyceride have led to the overall concept of a glucose–fatty acid cycle.

At the physiological level this cycle would operate when fat oxidation overnight alternates with the onset of carbohydrate oxidation and storage when food is eaten. This nutritional cycle (Fig. 7) is controlled by the presence or absence of glucose. When glucose is absent, fatty acyl-CoA is oxidized. In the presence of glucose, glycerol phosphate, an obligatory precursor of triglyceride synthesis, is increased, fatty acyl-CoA is removed to triglyceride and glucose is oxidized. Hormonal control is also exerted by increase of activity of enzymes hydrolysing triglycerides in adipose tissue by adrenalin, glucagon, adrenocorticotropic hormone (ACTH), growth hormone and others, and reduction by insulin.

In relation to the pathogenesis of diabetes mellitus it is suggested that the high levels of free fatty acids in plasma antagonize the action of insulin. Free fatty acids also stimulate secretion of insulin and thus could occur, as is seen in type II or non-insulin-dependent diabetes (p. 183), insulin resistance in the presence of high plasma insulin levels.

Polysaccharide synthesis and breakdown

It was seen earlier that one of the fates of glucose-6-phosphate is conversion to glucose-1-phosphate for glycogen synthesis. The next step is ill understood. Glucose-1-phosphate reacts with UTP (uridine triphosphate, a high energy compound made by the reaction of UDP with ATP). UDP-glucose results. From this glycogen can be synthesized, releasing UDP in the process. The reaction involves a marked fall in free energy (is strongly exergonic).

Glycogen breakdown in liver and muscles is brought about by phosphorylase to yield glucose-1-phosphate. Inorganic phosphate is required.

The synthesis and breakdown of glycogen appear to be under separate control. Glycogen synthetase is thought to be stabilized by the presence of glucose-6-phosphate although the latter plays no direct part in the synthesis. Consequently, if glucose is lacking and there will be little glucose-6-phosphate, glycogen will not be formed. When glucose is plentiful glucose-6-phosphate will accumulate and glycogen will be formed.

The control of glycogen breakdown is more complex. Adrenalin and glucagon exert control through phosphorylases.

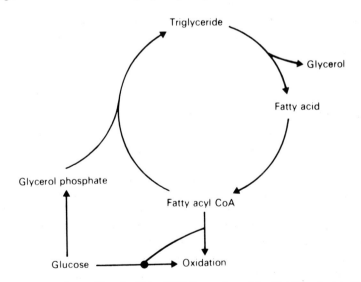

Fig. 7 The glucose fatty acid cycle. Haley 1966 Proceeding of the Nutrition Society 25: 61.

FAT METABOLISM

Glycerides form an important source of energy and when energy from carbohydrates is limited, as in starvation and diabetes mellitus, they are of primary significance. Resting muscle R.Q. is 0·7 oxidizing mainly fatty acids. Surplus fatty acids and carbohydrate are stored as triglycerides in adipose tissue.

Glyceride oxidation

Initially glycerides are broken down into glycerol and fatty acids. Glycerol can enter the glycolytic pathway of carbohydrate oxidation in the form of a-glycerophosphate to which it is converted by ATP.

Even-numbered fatty acids are oxidized to acetyl-CoA by going through a cycle repeatedly in which two carbon atoms are split off from the fatty acid chain. This is known as *β-oxidation* as it begins at the carboxyl end of the chain. The acetyl-CoA can be completely oxidized by way of the citric acid cycle. An acyl-CoA with two carbon atoms less than the original one is left and the cycle repeated until acetyl-CoA is left. In the case of the much rarer odd chain fatty acids the end product is propionyl-CoA which can enter the citric acid cycle by being converted to succinyl-CoA via methylmalonyl-CoA. Biotin is involved in the first step and vitamin B_{12} in the second.

Ketosis

If the level of oxaloacetic acid in the citric acid cycle is low the acetyl-CoA from fatty acid oxidation cannot be completely oxidized. Pyruvic acid is the main source of oxaloacetic acid but it will not be available if glycolysis is not taking place. This occurs in diabetes mellitus, starvation and high fat diets, where carbohydrate oxidation is reduced, fatty acid oxidation increased, and ketosis results.

Acetyl-CoA molecules react together to form ketone bodies: aceoacetic acid, β-hydroxybutyric acid and acetone which arise in the liver and appear in the blood and the urine.

Fatty acid synthesis

Fat is synthesized from carbohydrates but the reverse cannot take place. Two systems for fatty acid synthesis are known. The first is found outside the mitochondria and can synthesize fatty acids from acetyl-CoA. The binding of CO_2 to acetyl-CoA to form malonyl-CoA is performed by an enzyme which contains biotin. This stage requires ATP. Two carbon atoms at a time are added until the required chain length is reached, often palmitic acid.

The second system is within the mitochondria and is incapable of synthesizing the short chain fatty acids but, if the short chain acids are presented as substrates, it can add two carbon atom units to them and so lengthen the chain.

Both routes of fatty acids synthesis require NADPH and as the only known large-scale source is the alternative pathway of glucose oxidation (hexose monophosphate shunt), this explains why this pathway is associated with tissues where fatty acid synthesis is going on, i.e. liver, adipose tissue and the lactating mammary gland.

Regulation of lipogenesis

This process is concerned with the conversion of glucose and intermediates such as pyruvate and acetyl-CoA to fat. The rate is high on an adequate diet high in carbohydrate especially with a high sucrose content. It is depressed in restricted energy intake, a high fat diet and when there is deficiency of insulin as in diabetes mellitus.

The rate-limiting reaction in the lipogenic pathway is at the acetyl-CoA carboxylase step. Carnitine, which is synthesized from lysine and methionine, is essential for transport of long-chain fatty acids into mitochondria for β-oxidation.

Mobilization of fat

Lipid leaving adipose tissue cells is largely transported as unesterified fatty acids bound to plasma albumin. At the same time smaller amounts of glycerol appear in the plasma. The release is catalysed by a lipase and the turnover of fatty acids is very rapid. Fat mobilization is influenced by (1) *hormones* and (2) *the liver.*

1. *Hormones and lipid mobilization.* In outline the process consists of (1) conversion of triglycerides to free fatty acids within adipose tissue, (2) carriage by albumin in plasma, (3) oxidation and, in the presence of glucose, re-esterification to triglyceride of part of liberated fatty acids, (4) re-esterification into triglyceride and cholesterol ester, chiefly in kidney and liver and (5) discharge of triglyceride and cholesterol esters from liver as lipoproteins.

The hormones capable of bringing about mobilization include adrenaline, adrenocorticotropin, glucagon, thyrotropin and the lipid mobilizing factor of the hypophysis.

2. *The liver and lipid metabolism.* Besides synthesizing and oxidizing fatty acids, synthesizing triglycerides and phospholipids and converting fatty acids to ketone bodies, as already mentioned, the liver is the main source of plasma lipoproteins from endogenous sources. Hepatic triglycerides are the immediate precursors of those in VLDL (p. 52). Normally most of this comes from synthesis in the liver from acetyl-CoA derived from carbohydrate, but some derives from circulating free fatty acids and uptake of chylomicrons.

Triglyceride usually accumulates in the liver, but fatty liver results when this is excessive. This is of two main types. The first is associated with raised levels of plasma FFA due to mobilization from adipose tissue. It occurs in starvation, high-fat diet and diabetes mellitus. The second type results from a metabolic block in the production of plasma lipoproteins for a number of reasons. The fatty liver of kwashiorkor (p. 106) is of this nature. Liver poisons such as ethanol (p. 242) and carbon tetrachloride have the same effect. Deficiency of lipotropic factors, such as choline, involved in transmethylation causes fatty liver in animals, but has not been implicated in human disease.

Essential fatty acids

They are present in all lipid macromolecules but especially abundant in membranes of cells and intracellular organelles such as mitochondria, their low melting point and greater chain length probably making for stability. Arachidonic acid is the precursor of at least four classes of compounds that are being studied extensively in relation to many disease states. They are prostaglandins, thromboxanes, prostacyclins and leukotrienes.

Brown fat

Infants have an interscapular deposit of fat rich in mitochondria and highly vascularized. Heat produced locally warms the circulation and assists in temperature regulation by 'non-shivering thermogenesis'.

PROTEIN AND AMINO ACID METABOLISM

Protein turnover

The rate of protein turnover is the net result of protein synthesis and catabolism. It varies for different proteins and is influenced by the nutritional status of the body, for protein and other nutrients as well as energy. Isotope trace techniques have made possible estimates of turnover rate. Total protein turnover in the adult is about 2·5 g/kg/day, equivalent to 150 g of protein broken down in a 60 kg man. The daily obligatory nitrogen loss from the body is equivalent to only about 30 g protein which means that 80 per cent of the amino N produced by protein breakdown must be reutilized for synthesis. In the adult only 20 per cent of the dietary protein needs to be in the form of essential amino acids, although they form 40 per cent of tissue proteins, indicating that their reutilization is even greater (almost 90 per cent). Children require about twice the adult proportion of essential amino acids in the diet, for the laying down of new protein during growth.

Synthesis of non-essential amino acids

After ammonia is fixed into organic linkage amino acids are then built from carbon compounds which are available as products from carbohydrate metabolism, e.g. pyruvate and oxaloacetate. Each reaction in these synthetic pathways is catalysed by specific enzymes. Each pathway must be essentially irreversible, i.e. proceed with a relatively large loss of free energy, in order to provide a continuing supply of amino acids. Amino group transfer from glutamic acid provides a mechanism for synthesis of most of the other non-essential amino acids by transamination. This provides a means of redistributing nitrogen when a mixture of amino acids has been ingested which may not be optimum for the organism. The liver contains transaminases specific for transamination from glutamic acid to each of the a-amino acids with the possible exception of glycine, threonine and lysine. Pyridoxal phosphate, the coenzyme form of vitamin B_6, is present in all transaminases.

Amino acid degradation

The first stage in the degradation of amino acids is the removal of the a-amino group by deamination and this takes place primarily in the liver.

The main enzyme which can carry this out is L-glutamic dehydrogenase which can either deaminate glutamic acid to give a-ketoglutaric acid or carry out the reverse reaction. It is probable that most of the other amino acids are first acted on by appropriate transaminases which transfer the amino group to ketoacids.

Urea synthesis

The liver converts ammonia to urea. When each of the individual amino acids is added to a liver slice preparation one atom of amino acid nitrogen gives rise to one atom of urea nitrogen, except in the case of ornithine and arginine when about ten times as much urea is produced. In the ornithine cycle of urea formation, first proposed by Krebs, arginine is repeatedly synthesized from ornithine, broken down to give urea and the reforming of ornithine. Citrulline is intermediate between arginine and ornithine. Most of the nitrogen from amino acids appears in the urine as urea.

Fate of the carbon skeleton

Urea formation is irreversible and therefore the a-ketoacids that remain are utilized for energy production. Those which form pyruvic acid can be converted to glucose while those which form acetyl-CoA or acetoacetic acid give rise to ketone bodies or fatty acids.

Amino acids are important precursor substrates in the gluconeogenic process. In the postabsorptive state (12-hour fast) amino acids, among which alanine predominates, are released by muscles and the gut and taken up by the liver. Approximately 75 per cent of glucose production comes from glycogen, 10 to 15 per cent from pyruvate and lactate, 5 to 10 per cent from alanine, 5 per cent from other glycogenic amino acids and 2 per cent from glycerol. Of the 225 g produced in 24 hours, 125 g are used by the brain, 50 g by muscles and 50 g by blood cells. As fasting extends beyond 12 hours gluconeogenesis becomes relatively more important.

A glucose-alanine cycle has been proposed as shown in Figure 8. The cycle is probably of importance not only in gluconeogenesis but also in nitrogen metabolism, as alanine acts as a non-toxic alternative to ammonia in the transfer of amino groups from muscle to liver. Twenty-five to 30 per cent of this net transfer occurs in blood cells and the rest in plasma.

Amino acids as precursors of other compounds

Among the most important of these are those listed below:

1. Porphyrins which are important in haemoglobin metabolism and some enzymes.

2. Nucleic acids. These compounds direct cellular metabolism, carry genetic information, and control the synthesis of enzymes.

3. Hormones such as those of the thyroid, adrenal medulla and melanin; all formed from tyrosine.

4. Serotonin (5-hydroxytryptamine), which acts on vascular and extra-vascular smooth muscle, is formed from tryptophan.

5. Histamine, produced by the decarboxylation of histidine.

6. Creatine, synthesized from arginine, glycine and methionine. It is present in muscle as a high energy phosphate compound, phosphoryl-creatine. It appears to act there as a store of energy additional to ATP which

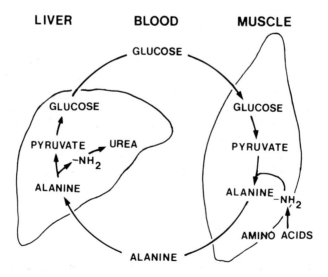

Fig. 8 The glucose alanine cycle. (Reprinted from Felig, Wahren 1974 Federation Proceedings **33**: 1092.)

can be used to regenerate ATP extremely rapidly but is not part of the contractile system itself. Creatinine is the final product of its degradation, and its excretion in urine is proportional to muscle mass if renal function is normal.

Amino acids in urine. Excretion of greater amounts than normal may occur (1) as an overflow phenomenon when circulating levels are high or (2) from a defect in tubular reabsorption (p. 192).

VITAMINS

Vitamin A

Photoreception in the rods and cones of the retina is a complicated process. In brief, the photosensitive pigment in man is rhodopsin, which consists of retinal and a protein, opsin. The pigment is bleached as an essential part of the process of photoreception in dim light and requires retinal, from the oxidation of retinol, for its regeneration. An analogous system in the cones, with retinal combined with another protein to form iodopsin, is the basis for the perception of light of high intensity and of colour.

Elsewhere in the body retinal is essential for the normal proliferation and differentiation of many epithelial tissues. Deficiency leads to loss of goblet cells, keratinization of epithelia and predisposes to infections (p. 111); it may be an important determinant of morbidity and mortality among young children in developing countries (p. 224), and may predispose to epithelial cancers (p. 110).

Thiamin

Thiamin pyrophosphate (TPP, cocarboxylase) is the coenzyme of carboxylase, involved in the decarboxylation of a-keto acids, such as pyruvic and a-keto-glutaric. In mammalian metabolism pyruvate is oxidatively decarboxylated and the activity of the thiamin derivative is linked with that of lipoic acid and coenzyme A. As a result a key compound for many metabolic pathways is formed, acetyl-CoA. The oxidation involves NAD derived from niacin, and CoA contains panthothenic acid. Furthermore, thiamin plays a part in activating transketolase, an enzyme involved in the direct oxidative pathway for glucose (see p. 116). Although less than 10 per cent of all glucose is normally utilized by this path, it is the only way the body can produce ribose for the synthesis of RNA; it is also an intermediate in the synthesis of fatty acids.

Riboflavin

All flavoproteins consist of specific proteins (apoenzymes), containing either flavin mononucleotide (FMN, riboflavin phosphate) or flavin adenine dinucleotide (FAD) as prosthetic groups, or coenzymes. At least three flavoproteins with enzymatic activity have been shown to contain FMN, namely: Warburg's yellow enzyme, cytochrome c reductase and L-amino-acid oxidase.

These enzymes are involved in many biological oxidation-reduction reactions. They oxidize (dehydrogenate) L-amino-acids, D-amino-acids, xanthine and hypoxanthine. They accept hydrogen from nicotinamide-adenine dinucleotide systems (NAD and NADP) and pass it on to the cytochrome system and thus to oxygen. Flavoproteins are relatively unstable, especially when tissue protein is depleted by physiological stress, dietary deficiency or disease. Under these conditions increased levels of riboflavin are lost in the urine.

Niacin

Through the role of NAD and NADP in oxidation-reduction reactions the derivatives of niacin play a vital function in a series of reactions essential to life. Among these are: (1) the synthesis of high energy phosphate compounds, (2) glycolysis (3) pyruvate metabolism, (4) pentose biosynthesis, (5) glycerol and fatty acid metabolism, and (6) obtaining energy from protein.

Vitamin B_6

Pyridoxine appears to have no direct role in energy metabolism but is concerned primarily in protein metabolism. Among the known metabolic processes in which pyridoxal phosphate is concerned are the following:

1. Transamination. The exchange of amino groups between a-ketoglutarate and a variety of amino acids yielding glutamate and the corresponding keto acid (p. 71).

2. Decarboxylation of amino acids to form special amines, such as histamine from histidine, serotonin from 5-hydroxytryptophan, β-alanine from aspartic acid, taurine from cystic acid or other derivatives of cystine, γ-aminobutyric acid from glutamic acid.

3. Formation of melanin.

4. Metabolism of tryptophan (see Fig. 5). In addition to decarboxylation and transamination, tryptophan is metabolized by pyridoxal phosphate enzymes in at least three further ways:

   (a) Tryptophanase catalyses the breakdown of tryptophan to indole, pyruvate and ammonia.

   (b) Tryptophan is metabolized in the animal through kynurenine. Pyridoxal phosphate is the coenzyme of two steps along this pathway.

   (c) Pyridoxal phosphate is involved in formation of tryptophan from indole and serine (in E. coli, not man).

5. Transmethylation by methionine.

6. Pyridoxal phosphate is a cofactor of δ-amino levulinic acid synthetase, which is probably the rate-limiting enzyme in porphyrin biosynthesis.

7. The pyridoxine-containing enzyme phosphorylase facilitates the release of glycogen from liver and muscle as glucose phosphate.

Pantothenic acid

Pantothenic acid is present in all living cells, mostly in the form of coenzyme A (CoA). Two carbon fragments from the breakdown of glucose, and some amino acids combine with CoA to form acetyl-coenzyme A (acetyl-CoA) which can be oxidized in the citric acid cycle (p. 65) or lead to fatty acid synthesis via malonyl CoA.

Biotin

Biotin in particular plays a role in (1) carboxylation and decarboxylation of oxaloacetic acid, (2) biosynthesis of aspartic acid (3) metabolism of serine, threonine and citrulline, and (4) formation of cis unsaturated fatty acids.

Folic acid

In the tetrahydro form folates act as coenzymes in all metabolic systems where there is a transfer of a one-carbon unit. These include steps in early purine and pyrimidine biosynthesis, the generation and utilization of formate and amino acid conversions. The latter include serine to glycine (requiring pyridoxine), histidine to glutamic acid and homocysteine to methionine (see vitamin B_{12} below).

Vitamin B_{12}

Vitamin B_{12} can effect the reduction of ribose to deoxyribose, converting uracil ribotide to uracil deoxyribotide prior to the addition of a single carbon unit by folic acid coenzyme to form thymine deoxyribotide. Methylcobalamin is required for the remethylation of homocysteine to methionine. The isomerization of methyl malonyl CoA to succinyl CoA is under the control of deoxyadenosylcobalamin. Recently it has been shown that vitamin B_{12} is necessary for the synthesis of thymidylate synthetase, an enzyme involved in the *de novo* synthesis of DNA for which folic acid acts as coenzyme.

Vitamin C

L-Ascorbic acid is readily oxidized and reversibly reduced; both forms are usually found in tissues possessing high metabolic activity, suggesting a role in reactions involved in electron transfer in the cell.

It has long been known that in the absence of vitamin C normal fibrous collagen is not formed, being replaced by a non-fibrous collagen precursor. In connective tissue it acts as a reductant and with molecular oxygen, ferrous iron and a 2 ketoacid it activates enzymes responsible for the hydroxylation of protocollagen proline and lysine to collagen hydroxyproline and hydroxylysine. Ascorbic acid also antagonizes the conversion of folic acid to folinic acid by folic acid reductase, promotes the release of free folic acid from conjugates in food, and facilitates iron absorption.

The claims of Linus Pauling that doses of vitamin C of up 4 g daily (nearly 100 times the RDA) decrease the incidence and severity of the common cold have not been conclusively substantiated or disproved by several recent studies. More recent claims for effectiveness in preventing certain forms of cancer are even more controversial. Prolonged high level dosing may result in iron overload due to enhanced iron absorption (p. 160) and urinary stone formation. The majority of medical opinion regards his case as 'non proven' at the present time.

Vitamin D

As was mentioned earlier (p. 58) $25(OH)D_3$ undergoes one of two hydroxylations in the kidney. It has recently been shown that provitamin D_3 (7-dehydrocholesterol) is converted by ultraviolet radiation on the skin to provitamin D_3 and stored there as such until it is thermally isomerized to vitamin D_3 and transported to the liver on vitamin D-binding protein. It is there hydroxylated to $25(OH)D_3$ which undergoes enterohepatic circulation, is reabsorbed from the gut and is the major circulating form. At physiological doses $25(OH)D_3$ does not function directly in any of the known systems responsive to vitamin D_3.

$25(OH)D_3$ goes to the kidney where it undergoes one of two hydroxylations. If there is need for calcium or phosphate the kidney is stimulated to produce $1,25(OH)_2D_3$, which acts as a calcium and phosphate mobilizing hormone. If supplies of calcium and phosphate are adequate the l-hydroxylase is shut down and 24-hydroxylase produces $24,25(OH)_2D_3$ whose role is unclear at present. 24-hydroxylase is repressed by parathyroid hormone. Low calcium probably results in increased renal clearance of phosphate and change in its intracellular concentration in proximal tubules is thought to be the most immediate stimulus to $1,25(OH)_2D_3$ formation.

The actions of vitamin D, or more appropriately its metabolite(s), are summarized in Table 3.

Table 3 Actions of vitamin D and its metabolite(s)

Intestine	Enhances Ca transport
	Enhances PO_4 transport
Bone	Enhances bone resorption
	Stimulates normal mineralization
	Affects collagen maturation
Muscle	Maintains normal function (? mechanism)
Parathyroid glands	? Inhibits PTH section
Kidney	Variable effect on reabsorption of Ca
Other	Permits normal growth

Figure 9 shows the 'butterfly' model that has recently been proposed to describe the major known interrelationships of vitamin D, parathyroid hormones and calcitonin. Other short feedback loops probably occur but are incompletely understood at present.

Vitamin E

The role of vitamin E at the molecular level is little understood. It appears to act as a lipid antioxidant, preventing the formation of peroxides from polyunsaturated fatty acids. This may possibly be related to its role in maintaining stability of biological membranes such as those of lysosomes in liver and muscle and of the erythrocyte. Vitamin E appears to be required for synthesis of haem as activity of one of the enzymes involved, delta aminolevulinic acid dehydratase, is diminished in deficiency. Selenium is an integral part of the enzyme glutathione peroxidase that is thought to destroy peroxides derived from unsaturated fatty acids. This may explain the similarity of action of selenium and vitamin E *in vivo*.

Vitamin K

In vitamin K deficiency an abnormal prothrombin is formed by the liver which cannot bind calcium, a necessary step in the conversion *in vivo* of prothrombin to thrombin and initiation of the blood clotting mechanism.

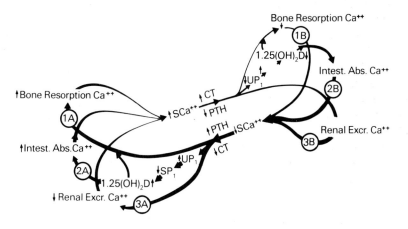

Fig. 9 The model consists of three overlapping control loops (negative feedback) that interlock and relate to one another through the level of blood concentrations of ionic calcium, parathyroid hormone, and calcitonin. The loops are numbered 1, 2 and 3; the limbs of the three loops that describe physiological events that increase blood concentrations of calcium are designated 'A' (left) and the limbs that describe events that decrease blood concentrations of calcium are designed 'B' (right). Thus, loop 1 represents bone resorption; limb 1A increased bone resorption; and limb 1B decreased bone resorption. Loop 2 represents intestinal absorption of calcium; limb 2A increased; and limb 2B decreased absorption. And loop 3 represents renal excretion of calcium; limb 3A decreased; and limb 3B increased excretion. (Fig. 1 from Arnaud C D 1978 Federation proceedings 37: 2557.)

Recently evidence has been obtained that vitamin K acts by inducing carboxylation of glutamyl residues in abnormal prothrombin, converting it to prothrombin and resulting in a new amino acid, gamma carboxylglutamic acid, responsible for calcium binding. Formation of factors VII, IX and X is also affected.

ELEMENTS

Almost every aspect of the life process is concerned. Pre-eminently, elements are deeply involved in the various homeostatic mechanisms of the body.

Maintenance of acid–base balance

Cellular processes can go on only within a very narrow pH range around neutral reaction. Certain elements play an important role in maintaining acid–base balance. Chlorine, sulphur and phosphorus are acidic while calcium, sodium, potassium, iron and magnesium are basic.

Most mixed diets contain a slight excess of acid-forming elements. This is counteracted by the excretion of carbon dioxide through the lungs and a slightly acid urine. A strict vegetarian diet is basic, a high protein diet has a predominantly acidic residue in the mineral ash and prolonged intake of sodium-containing antacids with a milk diet predisposes to alkalosis. Excesses of acid or alkali can be neutralized in several ways by the body. The blood contains buffers, such as carbonate, phosphate and proteins that can react with excess of either acid or base to keep the blood and fluids bathing the tissues nuetral. Bone can release phosphate to remove hydrogen ions from surrounding fluids. If the action of the buffers is insufficient carbonic acid can be formed from carbon dioxide and water of metabolism instead of their being excreted. Acidosis may be neutralized by reserve base formed from ammonia from deamination of protein and water.

Catalytic action

Many mineral elements act as catalysts between enzymes and their substrates. Transport of substances across membranes is also often element-dependent.

Components of body compounds

Hormones, enzymes and other vital compounds contain mineral elements. Notable among these are iodine in thyroxine, zinc in insulin, iron in haemoglobin, chlorine in hydrochloric acid of the gastric juice, metalo-enzymes like cytochrome oxidase (iron and copper), xanthine oxidase (molybdenum), glutathione peroxidase (selenium) and vitamins; thiamin (sulphur) and vitamin B_{12} (cobalt).

Water balance

The extravascular compartment acts as a buffer between the blood and the intracellular compartment. Fluid movement between compartments is determined to a large extent by the concentration of minerals on either side of the separating membranes. Sodium, in highest concentration extracellularly, and potassium concentrated intracellularly, play major roles in this process.

Transmission of nerve impulses

During stimulation of nerve fibres there are changes in permeability of the membrane of nerve cells facilitating the entry of sodium and exit of potassium. This brings about a temporary alteration in the electrical charge and membrane permeability and so the process passes down the fibre. Changes in mineral concentration affect transmission of the nerve impulse. The effect of such changes on muscular contraction is seen in tetany when a fall in extracellular calcium concentration in relation to magnesium, sodium and potassium increases excitability. Calcium regulates the release of acetylcholine which is responsible for the transmission of impulses from one nerve cell to another.

Muscle contractility

Constancy of composition of the interstitial fluid, in which muscle fibres are bathed, is important for their normal contractility. Calcium exerts a stimulating effect and sodium, potassium and magnesium promote relaxation.

Phosphorus

In addition to the functions already mentioned, phosphorus is a component of nucleic acids and of several B group vitamins. Phosphate ester is an essential step in the breakdown of carbohydrate. Adenosine triphosphate (ATP) is a concentrated source of energy for all cells, as is creatine phosphate in muscle. Cyclic adenosine monophosphate (cyclic AMP) and cyclic guanine monophosphate (cyclic GMP) are intracellular messengers. 2, 3-diphosphoglycerate (2,3-DPG) shifts the oxygen dissociation curve of haemoglobin to the right, increasing oxygen availability to the tissues.

7. NUTRITION AND THE LIFESPAN

THE FETUS

Intrauterine growth has been studied by measurements made of infants born at various gestational periods and, more recently, *in utero* by ultrasound. Gestation is usually estimated in weeks from the first day of the last menstrual period before conception. Centile charts have been constructed relating fetal measurements to gestational age but these are only approximations as the conceptual age and the period of actual embryonal and fetal growth may be one to three weeks less than the estimated gestational age. Many factors besides nutrition before and during pregnancy may influence fetal growth, including maternal height, weight gain to midpregnancy, parity, age, ethnic group, genetic factors, socioeconomic factors and smoking during pregnancy. Recent studies have suggested that measurement of enzyme levels in maternal serum or leucocytes may be predictive of fetal growth.

The body of the 1 kg fetus at about 26 weeks contains about 86 per cent water, 85 g protein, 10 g fat, 6 g calcium, 3·4 g phosphorus 64 mg iron and 220 mg magnesium. With a threefold increase of weight by birth most of these measurements have also increased about threefold, but fat increases 30-fold and water decreases to about 70 per cent. This great increase in fat may not be physiological, especially as there is a further increase in early infancy (see below). Maternal overweight may be partly responsible.

Sampling of venous and arterial cord blood has shown that the amino acid requirements of the fetus differ from those of the adult. Nine amino acids are significanlty retained: aspartic acid, tryptophan, methionine, phenylalanine, serine, cysteine, lysine, glycine and threonine; while four are released from fetal tissues: arginine, glutamic acid, proline and glutamine. Sodium and potassium are provided far in excess of fetal requirements by the maternal circulation, while calcium, phosphorus and magnesium are usually adequate. Iron and zinc are usually in short supply unless supplementation is provided. Copper accumulates in the fetal liver. Water-soluble vitamins readily cross the placenta but vitamin A is lower in fetal than in maternal blood. It is not known whether the fetal kidney can synthesize $1,25(OH)_2D$ or whether it is transported across the placenta.

THE INFANT AND YOUNG CHILD

Growth and development

Growth as reflected in increase in weight and height occurs throughout the early years of life and accounts for the relatively greater nutritional requirements in this period (p. 86). These increases are greatest in the first 1 to 1½ years but even so the velocity of gain is decreasing rapidly from that attained by the fetus. Chemical maturation takes place, especially during the first year (p. 7).

Centile growth charts for weight and height are in routine use in paediatric practice and those for other measurements, such as skinfolds and head circumference, are used in research. However, charts that plot velocity of growth, rather than 'distance' achieved, more sensitively reflect physical performance.

During early infancy the proportion of body weight as adipose tissue in groups used to provide 'reference' data has tended to reach unphysiologically high levels, as reflected in current weight and skinfold standards. Energy requirements for this age group have also been proportionately too high. This has almost certainly been related to overfeeding of artificially fed infants that were used for developing the growth standards. There is need for the development of new standards using breast fed infants of mothers who are neither overweight nor undernourished.

Breast milk versus cow's milk

While it is general knowledge that infants can be reared satisfactorily on modified cow's milk as well as the human breast there are important chemical and other differences between the two methods. Table 4 shows the major differences in composition.

Table 4 Composition of cow's milk compared with human milk and a modified infant formula (breast milk substitute). (All per 100 ml)

	Human* (mature)	Cows' (full cream)	A modified milk formula† (powder diluted as directed)
Energy (kcal)	70	67	69
Protein (total) (g)	1·1	3·5	1·5
Casein (% protein)	40%	80%	40%
Carbohydrate (g)	7·3	5·0	7·2
Fat (total) (g)	4.0	3·7	3·6
Saturated fat (% fat)	46%	66%	44%
Linoleic (% fat)	7–11%	3%	17%
Sodium (mmol)	0·7	2·2	0·71
Calcium (mg)	35	120	49
Phosphorus (mg)	15	95	30
Iron (mg)	0·075	0·050	0·9
Vitamin C (mg)	3·8	1·5	6·9
Vitamin D (μg)	0·8	0·15	1·1

* The composition of breast milk varies considerably with stage of lactation, between individuals, and with maternal nutrition.
† Mean of Cow and Gate Premium and SMA-S26.
(reproduced from The Australian Nutrition Foundation Inc.)

Breast milk varies in composition during each feed, in the course of the day, over the period of lactation, between women and even in the same woman between the two breasts and in different pregnancies. Colostrum secreted during the first five days postpartum contains more protein, fat-soluble vitamins, less sugar and much less fat than mature milk.

Breast feeding is always cheaper, safer with regard to hygiene (p. 176) and more convenient. The psychological satisfaction to the mother is greater and this may have a beneficial influence on the baby.

Human milk provides the infant with antimicrobial factors such as IgA, lactoferrin and lysozyme. Free amino acids are higher in human milk, including taurine which infants cannot synthesize from cysteine and present in high concentration in the developing nervous system.

Infant feeding

In recent years there has been evidence of a welcome popular return to breast feeding in technologically developed societies, especially among the better educated. The abandonment of the practice with rapid social change in developing countries continues to bring a great tide of infant malnutrition in its wake (p. 102). A strict four-hourly regime should not be slavishly adhered to, neither should the baby be fed on the slightest demand. Most babies appear to know how much and how often they require nourishment and a natural routine is usually easily established.

Exclusive breast feeding has been shown to have a contraceptive effect, due to inhibition of ovulation by the raised amounts of prolactin in the circulation under the powerful reflex influence of the suckling stimulus. It has been calculated that more births are prevented by the practice of prolonged breast feeding in developing countries than by all forms of artificial contraception together. The consequent spacing out of children results in their having the benefit of improved mother care. An extreme example is the Kung hunter-gatherers of southern Africa among whom hyperprolactinaemia and amenorrhoea are commonly maintained for nearly two years; this requiring breast feeding six times a day for at least 80 minutes.

In cow's milk the protein is high and most consists of casein which tends to form indigestible curd on hydrolysis in the infant's stomach. Electrolytes are high and the milk, usually in the form of dried or evaporated milk, is diluted and sugar added to bring the energy value to about 67 kcal (0.28 MJ) per 100 ml before feeding. With artificial feeding the danger of giving over-concentrated feeds, or of giving a feed instead of glucose water to counteract fluid loss, has to be guarded against. Obesity (p. 151) or even hypernatraemia (p. 158) may result from these malpractices. However, with greater public awareness there has been a notable decline in these problems in recent years.

Weaning is generally considered to commence when foods other than milk are given. This should not be before 3 to 4 months as requirements can fully be met by milk until this stage. Earlier introduction unnecessarily increases the solute load, and much longer delay of the use of family foods in developing countries results in protein deficiency and kwashiokor (p. 102). These supplementary foods should be introduced gradually and in a puréed form at first to accustom the infant.

LATER CHILDHOOD

This period is relatively free from nutritional hazards usually — growth is less than in earlier childhood and during adolescence, and infections are few. For many children, about one in six of all meals will be taken at school. In some countries, as in the UK until 1980, there is statutory provision for nutritious school lunches, in some cases containing about one-third of energy needs, 40 per cent of protein requirements and being rich in some vitamins and elements. This is the time when mothers largely control their children's eating and to a considerable extent determine their life-long dietary patterns that will influence future health. The advice given in Figure 10 can be recommended —for all ages.

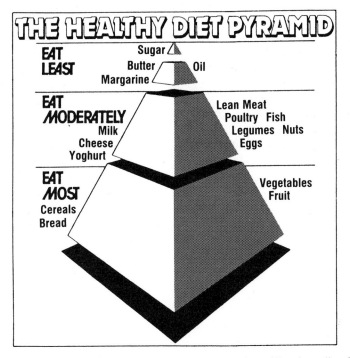

Fig. 10 Dietary advice for young children. (reproduced from The Australian Nutrition Foundation Inc.)

ADOLESCENCE

The adolescent growth spurt, the only time in extrauterine life when the velocity of growth actually increases, usually commences in the 9th or 10th year. The maximum acceleration in girls is between 10 to 12 years and 2 years later in boys. While the linear spurt contributes only 15 per cent to final adult height, the weight spurt contributes almost 50 per cent to final weight and nutrition therefore plays a key role in doubling body mass during adolescence. Furthermore, nutritional requirements are consequently related more closely to biological than to chronological age. Energy and protein requirements are higher than at almost any other time in life (p. 89). Because of the marked increase in skeletal growth at this time, calcium, phosphorus and vitamin D requirements are considerable. Iron requirements rise sharply in the adolescent female with the onset of menstruation. Haemoglobin values have been shown to differ in the sexes. Between 6 and 12 years they rise from 12·8 to 14·0 g in boys and 13·2 to 13·7 g in girls. By 18 years the value has risen to 15 g in boys and that for girls has fallen to 12·9 g.

PREGNANCY

During normal pregnancy there is an average weight gain of about 12·5 kg, though normal women may lose weight or gain over 20 kg. The mean weight gain is made up of fetus (3·5 kg), placenta (0·65 kg), amniotic fluid (0·8 kg), uterus (0·9 kg), breasts (0·4 kg), interstitial fluid (1·2 kg), maternal blood (1·8 kg) and 3·25 kg of maternal fat and protein storage. The fat is usually laid down over the hips and thighs in the first two trimesters and is usually lost later, a process aided by the energy cost of lactation. Among normal women the baby's birthweight is related both to the mother's weight before pregnancy and to her weight gain during pregnancy. Moreover, the mother's weight also affects the baby's growth after birth. Mothers are traditionally encouraged to 'eat for two'. Slimming is discouraged for overweight women for fear that fetal growth may be impaired. There is evidence to suggest that many infants in the west born to overweight and glucose intolerant mothers have excess fat at birth (see above).

Plasma volume increases throughout pregnancy, reaching an increase in volume of about 1350 ml by weeks 34–26, a 50 percent increases above the non-pregnant value of 2600 ml. Erythrocyte mass also increase but only by 250 ml, or about 20 per cent, of a non-pregnant value of 1400 ml. Supplemental iron raises this increase to 400 ml. As a consequence erythrocyte count, haemoglobin concentration and haematrocrit decline progressively in normal pregnancy until late second or early third trimester after which they rise slightly due to a relative decrease in plasma volume increase.

LACTATION

Energy requirements of the growing infant are the limiting factor in relation to the optimal duration of exclusive breast feeding. Human milk provides about 290 kJ (70 kcal)/100 g. The average woman produces about 700 ml of breast milk daily and consequently most mothers can meet their infant's requirements for energy only up until about the age of 4 months, at about which age supplementation with more energy dense semisolid foods should commence. Most women are physiologically capable of breast feeding satisfactorily. Complaints about having 'insufficient milk' usually reflect inhibition of the 'let down' reflex. Suckling of the infant stimulates sensory receptors in the nipples that send impulses up the spinal cord to the hypothalamus where they trigger the release from the posterior pituitary of oxytocin. This hormone in the blood stimulates myoepithelial cells in the alveoli of the breast and milk is ejected. This 'let down' reflex is markedly affected by the emotional state of the mother and can be easily inhibited by anxiety and insecurity. It might have been expected that the uncertainties of slum dwelling in the third world might have resulted in widespread 'breast failure', but in a recent study in a large slum in Bombay, breast feeding continued successfully to the end of the first year in over 90 per cent of mothers questioned.

OLD AGE

Ageing is associated with a decline in average values for many physiological functions. Between ages 30–80 years a decline of 30 per cent is reported in resting cardiac output, 50 per cent in renal blood flow, and 60–70 per cent in maximum breathing capacity and oxygen intake. However, values for individuals vary greatly. Most nutritional biochemical values are lower in the aged than the young but it is not clear whether they represent subclinical deficiency or are normal in respect of the reduced activity.

Average total energy expenditure falls with advancing age as does energy consumption and this reflects loss of lean body mass and reduction in physical activity. Recommended daily allowances in Tables 5 and 7 for older ages should be compared with those for young adults.

Many lifespan studies in the rat have shown that restriction of food intake leads to prolongation of the lifespan. Restriction of protein intake is accompanied by a reduced incidence of tumours and renal, cardiac and prostate gland diseases. These experiments serve to emphasize the importance of prudence in food consumption for man throughout life.

8. NUTRITIONAL REQUIREMENTS

For several decades and in most industrial and some developing countries expert groups have met at intervals to advise on the amounts of the known nutrients that should be provided daily in the diet. These figures are based on studies in which the amounts of nutrients necessary to prevent ill health and deficiency were determined. These are often termed the RDI — recommended dietary intake. This is not the same as RDA — recommended dietary allowance. For all nutrients the RDA is 'the level of intake considered to be adequate to meet the known nutritional needs of practically all healthy persons'. How a figure is put on this level varies from nutrient to nutrient; for energy it is the average requirement for the group (because in excess of this would predispose to obesity), but for protein it is the mean ± 30 per cent (variance of requirement is known to be 15 per cent) and this covers the needs of 97·5 per cent of the population, and for other nutrients where the variance is not known it is estimated and used in a similar way.

The nutritional needs of individuals vary, in some instances by as much as 100 per cent, and the same person will not have exactly the same requirement under all circumstances. RDAs are not meant to be applied to individuals, but only to large groups for the purpose of assessment and planning. The whole concept of RDAs is in a state of flux at present and, without an agreed consensus, one can only stay with the existing system. The latest published figures for the United States are those for 1980 and are given in Tables 5 and 6. A further revision was due to be published after five years but disagreements over the purposes of RDAs have prevented this. The committee was proposing to lower by about 30 per cent the adult RDAs for vitamins A and C,

Table 5 Recommended daily allowances,[a] revised 1980. (Food and Nutrition Board, National Academy healthy people in the USA)

| | | | | | | | *Fat-soluble vitamins* | | |
	Age (years)	Weight (kg) (lbs)		Height (cm) (in)		Protein (g)	Vitamin A (μg R.E.)[b]	Vitamin D (μg)[c]	Vitamin E (mg a T.E.)[d]
Infants	0.0–0.5	6	13	60	24	kg $\times$ 2.2	420	10	3
	0.5–1.0	9	20	71	28	kg $\times$ 2.0	400	10	4
Children	1–3	13	29	90	35	23	400	10	5
	4–6	20	44	112	44	30	500	10	6
	7–10	28	62	132	52	34	700	10	7
Males	11–14	45	99	157	62	45	1000	10	8
	15–18	66	145	176	69	56	1000	10	10
	19–22	70	154	177	70	56	1000	7.5	10
	23–50	70	154	178	70	56	1000	5	10
	51+	70	154	178	70	56	1000	5	10
Females	11–14	46	101	157	62	46	800	10	8
	15–18	55	120	163	64	46	800	10	8
	19–22	55	120	163	64	44	800	7.5	8
	23–50	55	120	163	64	44	800	5	8
	51+	55	120	163	64	44	800	5	8
Pregnant						+30	+200	+5	+2
Lactating						+20	+400	+5	+3

[a] The allowances are intended to provide for individual variations among most normal persons as they live in the United States under usual environmental stresses. Diets should be based on a variety of common foods in order to provide other nutrients for which human requirements have been less well defined. See Table 7 for heights, weights and recommended intake.

[b] Retinol equivalents. 1 Retinol equivalent = 1 μg retinol or 6 μg β carotene. See text for calculation of vitamin A activity of diets as retinol equivalents.

[c] As cholecalciferol. 10 μg cholecalciferol = 400 iu vitamin D.

[d] a-tocopherol equivalents. 1 mg d-a-tocopherol = 1 a T.E. See text for variation in allowances and calculation of vitamin E activity of the diet as a-tocopherol equivalents.

[e] 1 N.E. (niacin equivalent) is equal to 1 mg of niacin or 60 mg of dietary tryptophan.

of Sciences—National Research Council. Designed for the maintenance of good nutrition of practically all

	Water-soluble vitamins						Minerals					
Vitamin C (mg)	Thiamin (mg)	Riboflavin (mg)	Niacin (mg N.E.)ᵉ	Vitamin B_6 (mg)	Folacinᶠ (μg)	Vitamin B_{12} (μg)	Calcium (mg)	Phosphorus (mg)	Magnesium (mg)	Iron (mg)	Zinc (mg)	Iodine (μg)
35	0.3	0.4	6	0.3	30	0.5ᵍ	360	240	50	10	3	40
35	0.5	0.6	8	0.6	45	1.5	540	360	70	15	5	50
45	0.7	0.8	9	0.9	100	2.0	800	800	150	15	10	70
45	0.9	1.0	11	1.3	200	2.5	800	800	200	10	10	90
45	1.2	1.4	16	1.6	300	3.0	800	800	250	10	10	120
50	1.4	1.6	18	1.8	400	3.0	1200	1200	350	18	15	150
60	1.4	1.7	18	2.0	400	3.0	1200	1200	400	18	15	150
60	1.5	1.7	19	2.2	400	3.0	800	800	350	10	15	150
60	1.4	1.6	18	2.2	400	3.0	800	800	350	10	15	150
60	1.2	1.4	16	2.2	400	3.0	800	800	350	10	15	150
50	1.1	1.3	15	1.8	400	3.0	1200	1200	300	18	15	150
60	1.1	1.3	14	2.0	400	3.0	1200	1200	300	18	15	150
60	1.1	1.3	14	2.0	400	3.0	800	800	300	18	15	150
60	1.0	1.2	13	2.0	400	3.0	800	800	300	18	15	150
60	1.0	1.2	13	2.0	400	3.0	800	800	300	10	15	150
+20	+0.4	+0.3	+2	+0.6	+400	+1.0	+400	+400	+150	ʰ	+5	+25
+40	+0.5	+0.5	+5	+0.5	+100	+1.0	+400	+400	+150	ʰ	+10	+50

ᶠ The folacin allowances refer to dietary sources as determined by *Lactobacillus casei* assay after treatment with enzymes ('conjugases') to make polyglutamyl forms of the vitamin available to the test organism.

ᵍ the RDA for vitamin B_{12} in infants is based on average concentration of the vitamin in human milk. The allowances after weaning are based on energy intake (as recommended by the American Academy of Pediatrics) and consideration of other factors such as intestinal absorption; see text.

ʰ The increased requirement during pregnancy cannot be met by the iron content of habitual American diets nor by the existing iron stores of many women; therefore the use of 30–60 mg of supplemental iron is recommended. Iron needs during lactation are not substantially different from those of non-pregnant women, but continued supplementation of the mother for 2–3 months after parturition is advisable in order to replenish stores depleted by pregnancy.

Table 6 Recommended dietary allowances, revised 1980. (Food and Nutrition Board, National Academy of Sciences—National Research Council, Washington, DC. Estimated safe and adequate daily dietary intakes of selected vitamins and minerals[a])

	Age (years)	Vitamins			Trace Elements[b]						Electrolytes		
		Vitamin K (µg)	Biotin (µg)	Pantothenic Acid (mg)	Copper (mg)	Manganese (mg)	Fluoride (mg)	Chromium (mg)	Selenium (mg)	Molybdenum (mg)	Sodium (mg)	Potassium (mg)	Chloride (mg)
Infants	0–0.5	12	35	2	0.5–0.7	0.5–0.7	0.1–0.5	0.01–0.04	0.01–0.04	0.03–0.06	115–350	350–925	275–700
	0.5–1	10–20	50	3	0.7–1.0	0.7–1.0	0.2–1.0	0.02–0.06	0.02–0.06	0.04–0.08	250–750	425–1275	400–1200
Children	1–3	15–30	65	3	1.0–1.5	1.0–1.5	0.5–1.5	0.02–0.08	0.02–0.08	0.05–0.1	325–975	550–1650	500–1500
and	4–6	20–40	85	3–4	1.5–2.0	1.5–2.0	1.0–2.5	0.03–0.12	0.03–0.12	0.06–0.15	450–1350	775–2325	700–2100
adolescents	7–10	30–60	120	4–5	2.0–2.5	2.0–3.0	1.5–2.5	0.05–0.2	0.05–0.2	0.1–0.3	600–1800	1000–3000	925–2775
	11+	50–100	100–200	4–7	2.0–3.0	2.5–5.0	1.5–2.5	0.05–0.2	0.05–0.2	0.15–0.5	900–2700	1525–4575	1400–4200
Adults		70–140	100–200	4–7	2.0–3.0	2.5–5.0	1.5–4.0	0.05–0.2	0.05–0.2	0.15–0.5	1100–3300	1875–5625	1700–5100

[a] Because there is less information on which to base allowances, these figures are not given in the main table of the RDA and are provided here in the form of ranges of recommended intakes.

[b] Since the toxic levels for many trace elements may be only several times usual intakes, the upper levels for the trace elements given in this table should not be habitually exceeded.

Table 7 Mean heights and weights and recommended energy intake[a] (Recommended dietary allowances, revised 1980)

Category	Age (years)	Weight (kg)	Weight (lb)	Height (cm)	Height (in)	Energy needs (with range) (kcal)	(MJ)
Infants	0.0–0.5	6	13	60	24	kg × 115 (95–145)	kg × .48
	0.5–1.0	9	20	71	28	kg × 105 (80–135)	kg × .44
Children	1–3	13	29	90	35	1300 (900–1800)	5.5
	4–6	20	44	112	44	1700 (1300–2300)	7.1
	7–10	28	62	132	52	2400 (1650–3300)	10.1
Males	11–14	45	99	157	62	2700 (2000–3700)	11.3
	15–18	66	145	176	69	2800 (2100–3900)	11.8
	19–22	70	154	177	70	2900 (2500–3300)	12.2
	23–50	70	154	178	70	2700 (2300–3100)	11.3
	51–75	70	154	178	70	2400 (2000–2800)	10.1
	76+	70	154	178	70	2050 (1650–2450)	8.6
Females	11–14	46	101	157	62	2200 (1500–3000)	9.2
	15–18	55	120	163	64	2100 (1200–3000)	8.8
	19–22	55	120	163	64	2100 (1700–2500)	8.8
	23–50	55	120	163	64	2000 (1600–2400)	8.4
	51–75	55	120	163	64	1800 (1400–2200)	7.6
	76+	55	120	163	64	1600 (1200–2000)	6.7
Pregnancy						+300	
Lactation						+500	

[a] The data in this table have been assembled from the observed median heights and weights of children shown in Table 5, together with desirable weights for adults for the mean heights of men (70 inches) and women (64 inches) between the ages of 18 and 34 years as surveyed in the US population (HEW/NCHS data). The energy allowances for the young adults are for men and women doing light work. The allowances for the two older groups represent mean energy needs over these age spans, allowing for a 2% decrease in basal (resting) metabolic rate per decade and a reduction in activity of 200 kcal/day for men and women between 51 and 75 years, 500 kcal for men over 75 years and 400 kcal for women over 75. The customary range of daily energy output is shown for adults in parentheses, and is based on a variation in energy needs of ± 400 kcal at any one age, emphasizing the wide range of energy intakes appropriate for any group of people. Energy allowances for children through age 18 are based on median energy intakes of children of these ages followed in longitudinal growth studies. The values in parentheses are 10th and 90th percentiles of energy intake, to indicate the range of energy consumption among children of these ages.

but objections were raised to this in the light of suggestive evidence that high intakes of these and some other micronutrients may be protective against certain cancers. It is not clear how this issue will be resolved, but it has brought the whole philosophy of RDAs under widespread scrutiny.

Tables 5 and 6 show RDAs for most known nutrients and Table 7 does the same for energy.

Energy

Energy allowances are usually considered in relation to the needs of a person living a normal life at rest; what is termed resting metabolism. The thermic effect of food and other minimal metabolic needs beyond basal metabolism are included. Allowances are calculated for reference man, 22 years old and weighing 70 kg and reference woman 22 years old and weighing 58 kg. The environmental temperature is 20°C and their physical activity is light. Their recommended daily allowances have been set at 3000 and 2200 kcal (12·57 and 9·22 MJ), respectively.

Adjustment in the energy allowance should be made for body size, and tables are available which enable this to be done in relation to 'desirable' weight, which may be considered to be the average weight of individuals of given sex and height at age 22.

The latest WHO/FAO expert group in their 1985 report on energy and protein requirments adopted a different approach. As the BMR is the largest component of energy expenditure all other components are calculated as multiples of the BMR. Linear equations are given for predicting BMR from body weight according to sex and age. Studies have already been published that show that these asumptions may introduce considerable errors. For this reason, and because of their convenience in practice, the earlier tables have been retained.

Protein

In considering protein requirements it is assumed that the diet is adequate in all other respects. The interrelationship with energy requirements is of special importance.

The basis of reference for protein requirements is usually the body weight. Two methods, the factorial method and nitrogen balance, have been used to estimate nitrogen requirements and the results are compared in the FAO/WHO Expert Committee report on Energy and Protein Requirements (1973).

Factorial method

The obligatory nitrogen losses on a protein-free diet from urine, faeces, skin and other small contributions total 54 mg/kg body weight (much lower than the 86 mg/kg by the 1965 FAO/WHO Expert Group). The former figure calculated on the basis of basal energy metabolism approximates to a total loss of 2 mg of N per kcal (0.48 mg of N per kJ). The same figure probably applies to women and children, except the very young. Since the coefficient of variation (standard deviation divided by the mean) $\times$ 100 is 15 per cent, a value 30 per cent larger ($+$ 2 s.d.) should encompass the losses of nearly all healthy persons in a normal population.

During infancy and childhood N requirements have to allow for growth as well as obligatory loss. In the 6 month infant the figures are 42 mg/kg/day for growth and 112 mg/kg/day for obligatory loss making a total of 154 mg/kg or about 3 times that of the adult. The figures decrease steadily with advancing maturity.

Balance studies

Direct evidence on N requirements is obtained from measurements of the lowest protein intake at which N equilibrium can be achieved in adults, and satisfactory growth and N retention in children. The figures obtained by this method in adults and children are consistently higher by about one-third than those obtained by the factorial method, suggesting that the efficiency of N utilization is considerably lower under balance conditions than when protein intake is low.

Amino acid requirements

These are summarized in Table 8. It should be noted that more recent evidence suggests that histidine is required by all age groups (p. 35).

The FAO/WHO Committee has suggested amino acid patterns (mg/g protein) in food consumed based upon the safe levels of protein intake for infants, children and adults (Table 9). The pattern for infants closely resembles that of breast milk. Those for children and adults bear a general resemblance to the patterns of egg and milk protein. For the purposes of biological testing either protein would seem to be suitable as reference standard.

The proportion of total amino acids that must be supplied as essential amino acids (the E/T ratio) falls with age (p. 70). The E/T ratio of egg protein is considerably higher than is required by the adult.

Table 8 Estimated amino acid requirements (mg/kg/day) (FAO/WHO, 1973)

Amino acid	Infants	Children aged 10 to 12 years	Adults
Histidine	28	—	—
Isoleucine	70	30	10
Leucine	161	45	14
Lysine	103	60	12
Methionine and cystine	58	27	13
Phenylalanine and tyrosine	125	27	14
Threonine	87	35	7
Tryptophan	17	4	3·5
Valine	93	33	10

Table 9 Comparison of suggested patterns of amino acid requirements with the composition of milk and egg protein (mg/g protein) (FAO/WHO, 1973)

Amino acid	Suggested patterns of requirement			Reported composition		
	Infant	School-child	Adult	Human milk	Cow's milk	Egg
Histidine	14	—	—	26	27	22
Isoleucine	35	37	18	46	47	54
Leucine	80	56	25	93	95	86
Lysine	52	75	22	66	78	70
Methionine + cystine	29	34	24	42	33	57
Phenylalanine + tyrosine	63	34	25	72	102	93
Threonine	44	44	13	43	44	47
Tryptophan	8·5	4·6	6·5	17	14	17
Valine	47	41	18	55	64	66

Dietary protein quality

The methods in use for evaluation have been discussed previously (p. 36). The amount of food eaten is determined largely by the requirement for energy. Consequently foods with low concentration of protein, such as cassava, yam, plantain, cannot be consumed in sufficient quantity to meet protein requirements.

Digestion or absorption may be incomplete and availability is usually over 90 per cent for amino acids of animal origin and may be less than 80 per cent for those from vegetable sources. Heat processing may reduce availability especially in carbohydrate rich foods and for lysine and sulphur amino acids. Thus biological tests of protein quality are essential.

Factors influencing protein requirements

Physical activity has not been shown to increase requirement for protein except for the additional protein laid down in muscle by athletes in training.

Nitrogen is lost in sweat but the amount is thought to be small. Infections result in increased loss of nitrogen, and other nutrients, in urine and by impaired absorption. Intake is also reduced.

The 1985 WHO/FAO report continued to use nitrogen balance as the basis for estimating protein requirements. Short term studies in different ethnic groups and 2 to 3 months nitrogen balances tended to confirm a slightly higher protein requirement than shown in Table 5. It was considered unnecessary to make allowance for differences in protein quality except for preschool children. A new feature was the allowance for the low digestibility of vegetable proteins.

Water

Water balance is closely related to thermal balance. A healthy, active male loses about 1000 kcal (4·19 MJ) day by evaporation from skin and lungs, 2000 kcal (8·38 MJ) by radiation and conduction from the skin, and 100 kcal (0·42 MJ) by increase in temperature of inspired air and excretion. Water requirements are directly proportional to the energy expendiure. An adult metabolizing 30 kcal (125·7 kJ)/kg/24 hr uses about 100 ml H_2O/100 kcal (419 kJ) or about 2·0 litres.

MULTIPLE CHOICE QUESTIONS

Answer each question true *or* false.

1. The following are statements about vitamin D:
    i) It is derived mainly from the diet
    ii) It circulates in the blood mainly as $1,25(OH)_2D$
    iii) Its action is facilitated by calcitonin
    iv) It controls calcium absorption through a calcium-binding protein
    v) The liver hydroxylates $25(OH)D$ to $1,25(OH)_2D$.

2. The following are statements about calcium:
    i) Normally about 20–30 per cent is absorbed
    ii) The normal plasma concentration is about 9–10 mg/100 ml (2·25–2·55 mmol/l)
    iii) In plasma most is present in protein-bound form
    iv) Phytic acid impairs absorption
    v) Efficiency of absorption increases in old age.

3. The following are statements about fat:
    i) Most dietary fat is triglyceride
    ii) Long-chain fatty acids are absorbed by the portal route

iii) Unsaturated fat is mainly of vegetable origin

iv) Some polyunsaturated fatty acid derivatives decrease blood coagulability

v) In the newborn adipose tissue is about 90 per cent lipid.

4. The following statements relate to energy:

i) Oxygen consumption is an indirect measure of energy expenditure

ii) Normal oxygen consumption is about 1 litre/min in the adult

iii) The average adult male daily energy requirement is about 12 MJ

iv) Creatinine phosphate is a source of energy for muscle

v) The energy efficiency of the body is about 80 per cent.

5. For which of these nutrients is the adult daily recommended dietary allowance less than 100 μg?

i) Iodine

ii) Vitamin B_{12}

iii) Folic acid

iv) Thiamin

v) Iron.

Explanation and answers on page 286.

FURTHER READING

1. Introduction
Baxter K, Fowden L (eds) 1982 Food, nutrition and climate. Applied Science Publishers, London & New Jersey
McLaren D S (ed) 1983 Nutrition in the community, 2nd edn. Wiley, Chichester
Schneider H A, Anderson C E, Coursin D B 1977 Nutrition support of medical practice. Harper & Row, New York, p 1–8
2. The body
Brozek J 1965 Human body composition. Pergamon, New York
Moore F D et al 1963 The body cell mass and its supporting environment. Saunders, Philadelphia and London
Widdowson E M, Dickerson J W T 1964: Comar C L, Bronner F (eds) Chemical Composition of the Body in Mineral Metabolism, Academic Press, New York, vol 2, part A, p 2
3. Food
Borgstrom G 1968 Principles of food science, Vol 1 : Food Technology, vol 2: Food Microbiology and Biochemistry. Macmillan, New York
Brown L R, Finsterbusch G W 1972 Man and his Environment: Food. Harper & Row, New York
Doughty J, Walker A 1982 Legumes in human nutrition. FAO Food and Nutrition Paper No 20. FAO, Rome
Food Protection Committee 1966 Toxicants occurring naturally in foods. National Research Council, Washington DC
Herbert V 1980 Nutrition cultism: facts and fiction. Stickley, Philadelphia
Hobbs B C, Gilbert R J 1978 Food poisoning and food hygiene, 4th edn. Arnold, London
Kent N L 1978 Technology of cereals, with special reference to wheat. Pergamon, Oxford
Kermode G O 1972 Food additives. Scientific American 226: no 3, 15–21
Levine A S, Labuza T P, Morley J E 1985 Food technology: a primer for physicians. New England Journal of Medicine 312: 628–34
Lowenberg M E, Todhunter E N, Wilson E D, Savage J R, Lubawski J L 1974 Food and man, 2nd edn. Wiley, New York

Nutrition Coordinating Committee, National Institutes of Health 1978 Symposium on role of dietary fiber in health. American Journal of Clinical Nutrition: 31 (Suppl) 1–291

Paul A A, Southgate D A T 1978 McCance and Widdowson's the composition of foods 4th edn. Revised and extended MRC Special Report no 297. Elsevier, Amsterdam

4. Nature and sources of nutrients

Passmore R, Eastwood MA 1986 Human nutrition and dietetics, 8th edn. Churchill Livingstone, Edinburgh

Rechcigl M Jr (ed) 1978 CRC Handbook Series in nutrition and food. Section E: Nutritional disorders, vol 3. CRC Press, Florida

5. Physiology of nutrients

Passmore R, Eastwood M A 1986 Human nutrition and dietetics, 8th edn. Churchill Livingstone, Edinburgh

Durnin J V G A, Passmore R 1967 Energy, work and leisure. Heinemann, London

Harper H A 1977 Review of physiological chemistry, 16th edn. Lange, Los Altos, California

Horrobin D F 1968 Medical physiology and biochemistry. Arnold, London

6. Metabolism of nutrients

Bothwell T H, Charlton R W, Cook J D, Finch C A 1979 Iron metabolism in man. Blackwell, Oxford

De Luca H F 1977 Vitamin D endocrine system. Advances in Clinical Chemistry 19: 125

Felig P, Wahren J 1974 Protein turnover and amino acid metabolism in the regulation of gluconeogenesis. Federation Proceedings 33: 1092

Harper H A 1977 Review of physiological chemistry, 16th edn. Lange, Los Altos, California

Havel R J, Goldstein J L, Brown M S 1980 Lipoproteins and lipid transport. In: Bondy PK, Rozenburg LE (eds) Metabolic control and disease. Saunders, Philadelphia, p 393–494

Horrobin D F 1968 Medical physiology and biochemistry. Arnold, London

Miller A T 1968 Energy metabolism. Davis, Philadelphia

Reeds P J, James W P T 1983 Protein turnover. Lancet i: 571–574

7. Nutrition and the life span

Cameron M, Hofvander Y 1983 Manual on feeding infants and young children, 3rd edn. Oxford University Press, Oxford

Heald F P 1982 Nutrition of the school child and adolescent. In: McLaren D S, Burman D (eds) Textbook of paediatric nutrition, 2nd edn. Churchill Livingstone, London

Jelliffe D B, Jelliffe E F P 1978 Human milk in the modern world: Psychosocial, nutritional and economic significance. Oxford University Press, Oxford

Joint WHO/UNICEF meeting on infant and young child feeding 1979. WHO, Geneva

Metcoff J 1982 Maternal nutrition and fetal growth. In: McLaren D S, Burman D (eds) Textbook of paediatric nutrition, 2nd edn. Churchill Livingstone, Edinburgh

Naismith D J 1977 Protein metabolism during pregnancy. In: Philip E E, Barnes J, Newton M (eds) Scientific foundations of obstetrics and gynaecology 2nd edn. Heinemann, London, p 503

Tanner J M 1978 Fetus into man: physical growth from conception to maturity. Open Books, London

Whitehead R G 1983 Nutritional aspects of human lactation. Lancet ii: 167–169

8. Nutritional requirements

FAO/WHO Expert Committee 1985 Energy and protein requirements. World Health Organization Technical Report Series no 724. WHO, Geneva

FAO/WHO 1974 Handbook on human nutritional requirements. WHO Monograph Series, no 61, WHO, Geneva

Food and Nutrition Board 1980 Recommended dietary allowances, 9th edn. National Academy of Sciences National Research Council, Washington DC

Truswell A S 1978 Minimal estimates of needs and recommended intakes of nutrients. In: Yudkin J (ed) Diet of man: needs and wants. Applied Science, London, p 5

Waterlow J C 1979 Uses of recommended intakes: the purpose of dietary recommendations. Food Policy, May 107–114

II

Primary and secondary nutritional disorders

'Whosoever was the father of a disease, an ill diet was the mother.'

GEORGE HERBET (1660)

9. INTRODUCTION

Malnutrition means disordered nutrition. Nutrition becomes disordered as a result of any deviation from normal. While gross deviations give rise to frank clinical signs and symptoms and definite biochemical abnormalities it is virtually impossible to draw a line between the 'normal' and the 'abnormal'.

Malnutrition may be classified in various ways as shown in Figure 11 and Table 10. This section is mainly concerned with primary nutritional disorders, that is to say those that are caused by dietary (nutriment) derangement. However, in many conditions primary and secondary factors operate. Primary and secondary forms of the same condition (e.g. nutritional and secondary rickets) have much in common and so are dealt with together in this section.

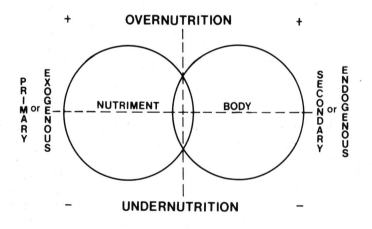

Fig. 11 Forms of nutritional disorders.

96

Table 10 Classification of malnutrition (McLaren D S 1976 Nutrition in the community. John Wiley & Sons Ltd)

1. Cause	primary (exogenous)
	secondary (endogenous)
2. Type	excess, toxicity (overnutrition)
	deficiency (undernutrition)
3. Nutrient	vitamins, elements, protein, energy sources
4. Degree	mild, moderate, severe
	or alternatively
	depleted stores, biochemical lesion, functional
	change,structural lesion
5. Duration	acute, subacute, chronic
6. Outcome	reversible, irreversible

Figure 12 shows the main types of malnutrition, together with some terms commonly used. In the general type of undernutrition or inanition the diet is deficient in all nutrients and energy. In undernutrition of special type while there may be sufficient food intake to allay hunger, the diet is deficient in certain essential nutrients and inadequate to meet the metabolic needs of the body. Thus the 'hunger' is 'hidden' and not alleviated by the usual demands made by appetite.

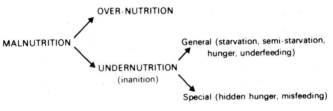

Fig. 12 Types of malnutrition.

The classification of undernutrition is confused. The general form is one degree or kind of PEM, whether occurring in hospitalized patients or famine victims (chapter 10) or in children of the third world (chapter 11).

10. PROTEIN ENERGY MALNUTRITION IN ADULTS

(Semistarvation, general inanition, hunger, underfeeding)

The organism subjected to a diminished food supply has considerable ability to adapt. Requirements are lessened as a result of lowered activity and, in the case of the young subject, there is diminished growth. Basal energy needs are first met by drawing on the small store of glycogen, but in a fast of several days or weeks adipose tissue and increasingly tissue protein, are catabolized.

Starvation is one of the most important forms of stress with which the physician needs to be familiar. It is not confined to special situations of deprivation encountered in prisoners and fasting volunteers. It constitutes the unhappy lot of vast masses of humanity and upon its control among the underprivileged nations hangs future peace and progress. Futhermore, any serious illness, of other than very short duration, has profound effects on metabolism, and nutrition. Inanition of this kind constantly forms a backdrop to the presentation of disease in hospital (section 3, p. 233).

General appearance

Emaciation is generalized but becomes most obvious where normally prominent depots of fat (e.g. buttocks) and muscle masses (thighs, back) waste and bones protrude. The skin becomes thin, dry, loose and inelastic, pale and cold with a tendency to cyanosis in cold weather. It is often pigmented in patches, of a brownish colour anywhere on the body, most commonly on the face, but not sufficiently marked to be confused with pellagra (p. 117). Sometimes heaping up of keratin around hair follicles (perifollicular hyperkeratosis) occurs of non-specific aetiology (p. 110). The hair is dry, staring and falls out easily. Apathy results in reduced energy expenditure and conservation of reserves.

The systems

Achlorhydria and diarrhoea are frequent, the latter ofter being terminal. There is bradycardia, lowered systolic and diastolic pressure, low venous pressure, reduced cardiac output and heart size. Vital capacity, respiratory rate, minute volume and efficiency are all reduced. Endocrine glands are affected irregularly; growth hormone is decreased but thyrotropic and adrenotropic hormones are unaffected. The lowering of basal metabolism is probably not due to diminished thyroid function. Corticosteroid excretion is normal. Gonadal atrophy leads to loss of libido and amenorrhoea in the female. Hypothermia is frequent and contributes to death. Neurological changes are rare in general starvation (but frequent in deficiency of thiamin, niacin and B_6 (p. 214). The intellect remains clear but the personality changes. Inability to concentrate, introspection, irritability and apathy are common. Anaemia is usually mild (normocytic, normochromic), with hypoplastic marrow. It can be accounted for by considerable plasma volume expansion and reduced erythropoiesis.

Work capacity is affected in prolonged starvation mainly due to loss of muscle, and ultimately severe limitation results from anaemia and cardio-respiratory failure. The most obvious change, weight loss, reflects the use of body constituents for energy. It may be as much as 50 per cent in the adult, especially in anorexia nervosa (p. 213), or even more in the child, In the early days water accounts for much of the loss. Of the organs, liver and intestine suffer first, later muscle and skin account for most of the loss. Brain, spinal cord and eyes are well preserved to the end.

The nature of famine oedema, dependent in type, is ill-understood. Plasma proteins are slightly, if at all, reduced. Total body water and extracellular space are increased, not actually but in relation to body weight. Loss of adipose tissue which is very low in water content accounts for much of this. This may lower tissue tension and facilitate oedema formation. Body sodium remains normal. Increase of proportion of extracellular water from the adult normal (about 23·5 per cent) to about 30 per cent seems to be critical for appearance of clinical oedema (Fig. 13). While renal function appears normal, nocturnal polyuria is troublesome.

Metabolism

The overriding demand is for energy. The energy released in starvation as shown in Figure 13 amounts to about 70 000 kcal (293·3 MJ) (over 80 per cent from 6.5 kg fat, 17 per cent from 3 kg protein, and only about 1 per cent from 200 g carbohydrate). With energy expenditure at about a basal rate of 1600 kcal (6·70 MJ)/day these reserves would theoretically last nearly 50 days. Total fast for several weeks has often been undertaken without any ill effects (Figure 13). Carbohydrate stores, as glycogen, in liver and muscle are soon exhausted. When less than 15 per cent of energy is derived from carbohydrate ketosis occurs. Fatty acids are released from the fat depots and lipolysis in the liver is increased resulting in large amounts of acetoacetyl CoA, precursor of ketone bodies. At the same time tissue protein is increasingly burnt for energy. It is not entirely clear whether or not protein is actually stored by the body; so called 'labile protein'. In acute starvation the daily loss of nitrogen in urine diminishes steadily for about 1 week and thereafter the loss is almost steady. Most of this diminution is accounted for by urea, and so the urea/total nitrogen ratio falls from a normal of about 90 per cent to below 70 per cent. Protein synthesis is depressed and certain amino acids become available for energy purposes.

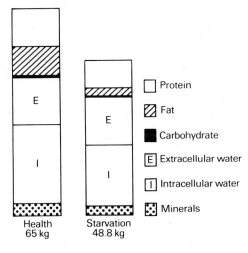

Fig. 13 Body composition changes in starvation.

In prolonged starvation glucose turnover is curtailed by nearly 50 per cent to less than 90 g per day. Much of this is accounted for by marked reduction in output of alanine from muscle and consequent hypoalaninaemia. Another adaptive change is decrease in energy expenditure. About one third of conservation is achieved by a lowered BMR early on by reduction in oxygen consumption of liver and later by decrease of metabolizing mass. Most of the remaining saving is due to decreased cost of activity, accounted for both by a decrease in the amount of spontaneous activity and also lessened cost of the activity related to loss of body weight.

Minerals tend to be conserved by diminution of urinary excretion and vitamin requirements appear to be reduced.

A study in obese patients undergoing prolonged fast showed that β-hydroxybutyrate and acetoacetate can replace glucose as the main fuel for brain metabolism.

Treatment

Rehabilitation of undernourished groups is often more an administrative than a medical problem. In the early stages limitation of the food intake may be necessary until impaired function of the gastrointestinal tract has been overcome. Bland foods only can be tolerated. A recommended formula consists of 42 per cent dried skim milk, 32 per cent edible oil, 25 per cent sucrose plus K, Mg and vitamin supplements, reconstituted to give 10–12 per cent dried skim milk. Intake is gradually increased until about 5000 kcal (20·95 MJ)/day may be consumed and weekly weight gain of 1·5–2·0 kg attained. If diarrhoea persists in the absence of infections temporary lactose intolerance may be suspected. Yogurt, in which lactose is partially hydrolysed to glucose and galactose, is well tolerated. Severely debilitated patients require intragastric feeding in order to obtain a satisfactory positive energy balance. Soft nasal tubes are well tolerated and parenteral feeding should be resorted to only when strictly indicated (p. 238).

Acute protein deficiency

This is a much less common form of PEM than starvation in hospitalized patients. It has also been called acute hypoalbuminaemia and, less appropriately, 'kwashiorkor-like syndrome'. It is precipitated by severe stress and by sepsis. Transport proteins fall precipitately; wasting, fatty liver, oedema and skin changes are not seen. Mortality can be high and the outlook depends upon the treatment of the underlying cause rather than the nutritional state.

11. PROTEIN ENERGY MALNUTRITION IN CHILDREN
(PEM: marasmus and kwashiorkor)

This is at present the generally accepted term for the widespread form of malnutrition affecting primarily young children in developing countries. It is best considered as a spectrum of disease with its severe forms manifesting themselves clinically as marasmus and kwashiorkor. Cases with mixed features are often termed marasmic-kwashiorkor. It is estimated that several million new cases occur annually.

There is no precise way of defining subclinical forms that are characterized by retardation of growth and development. They are sometimes referred to as 'mild-moderate' forms of PEM. A large proportion of the several hundred million preschool children in the developing world are affected to some degree.

There is deficiency of energy and all nutrients in marasmus, while kwashirokor results from deficiency of protein and to a less extent other nutrients in the presence of adequate or even excess energy intake. Marasmus is really starvation in the child. It is widespread among the low socioeconomic groups of most developing countries and is much more common than kwashiorkor. Kwashiorkor (which in the Ga language of Ghana means: 'the disease the first child gets when the next one is on the way') is primarily a condition of early life but older children and adults may be affected whenever there is prolonged consumption of a diet low in protein and high in carbohydrate. Thus all ages are at risk among the approximately 200 million people (mainly in Africa, the Caribbean and Pacific islands) who subsist on starchy roots, plantain, and the like.

Pathogenesis

That marasmus and kwashiorkor, in their typical and extreme forms, have basically different causations is suggested by the significant difference in their age incidence reported in many places. Marasmus is primarily a disease of infancy (the first 12 months) while kwashiorkor is most common in the second and third years of life. In Figure 14 a scheme is outlined showing tracks which lead from early weaning to marasmus and from prolonged breast feeding to kwashiorkor. The urbanizing influences which foster marasmus include economic pressure on the mother to go out to work and progaganda which encourages artifical feeding for social and not medical reasons. Government subsidy of milk distribution schemes may have the same effect. The importance of the breast with correct supplementary feeding for the adequate nutrition of the child needs to be emphasized.

The interplay of malnutrition and infection is of paramount importance in the pathogenesis of PEM (p. 224). As precipitating and aggravating factors gastroenteritis may be singled out in relation to marasmus and stress laid on measles and pertussis predisposing to kwashiorkor. Figures 15 and 16 indicate the contrasting pathophysiology of the two states.

Clinical and epidemiological features

Marasmus. Growth retardation and wasting of subcutaneous fat and muscle

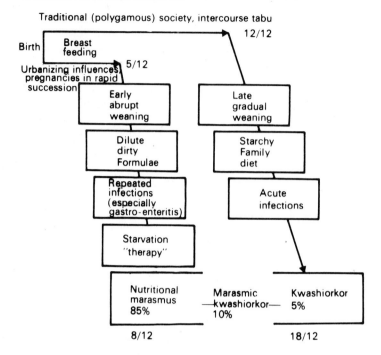

Fig. 14 Flow diagram of pathogenesis of marasmus and kwashiorkor. (McLaren D S 1966 *Lancet* **ii:** 485.)

are constant features. Weight is more affected than skeletal measurements such as length, head circumference, and chest circumference. The wasting can be quantified by measurement of the circumference of the mid-upper arm and skinfolds in biceps, triceps, scapula and umbilical areas. It is often evidenced by the wizened 'monkey facies'. Oedema is absent but mild skin and hair changes and enlarged liver, all common in kwashiorkor, are occasionally present. The infant is often bright-eyed, alert and hungry but too much stress should not be placed on psychomotor differences between marasmus and kwashiorkor. Gastroenteritis, often in repeated attacks, occurs especially throughout the summer months and leads to dehydration.Respiratory infections are common precipitating factors during the winter. Tuberculosis, severe parasitism and other chronic diseases lead frequently to emaciation and in practice marasmus of purely nutritional or dietary origin does not exist. Vitamin deficiencies, especially rickets and xerophthalmia, may be associated.

Kwashiorkor. Constant features are growth failure, preservation of subcutaneous fat with wasting of muscles, oedema and psychomotor change. As in marasmus, weight is more affected than skeletal growth but the extremes of weight deficit seen in marasmus (up to 60 per cent) do not occur, probably due to the presence of oedema and the older age. Although it has been

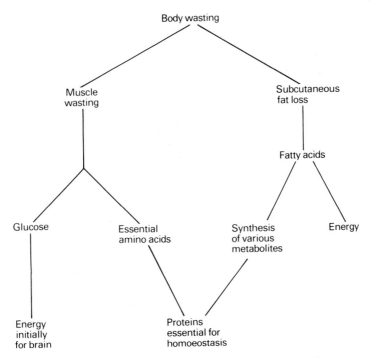

Fig. 15 Basic adaptation to total calorie deficiency. (Fig. 1 from Whitehead R G, Alleyne G A O 1972 British Medical Bulletin 28: 72.)

customary to attribute oedema to the fall in plasma oncotic pressure consequent upon hypoalbuminaemia, recent work failed to show a response proportional to protein refeeding and potassium deficiency may play a part. It is usually dependent but, together with preservation of the buccal pads of fat, gives the not-uncommon appearance of 'moon-face'. Other causes of oedema such as severe anaemia, often due to ankylostomiasis, or nephrosis have to be differentiated. Characteristically the child is apathetic, anorexic, miserable, withdrawn and has a weak, monotonous, whimpering cry.

The skin lesions are charcteristic but a diagnosis of kwashiorkor can be made in their absence. They are more frequent and severe in dark skinned races with depigmentation as the basic change. Desquamation, extensive in severe cases, leads to the characteristic 'enamel paint', 'flaky paint' or 'crazy paving' dermatosis. The most commonly observed appearance in fair-skinned children is a fine desquamation and hyperpigmentation called 'mosaic or crackled skin' especially prone to affect the forehead. Unlike the skin lesions of pellagra, those of kwashiorkor are not prominent on the parts of the body exposed to sunlight. The dermatosis resembles that of the zinc-dependent disease acrodermatitis enteropathica (p. 146) and there is some evidence that they relate to zinc deficiency. Hair changes consist of depigmentation, straightening if the normal hair is curly, fineness of texture and loose

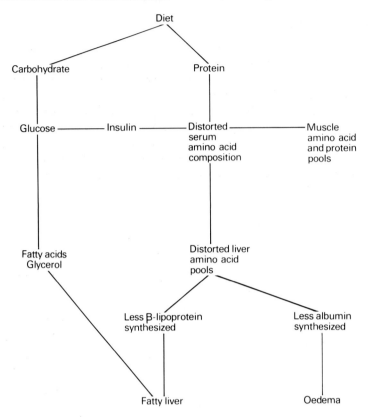

Fig. 16 Basic disturbances in homoeostasis during the development of classical kwashiorkor. (Fig. 2 from Whitehead R G and Alleyne G A O 972 British Medical Bulletin 28: 72.)

attachment of roots as evidenced by sparseness and the ease with which the hair may be plucked. Especially striking is the 'flag sign', with alternating light and dark bands recording periods of bad and good nutrition. The liver is usually large and fatty, but if splenomegaly is also present may be due to malaria. Anaemia is frequent, sometimes severe and may be complex in nature. Iron deficiency is common but megaloblastosis is not rare, usually due to folic acid deficiency but sometimes reported to respond to protein or other vitamins, such as B_{12}, riboflavin or E. Xerophthalmia is a frequent complication in some parts of the world (mainly S. and E. Asia) but in other places where vitamin A intake is fair although protein deficiency is severe it is uncommon.

Adult kwashiorkor is uncommon. Additional features include hypogonadism, gynaecomastia, and pancreatic dysfunction. Pregnancy and prolonged lactation may be precipitating factors; as may alcoholism and short-circuiting operations in a secondary form.

Laboratory findings

Mild-moderate PEM. These include a lowering of the urea nitrogen/creatinine ratio and hydroxyproline/creatinine ratio in urine occurring in all forms, and lowering of plasma transferrin and rise in plasma amino acid ratio (four non-essential/four essential) in 'prekwashiorkor' only. Probably more meaningful, and certainly more practical in the field, are cross-sectional and longitudinal records of weight, skeletal and skinfold measurements. (p. 269).

Severe PEM. Those tests mentioned above are markedly abnormal in frank kwashiorkor. In even severe marasmus levels of blood constituents tend to remain remarkably normal, suggesting considerable adaptation to nutritional stress. (Table 11).

Table 11 Some characteristics of marasmus and kwashiorkor

	Marasmus	Kwashiorkor
General features		
Occurrence	World-wide	Limited
Usual age	Infancy	Second and third years
Adaptation to stress	Good	Poor
Response to treatment		
immediate	Poor	Good (occasional sudden death)
ultimate	Fair	Good
Long-term effects		
mental	Severe	Less severe
physical	Severe	Mild
liver damage	Nil	Nil
Clinical signs		
Oedema	Absent	Present
Dermatosis	Rare	Common
Hair changes	Common	Very common
Hepatomegaly	Common	Very common
Mental changes	Uncommon	Very common
Wasting of fat and muscles	Severe	Mild
Stunting	Severe	Moderate
Anaemia	Common and severe	Mild
Vitamin deficiencies	Uncommon	Common
Laboratory findings		
General		
Total body water	High	High
Extracellular water	Some increase	More increase
Body potassium	Some depletion	Much depletion
Malabsorption	Some	More
Fatty infiltration of liver	Absent	Severe
X-ray bone loss	Mild	Mild
Renal function	Impaired	Impaired
I.V. glucose tolerance	Normal	Impaired
Response to adrenaline	Exaggerated	Lowered

Table 11 Some characteristics of marasmus and kwashiorkor (continued)

	Marasmus	Kwashiorkor
Serum		
Albumin, transferrin etc.	Slightly low	Very low
Enzymes (in general)	Normal	Low
Copper, zinc, sodium	Normal	Low
Non-essential/essential amino acids	Normal	High
Triglycerides	Normal	Normal
Cholesterol	Normal	Low
Non-esterified fatty acids	Normal	High
β-Lipoprotein	High	Low
Insulin	Low	Low
Growth hormone	Low or normal	High
Glucose	Low	Very low
Urine		
Urea/total N	Above 65 per cent	Below 50 per cent
3 methyl histidine	Very high	High
Hydroxyproline index	Low	Low
Liver		
Urea cycle enzymes	Low	Low
Amino acid-synthesizing enzymes	High	High

Pathology

The lesions depend on the severity of malnutrition and changes seen in most systems are common to kwashiorkor and marasmus. The liver, however, in marasmus is shrunken, having lost about 40 per cent of its substance but not fatty, while in kwashiorkor gross fatty infiltration is the rule. Small fat droplets usually appear first in the periportal area of the liver lobule and spread progressively to the central vein area with coalescence to form large globules. With treatment, fat disappears in the reverse order and is accompanied by lymphocyte and plasmacyte activity in the sinusoids. A proliferation of reticulin fibres radiating from the portal tract gives a starlike pattern which was earlier mistaken for incipient cirrhosis.

In marasmus there is marked wasting of all tissues and organs. The muscles are atrophic and pale with extreme wasting of the subcutaneous and visceral fat accentuating the bony eminences. The intestine has been described as tissue-paper thin. In kwashiorkor the depots are usually well preserved and the tissues are oedematous. Non-specific changes of atrophy, cloudy swelling and fatty degeneration are seen in the pancreas, kidney and some of the endocrine glands.

Treatment

Results depend upon the severity of malnutrition and the presence of complications such as dehydration, electrolyte imbalance, vitamin deficiencies, infections and infestations. Best results are obtained in special units where individual nursing and feeding care is given and dangers of cross-infection are kept to a minimum. Such units are few and far between in developing countries. Mothers should be admitted to assist and to learn.

In the acute phase rehydration should be cautious; large infusions are dangerous in a wasted child, weakening the myocardium and causing pulmonary oedema.

The degree of dehydration can be assessed clinically as follows:

Absent: *no dehydration.*

Grade 1: *mild dehydration.* An irritable baby with skin pallor and light red lips and sunken eyes.

Grade 2: *established dehydration.* An ill baby with pale face, sunken black-ringed eyes, dry mouth and whose fontanelle (when patent) is sunken. Skin turgor and elasticity diminished, peripheral pulses palpable.

Grade 3: *shock superimposed on established dehydration.* Limp baby with signs of established dehydration and in addition pale or mottled extremities and impalpable peripheral pulses.

Hyponatraemia, raised blood urea, potassium depletion and metabolic acidosis are common findings. Fluid and electrolyte balance is restored and maintained by nasogastric drip of a mixture of one part Darrow's solution (providing sodium 60 mEq/1, potassium 18 mEq/1, chloride 53 mEq/1, lactate 25 mEq/1) and one part of 5 per cent glucose. The basic amount to be given is 150 ml/kg/day and this is increased by 50 ml/kg for grade 1 depletion, and 100 ml/kg for cases of grade 2 and 3 depletion, in the first 24 hours. The intravenous route is reserved for grade 3 and those who do not respond to oral therapy. Dilute milk feeds can usually be introduced after the first 24 hours. Oral glucose is very effective in promoting water reabsorption and controlling diarrhoea.

Magnesium deficiency may cause irregular twitching, coarse tremors and convulsions, and is treated with 0·5 ml 50 per cent $MgSO_4.7H_2O$ intramuscularly every day for a child weighing less than 7 kg, going on to oral sources after 1 week. Severe anaemia is infrequent but a 100 ml transfusion given over 4 hours is justified when the haemoglobin is below 4 per cent, together with oxygen therapy. Hypothermia is a danger, especially in winter. Round the clock feeding raises body temperature. Severe infections require appropriate antibiotic therapy. Other deficiencies often requiring treatment are of vitamin A, iron, and folic acid.

Cow's milk alone has to be given at 150 ml/kg, to achieve 100 kcal (419 kJ)/kg/day. This provides 5·4g protein/kg resulting in marked solute diuresis and possible dehydration. A formula like human milk provides too much sodium and too little potassium. A modified milk formula has been recommended consisting of two parts whole cow's milk with one part of a 15 per cent dextrimaltose solution containing 1·5 per cent KC1. The diet should be introduced step-wise. Energy intakes of up to 150 or even 200 kcal

(838kJ)/kg/day should be achieved after the acute phase is over, for optimal catch-up growth. Arachis oil, or some other locally acceptable alternative (60g/l), should be added to provide a concentrated source of energy.

In the first few days the protein intake should not exceed 1 to 2 g/kg/day, increasing to 3 to 5 g/kg/day later. Much higher levels have not been shown to be advantageous and are accompanied by raised blood urea and possibly account for the so-called 'recovery syndrome' with non-fatty liver enlargement and some unexpected deaths. Nitrogen absorption is most efficient with milk protein, less so with vegetable sources, and retention is greater than normal even in seriously ill children. Full cream milk and vegetable oil supplements are usually well tolerated even during the early stages. Vegetable protein may have to be substituted for milk if a temporary lactose intolerance gives troublesome diarrhoea (see p. 185). Greater nitrogen retention is obtained with higher energy intakes, especially in marasmus. Within the first week a responsive case of kwashiorkor will lose his apathy, recover interest in his surroundings, and lose weight from loss of oedema. Then for several weeks, despite adequate food intake, there may be a 'lag phase' of stationary weight, most marked in marasmus. During this time body composition approaches normal with further loss of water. Thereafter weight gain, skeletal and skinfold measurements, and excretion of hydroxyproline and creatinine are good indices of progress. Serum albumin becomes normal after a month in kwashiorkor.

Prognosis

Short-term. If all admissions are included then even in special care units the mortality is usually about 15 to 20 per cent. The mortality is about twice as high in males as in females and higher in younger children of the same nutritional type. In kwashiorkor, death often occurs within the first few days after admission whereas in marasmus, providing rehydration has been successful, death is less frequent and occurs later. Signs singled out as of sinister significance are petechiae, jaundice and stupor. In fatal cases raised serum bilirubin, decreased serum sodium and retinol have been found. Humoral and cell-mediated immunity are more impaired in kwashiorkor than in marasmus. Recently, HIV infection has been shown to be very common in malnourished children.

Long-term. Comparison of children treated for severe malnutrition in early childhood, usually kwashiorkor, with children of other families in the same poor environment or with siblings has in general failed to show poorer physical development in the previously malnourished. Long-term follow-up studies have shown that the fatty liver of kwashiorkor leaves no permanent liver injury when the malnutrition has been adequately treated. Some degree of malabsorption and pancreatic deficiency may be long-lasting defects.

Mental development following malnutrition in early life has received considerable attention in recent years. In experimental animals severe and prolonged deficiency of protein and energy intake either *in utero* or shortly after birth has produced some degree of permanent impaired behavioural performance. Human studies are restricted by ethical considerations, the complex nature of the malnutrition state and the importance of social factors. The few prospective studies with healthy sibling controls that have been undertaken suggest that severe and early PEM, especially of the marasmic type, even after full rehabilitation, results in some impairment of mental development, although not of gross degree. Of greater public health implication is the evidence that moderate PEM, never severe enough to be treated in hospital, can also significantly retard mental development if sufficiently prolonged.

Prevention

PEM in its gross forms occurs under circumstances of special privation, resulting from the combined influence of poverty, ignorance and disease. Single measures, such as so-called 'protein-rich' food mixtures (p. 276) or amino acid fortification (p. 277) cannot by themselves solve the problem. With the present trek to the cities kwashiorkor is becoming less common but is more than being replaced by marasmus. Greater awareness among health personnel of the nature of the problem and simple educational measures through mothercraft centres (p. 277) can bring about considerable improvement. The malnourished child is deprived in many ways other than its nutrition and is a sick member of a sick community. The whole society is the patient.

12. VITAMIN DEFICIENCIES AND DEPENDENCIES

VITAMIN A: XEROPHTHALMIA

Prevalence

Xerophthalmia remains the major cause of blindness and provides a considerable contribution to mortality in young children in many of the countries of South and East Asia, the Near East, and parts of Africa and Latin America. On the basis of epidemiological studies it has recently been estimated that about 250 000 children go blind annually, of whom about 50 per cent die, and 8-9 million develop non-corneal xerophthalmia annually worldwide. Epidemics of night blindness associated with conjunctival xerosis and Bitot's spots occur in remote places when crops fail.

Experimental deficiency

Adults on a vitamin A deficient diet develop dry skin and perifollicular hyperkeratosis after some months and impaired retinal function as shown by abnormal electroretinogram when plasma vitamin A falls below 20 $\mu g/$

100 ml and impaired dark adaptation thereafter. At least 600 μg retinol per day is required to reverse the eye changes and probably more for the hyperkeratosis. The requirement for β-carotene was 1200 μg per day but somewhat more is required to maintain optimum serum levels.

Clinical features

Although in many animal species changes have been described in most systems, in man the only organ characteristically affected is the eye. Perifollicular hyperkeratosis of the skin may occur (p. 98). The immune response is impaired (p. 224) and an association with certain cancers has been reported (p. 245). Failure in the utilization of iron has been described, often masked by haemoconcentration. Much interest has been aroused by recent reports that even mild deficiency may be associated with increased rates of infections of the gastrointestinal and respiratory tracts and a higher mortality. The claim has been made that periodic dosing with vitamin A will significantly reduce these.

The eye

Posterior segment

In the eye the posterior segment is first affected and impairment of rod function leading eventully to night blindness forms the basis for several biophysical tests including dark adaptometry, rod scotometry, and electroretinography. For results to be interpreted correctly other causes of rod dysfunction have to be ruled out. Subjective factors that cannot be adequately controlled influence the results obtained.

Use under field conditions of any of these tests is made difficult by the need for sensitive apparatus and fully co-operative subjects. They are inapplicable to the most affected age-group: the young child and careful enquiry of the mother concerning night blindness has been shown to give reliable evidence of early deficiency.

Changes in the fundus were first attributed to vitamin A deficiency nearly 50 years ago. These descriptions come mainly form the Far East. Yellowish spots are seen on ophthalmoscopy, usually in the peripheral fundus. Patients are often older children, complaining of night blindness and having xerosis conjunctivae and Bitot's spots. The evidence that they are caused by vitamin A deficiency is not entirely convincing and there are at least two non-nutritional conditions, retinitis punctata albescens and fundus albi punctatus, that the lesions closely resemble.

Anterior segment

This is affected later than the posterior segment. The conjunctiva, followed by the cornea, undergoes the changes of *xerosis*. The process consists of dryness, thickening, wrinkling, pigmentation and loss of wetability. Goblet cells atrophy and secretions dry up. The exposed bulbar conjunctiva in the interpalpebral fissure is most affected. Both eyes are usually affected equally. Prolonged exposure to smoke, dust, glare and infections may also cause dryness, and dark-skinned races usually have a 'muddy' appearance of the conjunctiva.

Bitot's spot consists of a heaping up of keratinized epithelial cells most commonly occurring on the temporal aspect of the bulbar conjunctiva in the interpalpebral fissure near the limbus. It usually takes the form of a small plaque of a silver-grey hue with a foamy surface. Exceptionally, the material may be scattered widely over the conjunctiva, sometimes having a vertical corrugated arrangement. When associated with generalized conjunctival xerosis it is usually part of the vitamin A deficiency eye syndrome. The subjects are usually young children, sometimes night blind, and there is response to vitamin A. In older children and adults Bitot's spots are often isolated lesions with no accompanying evidence of vitamin A deficiency. In these circumstances local irritation and trauma appear to play a major role.

The earlist corneal change is xerosis of the epithelium, giving this structure a hazy appearance. The stroma then becomes infiltrated with round cells, giving the cornea a milky bluish hue. In young children the deficiency state may proceed rapidly. The final stage consists of a softening of the corneal substance, known as *colliquative necrosis*. Once deformity and loss of substance of the cornea have taken place, use of the term *keratomalacia* is appropriate. By this stage some degree of irreparable damage has taken place. Extrusion of the lens and loss of vitreous may occur. When panophthalmitis supervenes the end result is often a shrunken globe: *phthisis bulbi*. If the cornea holds out against rising intraocular pressure there will be *ectasia corneae* and *anterior staphyloma*. In less severe cases and in those treated in time, healing may leave a leucoma, usually central, that may be susceptible to keratoplasty but the final result is often vitiated by *amblyopia ex anopsia*.

Laboratory findings

Vitamin A depletion is a long process, starting with exhaustion of the usually considerable liver stores, going on to a fall in plasma level and after this leading to rod dysfunction and ultimately to changes in epithelial tissues. Plasma vitamin A levels alone cannot be taken as an indication of early deficiency. They are maintained at or near normal levels until there is advanced depletion. In the presence of the eye lesions values are very low ($< 5\ \mu g/100$ ml). RBP is also low ($< 20\ \mu g/ml$). Liver levels are a good indication of vitamin A status but cannot be readily tested. Most malnourished children have nearly exhausted stores ($< 15\ \mu g/g$ fresh liver). Nearly all children with xerophthalmia have evidence of protein energy malnutrition.

Pathology

Epithelial structures, including besides the conjunctiva and cornea, the ducts of the exocrine glands, the respiratory and genitourinary tracts and parts of the gastrointestinal tract undergo keratinizing metaplasia. Division of the basal cell layer results in an atrophic, keratinized epithelium superficially but, when vitamin A is supplied once more, the basal cells retain their ability to produce normal cells. Colliquative necrosis is found only in the cornea and is possibly related to the reported role of vitamin A-dependent enzymes in mucopolysaccharide formation. Disturbance of lysosome membrane stability could account for the weakening of the epithelial barriers to infection as a result of release of hydrolysing enzymes.

Pathogenesis

Deficiency of vitamin A may be due primarily to dietary lack, or secondarily to disease causing impaired absorption or storage. Xerophthalmia mainly affects children under the age of 4 years, whose dietary intake of vitamin A has been grossly inadequate for a long time. Deprivation beings *in utero* with inadequate liver storage and continues through the first year with low intake from milk and cereals. Requirements are high at this time because of rapid growth and infections such as gastroenteritis and measles cause added stress. Even in sophisticated communities infants have been known to develop xerophthalmia when fed on non-milk formulae from which vitamin A had been inadvertently omitted. In adults and older children night blindness and conjunctival xerosis tend to occur in epidemics under conditions of special privation, i.e. sieges, fasts, imprisonment and famine.

Less often severe deficiency may complicate the clinical picture in malabsorption due to coeliac disease, sprue, obstructive jaundice, mucoviscidosis. Cirrhosis and other chronic diseases of the liver are occasionally accompanied by a vitamin A-responsive night blindness, but some cases have responded only to zinc (p. 145).

Diagnosis

Impaired rod function and early conjunctival changes should not be attributed to vitamin A deficiency without supporting laboratory data. Therapeutic response is decisive. Secondary infection often makes recognition of the corneal changes difficult. The presence of bilateral changes, not necessarily of the same degree, in a young child with a history of poor diet and other evidence of malnutrition should leave little room for doubt. Rapid response to vitamin A within the limits set by the pre-existing damage will confirm suspicions already aroused.

WHO has adopted the classification in Table 12 for clincial and field recording of cases and suggested the criteria in Table 13 for determining whether a public health problem exists in the vulnerable group of children under 5 years of age.

Table 12 Xerophthalmia classification

XN	Night blindness
X1A	Conjunctival xerosis
X1B	Bitot's spot with conjunctival xerosis
X2	Corneal xerosis
X3A	Corneal ulceration with xerosis
X3B	Keratomalacia
XF	Xerophthalmia fundus
XS	Scars

Table 13 Criteria suggested for diagnosis of a public health problem of xerophthalmia

XN	$> 1 \cdot 0$ per cent
X1B	$\geqslant 0 \cdot 5$ per cent
X2 + X3A + X3B	$\geqslant 0 \cdot 01$ per cent
XS	$\geqslant 0 \cdot 05$ per cent
plasma vitamin A	$< 10 \ \mu g/100$ ml $\geqslant 5$ per cent

Treatment

WHO recommends retinyl palmitate be given as follows:

Table 14 WHO treatment schedule

Form	Route	Dosage
Water miscible	Intramuscular	100 000 i.u. (33 mg)
Oil	Oral	100 000 i.u. (33 mg)
		200 000 i.u. (66 mg)
Treatment		
Immediately upon diagnosis		200 000 i.u. oral
		(100 000 i.u. Im if vomiting)
Day 2		100 000 i.u. oral (< 1 yr)
1–4 weeks later		200 000 i.u. oral (> 1 yr)

Prognosis

The milder eye changes leave behind no permanent damage but are indicative of depleted reserves and potential danger if these are not replenished. In very young children they may be associated with serious general malnutrition and high mortality. The corneal changes are always of grave significance.

Prevention

Wherever a problem of public health magnitude is indentified according to the criteria given above the incorporation of rich sources of the provitamin and vitamin into the diet should be encouraged. Wherever feasible fortification with vitamin A of such foodstuffs as cereal grains, sugar or tea should be considered. Young children may be specifically protected by periodic massive dose programmes consisting of 100 000 i.u. under 1 year and 200 000 i.u. 1 to 6 years of age by mouth every 6 months.

THIAMIN: BERIBERI, (CHILDHOOD, CARDIAC, NEURAL, CEREBRAL)

Prevalence

Beriberi is an important public health problem in some countries of South and East Asia where polished rice is the staple, and is not uncommon secondarily to chronic alcoholism in the west.

Experimental deficiency

In volunteers an intake of 0·075 mg/1000 kcal (4·10 MJ) produced severe symptoms in 1 to 2 months but with three times this amount only mild deficiency developed in 6 to 8 months. Anorexia was constant and from mild to very severe psychic and emotional symptoms occurred frequently. Paraesthesiae, aching and weakness of leg muscles were complained of. There was impairment of perception of light touch, pin prick, temperature variation and vibratory sensation. Reflexes were increased at first but later disappeared. Cardiovascular system symptoms included dyspnoea, irregularities of heart rhythm and discomfort in the thorax after exertion. The blood pressure tended to be low, the pulse slow, the skin of hands and feet dusky red with diminished circulation time, and occasionally oedema of the extremities and face developed. The electrocardiogram showed premature ventricular contractions, sinus arrhythmia, prolonged A–V conduction time and decrease in the amplitude of ventricular complexes.

Childhood beriberi

The highest incidence is usually found between the second and fourth months of life and high infant mortality about this time is suggestive. Where this occurs many adults and adolescents have evidence of peripheral neuropathy and mothers of affected infants usually give a history of numbness of feet during pregnancy and show signs of peripheral neuropathy when the child is admitted to hospital.

The affected child is usually breast fed by a thiamin-deficient mother. It often has aphonia or a characteristic cry together with evidence of cardiac failure and absent deep tendon reflexes.

Clinical improvement is rapid after intramuscular administration of 10 to 50 mg of thiamin hydrochloride but neurological recovery is slow.

Beriberi heart disease

Although not as common as formerly in rice-eating areas of Asia, due to diversification of diet, thiamin supplementation and parboiling of rice, it continues to occur among the poorest sections of the community. In North America and Europe it is not uncommon in the chronic alcoholic patient.

Clinical features

Cardiovascular beriberi takes one of two forms: the more common high-output state and the rare, but fatal, low output state.

High-output state. Signs and symptoms of biventricular heart failure are present. The right ventricle is more affected than the left, resulting in dyspnoea, orthopnoea and pulmonary rales. There is sinus tachycardia, a wide pulse pressure and, before heart failure supervenes, a sweating and warm skin. In the presence of heart failure, peripheral vasoconstriction results in cold and cyanosed extremities in an attempt to maintain arterial pressure.

Low-output state (Shoshin disease). This form is characterized by signs and symptoms of severe hypotension, lactic acidosis, and very low systemic vascular resistance. Peripheral oedema is absent.

Treatment

Although the life-saving effects of intravenous administration of 100 mg thiamin are well known haemodynamic studies during recovery are few.

Traditionally cardiac glycosides have been regarded as ineffective in beriberi heart disease.

Beriberi heart failure occurs especially in patients who continue hard physical work, maintaining a high cardiac work load. Consequently bed rest alone is quite effective and the protective action of rest is also evident in the rarity of heart failure in patients with severe peripheral neuritis.

Neurological aspects

These may accompany the cardiovascular manifestations to a varying degree but, especially when of mild degree, may also occur as isolated phenomena. To only a limited extent is it justifiable to consider 'wet' (cardiac) and 'dry' (neural) beriberi as separate entities.

Clinical features

The most characteristic features of the peripheral neuropathy are symmetrical foot drop, associated with great tenderness of muscles and a mild disturbance of general sensation over the outer aspects of the legs, the thighs, and in patches over the abdomen, chest and forearms. Other features such as ataxia with loss of position and vibration sense, amblyopia, and burning paraesthesiae in the feet occur frequently in patients with beriberi, especially associated with chronic alcoholism, but are more characteristic of chronic diabetic polyneuropathy, pellagra and other conditions.

With the severe dietary restriction associated often with alcoholism, *Wernicke's encephalopathy* results, together with varying degrees of poly-neuropathy. Any form of recurrent vomiting, as in pyloric obstruction or the 'pernicious' vomiting of pregnancy may precipitate encephalopathy, as can the administration of large amounts of glucose without thiamin coverage. The signs of encephalopathy usually develop as the result of the superim-position of acute thiamin lack on the background of chronic deficiency. The most acute symptom is mental confusion leading to coma, and if it is accompanied by bilateral 6th nerve weakness, then Wernicke's syndrome is present. If the deprivation is less, the 6th nerve weakness becomes merely nys-tagmus, and if less still then aphonia and mental confusion may be the first or perhaps only symptoms. The 6th nerve weakness is the symptom most easily relieved by thiamin, the mental confusion being difficult to reverse. *Korsakoff's psychosis* is a milder degree of the confusional state of Wernicke's syndrome, often appearing as the latter tends to subside.

Pathology

In severe involvement of the peripheral nerves there is Wallerian degener-ation beginning in the most peripheral part of the longest nerve fibres. Proximal to these areas there is segmental thinning of the myelin. The presence of such demyelination in long segments in the most peripheral parts of the peripheral nerves is especially characteristic of beriberi. In Wernicke's encephalopathy capillary damage results in degeneration and occasionally pin-point haemorrhages in the mammillary bodies, the related walls of the third ventricle, the aqueduct, and in the tegmentum of the medulla.

Laboratory findings

Elevated blood pyruvate and diminished thiamin excretion (< 50 µg/dy) are consistent but late changes. More sensitive is diminished erythrocyte transketolase activity, measured before and after addition of thiamin pyrophosphate (TPP effect). Variations in apoenzyme levels in some diseases may complicate interpretation of this test. TPP may be estimated directly in plasma.

Diagnosis

A careful dietary history including alcohol consumption, together with detailed investigation of the cardiovascular and neurological systems and prompt response to thiamin in the acute forms should provide the answer.

Prognosis

While immediate clincial response is often dramatic in even the most severe thiamin deficiency, ultimate recovery may be incomplete and relapses occur especially if precipitating factors persist. Recovery is usually long delayed after prolonged paralysis.

Treatment

The acute biochemical defect can usually be corrected in a matter of hours or a day or two, commencing with 100 mg thiamin intravenously, followed by 10 or 20 mg three or four times a day orally. To ensure maximal recovery liberal amounts of thiamin (10 to 15 mg daily) should be given for weeks or months.

Prevention

Reliance on polished milled rice as the staple diet underlies the problem of endemic beriberi. Home pounding or parboiling of rice prevents the disease but their advocacy is unlikely to succeed. A policy of enrichment with thiamin exists in some areas but is difficult to enforce. Introduction of new dietary items, especially pulses and vegetables, probably holds out the best hope. Alcoholism is causal in the west.

NIACIN (NICOTINIC ACID): PELLAGRA

Prevalence

With a greater diversification of foodstuffs eaten, pellagra has virtually disappeared from most of the less remote parts of the developing regions. Foci remain in parts of the Near East, Africa and south-east Europe, usually in populations subsising on maize not lime treated. Alcoholism is a precipitating factor in some parts.

Clinical features

The disease follows a chronic and relapsing course with a peak incidence at the end of winter. The significance of prodromal symptoms such as loss of weight, anorexia, soreness of the tongue and mouth, indigestion, diarrhoea, insomnia and mental confusion may easily be overlooked unless a careful history is taken. The skin lesions dominate the picture and without them the diagnosis is rarely made. The gastrointestinal and nervous systems are also affected and the well-known aid to memory recalls this—the disease of the 3Ds: 'dermatitis, diarrhoea and dementia'.

The skin. The dermatosis is usually preceded by prodromal symptoms, especially of the digestive system. The changes are characteristic and pathognomonic and their distribution is determined by exposure to the sun and by trauma. The dermatosis begins as an erythema on the dorsum of the hands, with pruritus and burning. It is characteristically symmetrical. There is slight oedema of the skin. In some patients, several days after the onset of the erythema blebs appear and run together to form bullae and then burst.

In the second stage the dermatosis becomes hard. rough, crackled, blackish and brittle. When the deficiency state is far advanced the skin becomes progressively harder, drier, more cracked and covered with scales and blackish crusts due to haemorrhages.

The usual sites are the face, neck, and dorsal surfaces of the hands and arms and the feet. The symmetry and clear line of demarcation from normal skin are especially striking.

On the forehead there is always a narrow border of normal skin between the erythema and the hair. The face is often slightly affected. The rash never appears there independently of lesions upon the hands and elsewhere.

Casal's 'necklace' extends as a fairly broad band or collar entirely around the neck. Men, women and children have the necklace and it is always accompanied by the characteristic dermatosis elsewhere.

The so-called 'pellagrous' vulvitis, and lesions of the perianal region and scrotum are part of the 'oro-oculogenital' syndrome of riboflavin deficiency (p. 120).

The gastrointestinal tract. Glossitis and stomatitis usually appear early. The affected tongue has a 'raw beef' appearance. The other oral structures may undergo similar changes with spread to the lower regions of the tract accounting for indigestion and diarrhoea. Achylia gastrica occurs in about 60 per cent of patients.

The nervous system. In the early stages periods of depression and apprehension occur, with insomnia, headaches and dizziness. Later, tremulous movements or rigidity of the limbs increase and then finally loss of the tendon reflexes, and numbness and paresis of the extremities progressively incapacitate the patient. In profound deficiency an encephalopathy has been described, resembling that of the Wernicke type, but responding to niacin.

Niacin deficiency secondary to metabolic disorders

Several cases of pellagra have been reported arising in patients receiving isoniazid. It appears to act by replacing nicotinamide in DPN. Pyridoxine deficiency is an even more frequent complication (p. 121).

A malignant tumour of the adrenal gland (phaeochromocytoma) may divert as much as 60 per cent of the body's tryptophan to form large amounts of 5-hydroxytryptamine and thus induce niacin deficiency.

The hereditary metabolic disorder, Hartnup disease, presents in childhood with pellagra and attacks of cerebellar ataxia (p. 197).

Laboratory findings

Deficiency levels of excretion of N'-methylnicotinamide of 0·2 mg per 6 hour or 0·5 mg per g creatinine have been derived principally from human deprivation studies.

Pathogenesis

Endemic pellagra is usually associated with a maize diet. Much of the niacin is lost in milling or is in a bound form (niacytin) unavailable unless the food is prepared with alkali, as in *tortillas* in Central America. Maize is also low in tryptophan, which is capable of conversion to niacin in the body. Pellagra associated with other than maize diets may possibly arise from amino acid imbalance. In one part of India it is found in relation to the consumption of millet (*Sorghum vulgare,* jowar) which has a high leucine content.

Treatment

Dramatic response of the glossitis, stomatitis and improvement in the patient's mental state are usually seen within 24 hours of a daily dose of 500 mg of nicotinamide. Healing of the skin lesions is slower, becoming apparent after 4 or 5 days. Balanced diet therapy is most important.

Prevention

Pellagra appears to be infrequent among maize eaters where lime treatment is practised or where beans, which are good sources of niacin and tryptophan, are eaten. With the spread of urbanizing influences diets may become more diversified and conditions less suitable for pellagra to arise. As part of the same trend, however, alcoholism may constitute an obstinate barrier to eradication.

RIBOFLAVIN: A-OR HYPORIBOFLAVINOSIS; OROGENITAL SYNDROME

Prevalence

According to dietary survey data riboflavin deficiency should be one of the most widespread nutritional conditions. Its manifestations in man, however, seem to be relatively trivial. This is probably because deficiency is usually mild. It usually accompanies other deficiencies such as pellagra, beriberi or protein energy malnutrition. Adolescents and pregnant women appear especially susceptible. Chronic alcoholics tend to become deficient in this and other B vitamins.

Experimental deficiency

In a group of patients with a riboflavin intake of less than 0·55 mg per day pallor and maceration of the mucosa in the angles of the mouth were followed by superficial linear fissures which became crusted. The skin in the nasolabial folds, alae nasi, ears and eyelids became mildly erythematous, scaly and greasy.

Riboflavin deficiency has been induced in patients with inoperable neoplastic disease by a riboflavin-deficient diet and the antagonist, galactoflavin. In addition to the changes in skin and mucous membranes a severe anaemia developed and was reversed by riboflavin administration. The anaemia was normochromic normocytic in type with reticulocytopenia.

Clinical features

In addition to the signs described in the early experimental work, magenta tongue, vascularization of the cornea, epithelial keratitis, nutritional amblyopia and scrotal dermatitis and vulvitis have all been reported to respond to riboflavin.

The dermatosis affecting the genital area may begin either as a patchy redness associated with scaling of the superficial epithelium or as a fine powdery desquamation without any colour change.

The term, 'oro-oculogenital' syndrome, is sometimes employed to cover all these signs but it has to be emphasized that no single one is pathognomonic.

Laboratory findings

Urinary excretion of less than 50 µg riboflavin in 24 hours is usually associated with clinical signs. An earlier indication of riboflavin deficiency is provided by determination of glutathione reductase activity in erythrocytes, comparable to the TPP effect for thiamin deficiency.

Treatment

Under experimental conditions, induced lesions, including far advanced scrotal dermatitis with severe inflammation, responded promptly to 6 mg riboflavin per day.

Prevention

As part of the general programme in nutrition education the encouragement of the consumption of legumes, pulses and animal products as available together with proper preparation of food and improved cooking methods is advocated.

PYRIDOXINE: DEFICIENCY AND DEPENDENCY

Prevalence

There is little evidence that natural dietaries are ever likely to be seriously deficient. Sporadic cases occur secondarily to malabsorption, alcoholism, drug antagonism or due to dependency.

Experimental deficiency

Adult subjects studied while receiving a diet low in vitamin B_6 together with the antagonist, 4-deoxypyridoxine, became irritable and depressed. Seborrhoeic dermatosis affected especially the nasolabial folds, eyebrows, cheeks and occasionally spread to neck and perineum. Glossitis, cheilosis, angular stomatitis and blepharitis affected several subjects as did peripheral neuropathy. Lymphopoenia was common.

Deficiency and dependency states

Cellular metabolism dependent on vitamin B_6 will be impaired if there is restricted availability of the coenzyme pyridoxal-5′-phosphate to the protein component of the enzyme, or *apoenzyme.* This can happen in two ways: (1) the tissue pool of pyridoxal-5′-phosphate may be smaller than normal; this constitutes *deficiency;* (2) the coenzyme pool may be adequate but either (a) chemical interference alters its availability to apoenzyme, or (b) one enzyme or more is altered with regard to apoenzyme interaction. Diseases manifesting a single enzyme defect and attributable to genetic modification in the apoenzyme are due to vitamin B_6 *dependency* (see Table 16).

Deficiency states

Table 15 outlines the various ways in which pyridoxine deficiency is known to arise.

Primary dietary deficiency is very uncommon. Other forms of deficiency are brought about by some condition that offsets an otherwise adequate intake of vitamin B_6 as indicated in Table 15. In these circumstances it is possible for some patients to have greater than normal daily requirements of vitamin B_6. This is not dependency

Clinical features

Nervous system. A convulsive disorder of infancy is the most serious. The special susceptibility of the brain in this age group is probably related to activity of glutamic acid decarboxylase. This enzyme is in high concentration in the grey matter. Decarboxylation produces γ-amino butyric acid (GABA)

Table 15 Mechanisms for reduction of effective pyridoxal phosphate pool size

Exogenous deficiency
Inadequate dietary intake of vitamin B_6
'Conditioned' deficiency (primary intake adequate)
1. Impaired delivery
   Defective intestinal absorption
   Defective cellular and intracellular and intracellular transport

2. Impaired phosphorylation
   Inhibition (e.g. deoxypyridoxine)
   Deficient pyridoxal kinase activity

3. Chemical inactivation of phosphorylated vitamin (e.g. isoniazid therapy)

4. Excessive loss of vitamin
   Renal clearance
   Excessive oxidation

Relative deficiency (primary intake inadequate in relation to demand)
1. Increased metabolic activity (pregnancy, fever, etc.)
2. Apoenzyme induction

Table 16 Conditions exhibiting vitamin B_6 dependency

Condition	Biochemical findings	Clinical findings	Apoenzyme probably affected
Pyridoxine-responsive convulsions	None	Seizures	Glutamic acid decarboxylase
Cystathioninuria	Cystathioninuria	Usually none	Cystathionase
Familial xanthurenic aciduria	Xanthurenic-acidura	Urticaria	Kynureninase
Pyridoxine-responsive anaemia	Defective haem synthesis	Hypochromic anaemia	δ-Amino levulinic acid synthetase
Homocystinuria	Defective methionine metabolism	Mental retardation throbo-embolism, ectopia lentis, osteoporosis	Cystathionine synthase

which has neuroinhibitory properties. Its concentration in brain is usually less in early infancy than in later life, possibly accounting for the poor ability of the infant to adapt to pyridoxine deficiency.

Haemopoietic system. Over 100 cases of pyridoxine-responsive anaemia have been reported. In addition, about one-third of patients with a refractory 'sideroblastic' anaemia have shown significant although variable response to pyridoxine therapy. Most cases have normoblastic erythropoiesis, but in about 1 in 6 erythropoiesis is frankly megaloblastic or megaloblastoid. The anaemia is usually severe, mean Hb being < 4 g/100 ml, and there is often hyperferraemia, iron overload and impaired liver function. Poor nutrition and excessive alcohol intake seem to play a role more often in the megalobastic than the normoblastic type. The familial occurence of haematological abnormalities in about one-third of the patients suggests the existence of an inborn error of metabolism.

Drugs. Vitamins B_6-responsive signs have been reported arising during the course of therapy with several drugs. Those of the hydrazide type, such as isoniazid used in the treatment of tuberculosis and the antihypertensive drug, hydrallazine, probably act by competitive inhibition of pyridoxal kinase and also by hydrazone formation and inactivation of pyridoxal-5'-phosphate (PLP). About 10 per cent of patients receiving either isoniazid or hydrallazine have paraesthesiae and rarely a frank sensorymotor neuropathy develops. In one instance bilateral optic neuropathy has been described arising in a patient with Wilson's disease who had been receiving DL-penicillamine therapy for more than two years. It is suggested that penicillamine complexes with the aldehyde group of pyridoxal, forming a thiazolidine compound.

Laboratory findings

The tryptophan load test (2 g) shows increased urinary excretion of xanthurenic acid (> 50 mg/day) and other intermediates on the niacin pathway. Plasma pyridoxine falls (< 25 mg/ml) as does urinary excretion of pyridoxine (< 20 µg/g creatinine) and pyridoxic acid (< 0.5 mg/day).

Single determinations of glutamic-oxalacetic transaminase (GOT) and glutamic-pyruvic transaminase (GPT) in blood are generally regarded as being non-specific.

Treatment of deficieny

Supplementation of the diet is of primary importance in order to replete the coenzyme pool. If the defiency is conditioned by some additional metabolic demand the amount required may be considerably in excess of the recommended allowance. Underlying causes such as hydrazide administration or malabsorption should be treated. Even so no cause may be found. This is especially true in infants and the possibility that there is genetic variation in nutritional requirements has still to be investigated.

Treatment of dependency

In pyridoxine dependency the requirements for vitamin B_6 are 2 to 11 mg as compared with those of the normal infant: less than 250 µg. Early recognition and therapy are essential to prevent death or subsequent mental retardation. It should be suspected in infants who have an early onset of convulsions in the absence of other aetiological factors, especially if there is a family history . If convulsions are not controlled within several minutes of parenteral dose (5 to

10 mg), then pyridoxine dependency can be ruled out. The state of dependency is apparently permanent.

FOLIC ACID (FOLACIN, PTEROYLGLUTAMIC ACID (PGA)) DEFICIENCY AND DEPENDENCY

Prevalence

Folic acid deficiency is possibly the most common vitamin deficiency in North America and western Europe today. This is certainly true in pregnancy, in which it is the most common cause of megaloblastic anaemia.

Haemopoietic system

Changes are seen in the erythroid cells, the myeloid cells, and the thrombocytes. The appearances found do not lend themselves to the quantification of the deficiency, and indistinguishable changes result from deficiency of folate or vitamin B_{12}. In the peripheral blood the red cell count is more reduced than the haemoglobin level. Macrocytosis and ovalocytosis occur early. Hypersegmentation of the neutrophil polymorphonuclear leucocytes, with increase in the number of strands between lobes as well as in the number of lobes, can be seen before the anaemia becomes severe.

In the marrow the erythroid cell precursors show a more 'stippled' appearance of the nuclear chromatin than normal. The myeloid cell precursors show early commencement of nuclear lobulation and elongation in comparison with corresponding stage of development of the cytoplasmic and granular elements. Among the earliest changes are abnormal metamyelocytes, and these are often the last feature to revert to normal after treatment.

Other systems

In recent years there have been reports of folate deficiency associated with peripheral neuropathy and/or myelopathy and with such conditions accompanying pregnancy as spontaneous abortion, abruptio placenta and fetal abnormalities. The anticonvulsant, phenytoin, is known to be a folic acid antagonist. The evidence for folic acid deficiency has usually been low serum folate levels and low formiminoglutamic acid (FIGLU) excretion, in the absence of megaloblastic anaemia. Recently folic deficiency has been shown to reduce synthesis of the neurotransmitter 5-hydroxytryptamine in the brain. This may relate to the deficiency commonly found in psychiatric patients.

Laboratory findings

Erythrocyte folic acid (normal 160 to 640 ng/ml whole blood) is the best indicator of status. Plasma folate (normal 3 to 21 ng/ml) reflects recent dietary intake.

Pathogenesis

Table 17 shows how folate deficiency may arise under different circumstances. Sometimes more than one factor operates. Combined deficiencies of folic acid, vitamin B_{12}, ascorbic acid, iron and other nutrients are more common than isolated deficiency. Oral contraceptives may inhibit the absorption of folic polyglutamate.

Diagnosis

The megaloblastic anaemias are morphologically indistinguishable but peripheral nerve or posterolateral column involvement strongly suggests vitamin B_{12} deficiency. While folate stores at birth may be exhausted in three to six months, those of vitamin B_{12}, last for three to six years. The physician should keep watch for folate deficiency in association with alcoholism, haemolytic anaemias, hookworm infestation, infancy, pregnancy, malignancies and tropical and non-tropical sprue. It seems to be more common in Britain than the United States, possibly due to the more prolonged cooking of food in the former.

Treatment

The usual dose is 1 mg/day orally. Divided doses of 15 mg folic acid orally are usually required to bring about a remission in tropical sprue. A dose of 1 to 5 mg daily orally is indicated in the megaloblastic anaemia of infancy. Temporary improvement of the anaemia and glossitis of pernicious anaemia and other vitamin B_{12}-deficiency anaemias occurs but unless vitamin B_{12} is given neurological degeneration is precipitated. Folinic acid is as potent as folic acid in these conditions but in a dose of 3 mg daily parenterally is of special value in the reversal of aminopterin toxicity.

Dependency

Several very rare enzyme defects leading to anaemia or mental retardation in early childhood respond to large doses of folic acid.

Table 17 Mechanisms of folic acid deficiency. (McLaren D S, Burman D 1976 Textbook of paediatric nutrition. Churchill Livingstone, Edinburgh.)

Primary
Poor diet; lacking fresh, slightly cooked food
Secondary
Indequate absorption: malabsorption syndromes (especially coeliac disease), drugs (cycloserine), specific malabsorption for folate (congenital, acquired), blind loop syndrome.
Inadequate utilization: folic acid antagonists (methotrexate, pyrimethamine, triamterene, diamidine compounds, trimethoprim), anticonvulsants?, enzyme deficiency (congenital, acquired), vitamin B_{12} deficiency, scurvy
Increased requirement: prematurity, infancy, malignancy (especially lymphoproliferative), increased haematopoiesis, increased metabolism, anticonvulsants
Increased excretion: vitamin B_{12} deficiency? liver disease?

VITAMIN B_{12} (COBALAMIN): DEFICIENCY AND DEPENDENCY

Pure vegetarians (*vegans*) tend to develop an uncomplicated B_{12} deficiency with subnormal serum concentration (less than 120 pg/ml), glossitis, paraesthesiae and subacute combined degeneration of the cord.

Vitamin B_{12} deficiency arises more commonly from a defect of metabolism than as a result of poor dietary intake although this latter form has to be borne in mind among the undernourished and largely vegetarian populations of developing countries. The fish tapeworm, *Diphylobothrium latum*, absorbs enormous amounts of vitamin B_{12} from its human host and may induce deficiency. It only becomes established if freshwater lake fish is eaten raw, as is common in Finland.

Pernicious anaemia

The haematological changes are identical with those described in folate deficiency but usually take much longer to appear. They do not correlate with those in the other systems and the neurological changes (see below) may long precede the haematological changes. There is usually atrophic glossitis, nausea, vomiting, diarrhoea alternating with constipation, histamine-fast achlorhydria, and achylia gastrica. A high level of indirect bilirubin due to increased destruction of erythrocytes and megaloblasts gives the skin and sclerae a characteristic lemon-yellow colour.

Pernicious anaemia in childhood

About 30 such cases have so far been reported. The majority are characterized by an early onset of vitamin B_{12} deficiency, usually before the age of $2\frac{1}{2}$ years. This appears to be due to a specific and congenital lack of intrinsic factor without loss of acid secretion and with normal gastric histology. It could be called 'congenital pernicious anaemia' . The other type develops later in childhood and the failure to secrete intrinsic factor is associated with achlorhydria and atrophic gastritis. This type might be designated 'juvenile pernicious anaemia'.

Subacute combined degeneration of the cord

This condition is characterized in varying degree by involvement of peripheral nerves, a dorsal funiculi syndrome and a pyramidal syndrome. Histamine-fast achlorhydria is usual as is megaloblastosis. Evidence of vitamin B_{12} deficiency is usually present and the symptoms show remarkable response to therapy. The recent demonstration that excretion of methy malonic acid (MMA) is greatest in patients with neurological changes suggests that altered propionate metabolism may be aetiologically involved.

Nutritional amblyopia (nutritional retrobulbar neuropathy). This has long been recognised as an occasional accompaniment of pernicious anaemia and has recently been shown to occur also in fish tapeworm infestation. Nutritional amblyopia was common in World War II Far East prisoners of war and one form is due to tobacco and alcohol excess.

The skin. Hyperpigmentation of the palms has been described in Indian children and Nigerian adults.

Laboratory findings

Signs and symptoms of deficiency usually do not appear until the body has been largely depleted of vitamin B_{12} but serum levels are depressed long before this. The value of a serum vitamin B_{12} determination by itself is limited. In pernicious anaemia the Schilling test is classically negative. In this test ^{57}Co-labelled vitamin B_{12} is given and urinary excretion measured. This is poor until the test is repeated with added potent source of intrinsic factor, when excretion is high in pernicious anaemia but still low in malabsorption. However, about 40 per cent of pernicious anaemia patients have low excretion in both stages of the test, indicating some intestinal damage which slowly disappears under vitamin B_{12} therapy.

Untreated pernicious anaemia patients excrete large amounts of methylmalonic acid (MMA) in the urine. MMA excretion appears to be a sensitive index of vitamin B_{12} body stores, for levels begin to fall as soon as therapy is commenced but do not reach zero until after haematologic abnormalities have been corrected and serum B_{12} levels reach normal.

Low serum vitamin B_{12} levels (< 150 pg/ml) have been found in normal individuals and cannot be taken alone as a reliable index of vitamin B_{12} status.

Pathogenesis

Table 18 indicates in outline the known ways in which a deficiency of vitamin B_{12} may develop. Except veganism and those cases that are caused by a single 'missing link' in the metabolic chain, vitamin B_{12} deficiency is usually part of a deficiency state involving other nutrients, especially folic acid.

Table 18 Pathogenesis of vitamin B_{12} deficiency (McLaren D S, Burman D 1976 Textbook of paediatric nutrition. Churchill Livingstone, Edinburgh.)

Primary deficiency
Inadequate diet: tropics, mainly vegetable, veganism
Secondary deficiency
Inadequate absorption: lack of intrinsic factor (congenital and juvenile pernicious anaemia, destruction of gastric mucosa, endocrinopathy), intrinsic factor inhibition, drugs, specific malabsorption for vitamin B_{12} (fish tapeworm, blind loop syndrome)
Inadequate utilization: antagonists, enzyme deficiencies, organ disease (liver, kidney, malignancy, malnutrition), transport protein abnormality
Increased requirement: hyperthyroidism, parasitization
Increased excretion: inadequate binding in serum, liver disease, renal disease

---

Diagnosis

Combined deficiency of vitamin B_{12} and of folic acid is frequent but when occurring separately certain points of difference may assist in the diagnosis. When the megaloblastic anaemia is dietary in origin, in contrast to pernicious anaemia, achlorhydria, achylia gastrica, neurological manifestations and jaundice are usually absent.

Treatment

Pernicious anaemia is usually treated with 1000 μg vitamin B_{12} subcutaneously followed by 500 μg monthly. Oral therapy over a wide range of dosage has given unpredictable response. A dose of 50 to 100 μg is advocated for patients with severe neurological disease, acute infections or advanced atherosclerosis. There is no objection to giving folic acid, so long as adequate vitamin B_{12} therapy is being provided.

Patients with sprue usually respond to parenteral doses of vitamin B_{12} (25 to 50 μg daily) larger than those necessary in pernicious anaemia, but the best results are obtained with folic acid. If there is a relapse on folate therapy vitamin B_{12} may then bring about a complete remission. A large dose (500 μg) of vitamin B_{12} will produce a haematologic response in folate deficiency.

Dependency

In recent years several disorders have been reported in which there is methylmalonicaciduria, but erythropoiesis is normal, and usually responding to massive doses of vitamin B_{12} (up to 100 μg/day). There is profound metabolic acidosis, long-chain ketonuria and MMA uria is increased by loading with valine, propionate or isoleucine indicating a block in the isomerization of MMCoA to succinyl CoA. Three specific disorders have been identified by Scriver; (1) partial impairment in biosynthesis of deoxyadenosyl coenzyme, (2) abnormality of the apoenzyme MMCoA carbonylmutase (resistant to vitamin B_{12}), and (3) deficient activity of both apoenzymes probably resulting from a defect at some stage in the pathway common to both coenzymes.

PANTOTHENIC ACID

Symptoms in man attributable to deficiency of this vitamin await substantiation. Claims of benefits in such diverse conditions as rheumatoid arthritis, postoperative paralytic ileus, diabetic neuropathy and some psychoses have been made on insufficient evidence.

Further investigation has failed to confirm that it is of use in a painful condition common in prisoners of war known as the 'burning feet' syndrome.

BIOTIN

Four volunteers were fed a diet containing minimal amounts of biotin and 30 per cent of the total energy intake in the form of egg white. The latter contains avidin, a biotin antagonist. Temporary fine scaly desquamation of the skin without pruritus appeared after 3 or 4 weeks. Several cases have been reported in patients consuming large quantities of raw eggs.

Biotin *dependency* states have been described involving carboxylase deficiencies with impaired immunity and developmental retardation. Response has been complete to large doses of biotin (10 mg) daily.

VITAMIN C (ASCORBIC ACID): SCURVY

Prevalence

Scurvy is rare in most countries today. Adult cases, usually old folk, appear in municipal hospitals from time to time from the slum areas of towns and cities. Outbreaks occur in desert places when the seasonal rains fail. Infants between the age of 6 and 12 months who are fed processed milk formulae unsupplemented with fruits and vegetables are very susceptible.

Experimental deficiency

The first symptoms reported in a human deprivation experiment were weakness, easy fatigue and listlessness, followed by shortness of breath and aching in bones, joints and muscles especially at night. In the skin there was keratosis of the hair follicles with slight surrounding haemorrhage.

Gum changes were most marked in those volunteers who showed evidence of gingivitis and parodontal disease at the start of the experiment. The earliest signs were reddening, swelling and tiny haemorrhages in the tips of the interdental papillae. Grosser changes observed in a few subjects consisted of purplish, swollen and spongy appearances of the gums with part of the tissue becoming necrotic with some bleeding.

The deficiency state

Infantile scurvy

The infant is well supplied with vitamin C at birth and the majority of cases present in the second half of the first year of life. With an increasing varied diet in the second year the incidence falls.

Clinical features. The presenting symptomatology is often dominated by the triad of irritability, tenderness of the legs and pseudoparalysis (failure to move or use the legs). The arms are less commonly involved. Manifestations of bleeding are relatively uncommon as presenting symptoms. The most common site is around erupting teeth.

The infant characteristically lies in the 'pithed frog' position of comfort with the legs flexed at the knees and the hips partially flexed and externally rotated. He is apprehensive and cries readily. Costochondral beading or 'rosary' can usually be palpated and is frequently visible also. Tenderness may be generalized or, when localized, is usually found in the legs. The gums are abnormal only in relation to erupted teeth where they may bleed after manipulation and are often red, turgid and overgrown. Subperiosteal haemorrhages can often be palpated at the distal end of the femur and proximal end of tibia, corresponding to the radiological changes.

Anaemia is commonly present, usually of the iron-deficiency type. Megaloblastic anaemia of infancy is frequent, due to a combined deficiency of folic acid and ascorbic acid. The child is often fevered on admission with a leucocytosis and an accompanying infection. Concomitant evidence of rickets may occasionally be found.

X-ray appearances. The earliest X-ray changes appear at the sites of most active growth: sternal end of ribs, distal end of femur, proximal end of humerus, both ends of tibia and fibula, and distal ends of radius and ulna. A zone of rarefaction immediately shaftward of the zone of provisional calcification gives rise to the 'corner fracture' sign. Atrophy of trabecular structure and blurring of trabecular markings cause a 'ground glass' appearance. Widening of the zone of provisional calcification causes a dense shadow at the end of the shaft and is also seen at the periphery of the centres of ossification. This ring-like appearance is seen best at the knee and is very characteristic of scurvy. As the deficiency proceeds, fractures may occur in areas of extending rarefaction and overlying zone of provisional calcification may be comminuted with the shaft and spur formation may occur. Epiphyses may separate and be displaced. Temporary healing often modifies the radiological appearance. With treatment, even the grossest deformities resolve, although radiological evidence may persist for several years. (Fig. 17)

Pathology. The mesenchymal tissues are chiefly affected, as shown by failure of deposition of intercellular substances by fibroblasts, osteoblasts and odontoblasts, resulting, respectively, in defective collagen, osteoid and dentine. Failure of deposition of intercellular cement substances leads to widespread rupture of capillaries and haemorrhage. Deposition of osteoid ceases throughout the shaft of long bones, the cortex is thinned, trabeculae are diminished in size and haemorrhages appear under the periosteum.

Diagnosis. The dietary history, presence of suggestive symptoms, typical physical findings and X-ray and laboratory tests must all be taken together. Confusion of the pseudoparalysis with poliomyelitis, attributing the bone changes to rickets, and the haemorrhagic phenomena to a blood disease, are the most common pitfalls.

Treatment. A dose of 200 mg orally daily for a week or 10 days gives dramatic improvement. The child will be asymptomatic in a few days, losing his irritability and gaining an appetite.

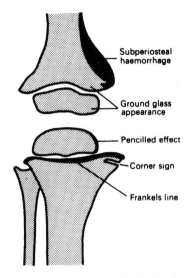

Fig. 17 X-ray appearances in scurvy. (Grewar 1965 Clinical Pediatrics 4:82)

Adult Scurvy

Elderly bachelors and widowers who cook for themselves or eat in restaurants are particularly prone. Women, even when living alone, are better able to fend for themselves, and fruit and vegetables have a more prominent place in their diet. Food fadists are especially at risk.

Clinical features. Patients with the disease show the early symptoms and signs described in experimental deprivation. Later, haemorrhages occur deep in muscles and into joints. Multiple splinter haemorrhages may form a crescent near the distal ends of the nail and are more extensive than those seen in bacterial endocarditis. In extreme deficiency the gums become swollen, purple, spongy, friable and bleed readily. Secondary infection, gangrene and loosening of teeth eventually supervene. The gum changes occur only when natural teeth or hidden roots remain in the mouth. Old scars break down and new wounds fail to heal.

Laboratory data. In healthy subjects plasma values vary tremendously, from 0 to 300 mg/100 ml and it is possible to relate such data to adequacy or dietary intake. Whole blood values are preferable.

Treatment. In persons suspected of having scurvy the usual dose is 100 mg 3 to 5 times a day by mouth, continued until 4 g have been administered, then 100 mg twice a day. In a critically ill patient 1 g can be given daily by intra-venous drip or in divided doses each of 100 mg , intramuscularly. Severe weakness and spontaneous bleeding cease within 24 hours, pain and fever disappear in 48 hours and gums, skin and haematomas heal over 10 to 12 days. Pigmentation of the skin may linger for months. Blood regeneration begins almost immediately.

VITAMIN D (CALCIFEROL): RICKETS AND OSTEOMALACIA

Prevalence

Vitamin D deficiency results mainly from a lack of exposure to ultraviolet rays and to some extent from inadequate dietary intake. There is new evidence that a dark skin impedes the action of ultraviolet light. Children of immigrant families coming to temperate zones from the tropics may be especially vulnerable. This appears to be less related to lack of exposure to sunlight than to impaired absorption of calcium from a diet high in wholemeal flour, as used in the making of chappatis by Asian immigrants to Britain. In them it is often a family disorder with most members affected, irrespective of age, including neonatal rickets in infants of osteomalacic mothers. Rickets is common in some developing countries where, although sunlight is plentiful, infants are closely wrapped or confined indoors. Osteomalacia is not uncommon in the elderly, associated with the use of some drugs, in kidney disease, or, following many pregnancies in rapid succession, may manifest itself as obstructed labour due to contracted pelvis.

Clinical features

Infants with early rickets are restless and sleep poorly, and the occipital hair is denuded by constant movement on the pillow. They fail to sit, crawl, or walk at the usual times. The fontanelles close late and craniotabes and frontal bossing occur. Later there is enlargement of the epiphyseal cartilages of the long bones particularly noticeable at the lower ends of the radius, ulna, tibia and fibula. Beading of the costochondral junctions gives the appearance of the rachitic rosary. If rickets is still active when the time for weight bearing comes bow-legs and arms and knock-knees result. Frequently at this time the diet becomes more varied, the child breaks away from the mother into the sun and the rickets heals 'spontaneously' and may leave no stigmas. Rickets may manifest in adolescence as pain on walking, impaired gait and genu valgum.

Rachitic tetany is caused by hypocalcaemia and may accompany either infantile or adult vitamin D deficiency (see p. 140).

X-ray appearances

These changes precede clinical signs and may become evident in the first few months of life. The diaphyseal ends of the bones, most characteristically the lower ends of the radius and ulna, lose their sharp, clear outline, become cup-shaped and show a spotty or fringe-like rarefaction. Due to failure of calcification the distance between the radius and ulna and the metacarpals appears increased. Shadows cast by the shaft decrease in density and the network formed by laminae becomes coarse. As healing begins, a thin white line of calcification appears at the epiphysis, becoming thicker and denser as calcification proceeds. Lime salts are deposited beneath the periosteum, the shaft casts a denser shadow and the lamellae disappear.

In osteomalacia weight bearing produces bowing of the long bones, vertical shortening of the vertebrae and flattening of pelvic bones and contraction of the outlet. Plasma 25(OH)D has recently been found to be low in a high proportion of elderly patients with fracture of the femoral neck (p.000).

Laboratory findings

The earliest evidence is obtained by determining vitamin and metabolites in plasma. 25(OH)D falls below 4 ng/ml and 1, 25(OH)D becomes undetectable. Serum calcium is usually maintained due to parathyroid action and only falls late on. Serum phosphorus is low as a result of diminished tubular reabsorption. Alkaline phosphatase is usually much increased (normal 5 to 15 Bodansky units) but may be unchanged in the presence of protein energy malnutrition.

Diagnosis

Tetany must be distinguished from convulsions due to other causes. Cases of rickets not due to deficiency of vitamin D are refractory to the vitamin and include renal rickets, renal tubular acidosis and the Fanconi syndrome (see Table 19).

Osteomalacia must be differentiated from other diseases characterized by widespread bone decalicification, e.g. hyperparathyroidism, senile or postmenopausal osteoporosis, adrenocortical tumour, multiple myeloma, Paget's disease.

Prevention

Simple rickets in sunny climates can be guarded against by judicious exposure of the young child. In cooler sunless parts and especially in cities suffering from air pollution, fortified milk and supplements are necessary. Family

Table 19 Classification of rickets and osteomalacia

Deficiency of vitamin D	Lack of sunlight, low dietary intake of vitamin D, calcium deficiency (rare), high phytate or phosphate intake, malabsorption states
Defective production of 25-(OH)D$_3$	Liver disease (advanced parenchymal and cholestatic disease) Anticonvulsants
Defective production of 1,25-(OH)$_2$D$_3$	Vitamin D-dependent rickets, type I (defective 1-hydroxylation) Vitamin D-dependent rickets, type II (end organ resistance to 1,25-(OH)$_2$D$_3$) Familial hypophosphataemic (vitamin D-resistant) rickets (renal tubular defect in phosphate transport) Other disease — acquired hypophosphataemic rickets, chronic renal failure (renal osteodystrophy), Fanconi syndrome, renal tubular acidosis, diabetes mellitus, pseudohypoparathyroidism

planning will prevent the osteomalacia of pregnancy and supplements are advisable in old age. A voluntary campaign among Asian schoolchildren in Glasgow, making available 10 μg daily, has been successful and has been extended to pregnant women.

Treatment

Nutritional rickets. In the presence of an adequate and balanced intake of calcium and phosphorus, cure can be brought about by giving daily 40 μg vitamin D and should be continued for about 1 month. Occasionally a rapid cure is essential, as when weakness of the thorax menaces life, and then 100 μg/day should be given, reduced to 30 μg/day as soon as there is evidence of healing plasma 25(OH)D and 1, 25(OH)$_2$D begin to rise within a day or two. A rise of serum phosphorus is seen in about 10 days. After 3 weeks there is deposition of Ca and P in the bones. If tetany is present calcium should be given intravenously.

Secondary rickets

Refractory forms of rickets

Those forms of rickets which result from defective production of vitamin D metabolites do not respond to the usual doses effective in nutritional rickets. Some of these conditions have responded to massive doses of vitamin D but toxicity has sometimes resulted.

In some of the conditions in which there is evidence of defective production of 25(OH)D$_3$, 50 μg/day of this compound has augmented 25(OH)D plasma levels and resulted in clinical improvement.

Hereditary vitamin D-dependent (pseudodeficiency) rickets, an autosomal recessive syndrome, is characterized by severe rickets, low or normal serum calcium, hypophosphataemia and generalized amino-aciduria, has responded to a wide range of vitamin D dosage (50–4000 μg/day), making safe long-term control difficult to achieve. In acute studies 1,25(OH)$_2$D$_3$ has been shown to be effective (1–2 μg/day i.v. or oral). Promising results have been obtained with the synthetic analogue 1-α (OH)D$_3$(1–3 μg/day). However, at present vitamin D therapy is advocated for routine use.

Familial hypophosphataemic (vitamin D-resistant) rickets is an x-linked dominant disorder that responds well to oral phosphate (1–4 g/day in five divided doses). Plasma calcium rises, parathyroid hormone levels fall, and there is healing of rickets and increased growth. 1-α (OH)D$_3$ (0.5–1.0 μg twice daily oral) alone has produced only temporary improvement.

Chronic renal failure osteodystrophy has responded for periods up to one year to date in some patients treated with 1-α (OH)D$_3$(1.5–2.0 μg/day). Calcium absorption has increased, positive calcium and phosphorus balances have been achieved, and modest increase in serum calcium, reduction in alkaline phosphatase and iPTH and improved skeletal X-ray and histological findings have been reported. Similar preliminary results have been obtained with small doses of $1,25(OH)_2D_3$.

VITAMIN E

Deprivation of adult male subjects over a period of 8 years produced progressive lowering of plasma tocopherol levels, increased susceptibility of erythrocytes to haemolysis in the presence of hydrogen peroxide, and decrease in erythrocyte life time. These changes were enhanced by increasing the daily consumption of polyunsaturated fatty acids, especially linoleic acid.

The vitamin E status of young children is especially precarious. Intake during pregnancy is variable, placental transfer inefficient and cow's milk is not a good source. Low birth weight infants are especially susceptible and, in a controlled study high dietary intake of polyunsaturated fatty acids, was associated with low serum tocopherol and hydrogen peroxide-induced haemolysis. Additional iron supplementation resulted in haemolytic anaemia indicating its potential danger in those circumstances. These infants may develop retrolental fibroplasia leading to blindness, or intraventricular or subependymal haemorrhage; responsive in some degree to vitamin E.

Malabsorption syndromes, especially with steatorrhoea, frequently have evidence of vitamin E deficiency in the form of creatinuria, ceroid deposition, increased serum creatine phosphate phosphokinase, low serum tocopherol, increased red cell haemolysis and decreased life span. Deficiency is very common in cystic fibrosis (p. 177). Vitamin E therapy may delay the progress of the retinopathy in a-β-lipoproteinaemia (p. 188). Spinocerebellar syndromes similar to that seen in this disease have responded to vitamin E in children with cystic fibrosis or chronic cirrhosis. In the presence of overt deficiency 100 to 600 mg vitamin E has been given daily.

Toxicity

Pharmacological doses in low birth weight infants have caused a high rate of sepsis and necrotizing enterocolitis with a high mortality.

VITAMIN K

Prolonged coagulation time of the blood, resulting in serious haemorrhages, occurs as a consequence of reduction of plasma prothrombin (factor II) activity. Coagulation factors VII (proconvertin), IX (Christmas factor), X (Stuart factor) and another recently identified factor are also affected. Deficiency may arise during prolonged antibiotic therapy when vitamin K-producing bacteria may be suppressed. Chronic disease may have the same effect. Exclusion of bile from the intestine, as in obstructive jaundice, may seriously impair absorption. When the liver is severely damaged, vitamin K administration by any route will not be effective. Dicoumarol, similar in structure, acts as a vitamin K antagonist. Phytonadione is the preparation of choice 10 mg in the adult, 2 mg in young children and 1 mg in the newborn, intramuscularly. Normal newborn infants have low plasma prothrombin levels which approach adult concentrations in subsequent weeks. When they are very low the serious condition known as *haemorrhagic disease of the newborn* results. Deficiency is more common in breast-fed infants; this milk has a lower concentration of vitamin K than cow's milk. Response to vitamin K either intramuscularly or by stomach tube is complete within 48 hours. All newborn should receive 1 mg prophylactically.

ESSENTIAL FATTY ACIDS

Growth failure and a skin rash occur in experimental animals and humans. Patients receiving total parenteral nutrition in which energy is supplied from non-lipid sources are susceptible. It sometimes occurs in severe malabsorption. Diagnosis is made by finding in plasma reduced amounts of linoleic and arachidonic acids and the presence in increased amounts of the abnormal metabolite 20:3 ω 9 from oleic acid. A ratio of 20:3 ω 9/20:4 or 0·4 or over is regarded as pathognomonic. Biochemical and clinical changes respond to i.v. administration of 100 to 300 g linoleate in the form of intralipid.

13. WATER, ELECTROLYTE AND ELEMENT DEFICIENCIES

Pure water depletion

This takes place when water intake stops without a concomitant loss of electrolytes. Obligatory losses of water continue through skin, lungs and kidneys. Electrolyte concentration consequently increases as extracellular fluid volume decreases and this compartment becomes hypertonic. Water leaves the cells in an attempt to restore osmotic equilibrium and thus dehydration occurs. Thirst, the earliest sign of water deprivation, occurs when as little as 2 per cent of the body weight is lost due to dehydration.

In mild depletion the kidneys excrete electrolytes to restore equilibrium. In severe depletion, oliguria occurs as antidiuretic hormone is secreted, stimulating the kidney to reabsorb more electrolytes and thus conserve water.

Pure salt depletion

Abnormal loss of body fluids with replacement of water only gives rise to pure salt depletion mainly in two clinical situations. The labourer who perspires excessively and drinks large quantities of water becomes salt depleted and so does the acutely ill patient who is vomiting, has diarrhoea, or has extensive losses of body fluids by a fistula or gastric or intestinal suction if replacement is by dextrose in water without salt. Unfortunately, unlike water depletion, there is nothing comparable to thirst to act as an alarm for salt depletion.

Table 20 Fluid and electrolyte dysequilibrium

| | | Change in fluid volume | | Change in osmolality |
		i.c.f.	e.c.f.	
Isotonic dehydration	Loss of water and Na^+ in isotonic ratio (vomiting, diarrhoea)	N	D	N
Hypertonic dehydration	Loss of more water than Na^+ (diabetes insipidus)	D	D	I
Hypotonic dehydration	Loss of more Na^+ than water (impaired renal function, adrenocortical insufficiency)	I	D	D

N = normal (no change), I = increase, D = decrease, i.c.f. = intracellular fluid, e.c.f. = extracellular fluid.

With replacement of water loss there is decrease in electrolyte concentration in the extracellular fluid with hypotonicity, transfer of water to cells to re-establish isotonicity, excretion of low specific gravity urine to conserve electrolytes but loss of water.

In actual practice pure water and pure salt depletion rarely occur; various possibilities can arise (Table 20).

Disorders of acid–base balance

These arise from an increased load of acidic or basic metabolites which cannot be accommodated by the normal excretory process (Table 21). For example, in uncontrolled diabetes the enhanced production of keto acids causes a metabolic acidosis. The accumulation of acid causes plasma bicarbonate to be converted to carbonic acid which stimulates the respiratory centre and causes hyperventilation with the expulsion of CO_2. Renal compensation is of minor importance with conservation of base by increased reabsorption of HCO_3^- and exchange of H^+ and NH^+ for Na^+ which is reabsorbed.

Metabolic acidosis also may result from a disproportionate loss of alkali. Bicarbonate ions are lost, resulting in increased dissociation of the weak acid H_2CO_3 and secondary increase in free hydrogen ion. Here renal compensation is of prime importance and respiratory compensation plays only a minor role. In metabolic alkalosis resulting from accumulation of base in the plasma, carbonic acid is converted to bicarbonate with resulting primary HCO_3^- excess and secondary H_2CO_3 decrease. The latter results in depression of the respiratory centre, hypoventilation and accumulation of H_2CO_3. Renal compensation consists of increased loss of base achieved by decrease in $H^+ - NH^+$ exchange and diminished resorption of HCO_3^-.

Table 21 Classification of disorders of acid-base balance

Acidosis (increased hydrogen ion concentration)
Primary excess of acid:
1. Hypercapnia (respiratory acidosis)
2. Ammonium chloride ingestion
3. Methyl alcohol intoxication
4. Diabetic acidosis
5. Lactic acidosis
6. Salicylate intoxication (late stage)
7. Renal insufficiency (glomerular insufficiency)
8. Ureterosigmoidostomy

Primary reduction of base:
1. Gastrointestinal loss of base (diarrhoea, ileostomy, biliary fistula)
2. Renal tubular acidosis
3. Dilutional acidosis

Alkalosis (decreased hydrogen ion concentration)
Primary excess of base:
1. Bicarbonate ingestion
2. Milk-alkali syndrome
3. Dissolution of bone
4. Contractual acidosis

Primary reduction of acid:
1. Hypocapnia (respiratory alkalosis)
2. Gastrointestinal loss of acid (vomiting or gastric drainage)
3. Potassium deficiency

Mixed disturbances of acid–base balance

(Levithin 1969, In: Duncan's diseases of metabolism , 6th edn. Bondy.)

Metabolic alkalosis may also result from an acid defect. Carbonic acid is lost, causing increased hydrolysis of HCO_3^- and secondary increase in hydroxyl ion. Respiratory is much less effective than renal compensation.

In general compensation is not complete and active therapy is needed.

To assist the clinical evaluation of the course of a patient with acid–base imbalance an answer should be sought to the following questions: (i) Has there been a normal intake of water? (ii) Has food intake been normal? (iii) Have there been any voluntary or medical restrictions or additions of food or dietary intake? (iv) Has there been any weight loss? (v) Has there been a loss of body secretions? (vii) Did the patient continue to take any fluids and/or food during this period of time?

Potassium deficiency

This develops primarily from abnormal loss of potassium from the body as this element is so abundant in almost all foods. Vomiting and diarrhoea or increased urinary excretion are the usual causes. Urinary loss may result from kidney disease as in renal tubular acidosis, from hyperaldosteronism or with most diuretics. Symptoms and signs are muscular weakness; leading to respiratory failure, paralytic ileus, and hypotension; and impaired renal concentration and cardiac arrhythmias with characteristic e.c.g. changes (S-T segment depression and increased V and T wave amplitude).

Progressive potassium depletion is associated with increasing alkalosis. This can be explained at least in part by the migration of hydrogen ion into the cell in exchange for the lost potassium. This leads to the generation of bicarbonate which accumulates as it is not excreted efficiently by kidneys. This impairment has been attributed to the potassium deficiency itself and the associated intracellular chloride deficiency. Treatment of hypokalaemia should consist of adminstration of both potassium and chloride.

As potassium is mainly intracellular, the plasma level does not reflect that in cells in a rapidly changing situation as in metabolic alkalosis with poor renal function. Where the whole body counter is available ^{40}K can be measured and the degree of depletion determined. Application of this method to localized areas of the body has shown the brain to be particularly deficient in potassium in protein energy malnutrition.

Fluid and electrolyte therapy

There are three objectives: (1) supply daily needs of the patient, taking into account current loss via urine, skin and lungs; (2) replace the deficit of total cations, bicarbonate and chloride from abnormal losses as assessed from clinical history and laboratory tests; (3) replace current abnormal losses if any. Each patient has to be assessed individually. A nutritional programme has to be planned on the basis of carefully kept records of intake and output and a daily cumulative summary of water and electrolyte balance.

Immediate needs can be met by use of one of the repair solutions shown in Table 22. Overfeeding is as serious as underfeeding. The major problem is to avoid gross distortion of the composition of the body fluids. This can usually be prevented if the condition of the patient permits administration by oral or rectal routes.

Table 22 Composition of some repair solutions

Solution	mmol/l	Na^+	K^+	Cl^-	HCO_3^-
Dextrose 5 per cent	278	—	—	—	—
Physiological saline	308	164	—	154	—
1/6M Na lactate	328	164	—	—	164
NH₄Cl (0.9 per cent)	336	—	—	168	—
Darrow's electrolyte	312	121	35	103	53

CALCIUM

When dietary intake is very low blood calcium is usually maintained within normal limits by secretion of 1, 25 $(OH)^2D$ and parathyroid hormone. Very occasionally rickets may be due to true calcium deficiency. Low calcium status may play a part in osteoporosis (p. 217) and hypertension (p. 206).

Hypocalcaemia (blood Ca < 2.25 mmol/l or 9.0 mg/100 ml) is found in a number of conditions which lead to disturbed calcium metabolism (see Table 23). Symptomatic hypocalcaemia (tetany), consists of muscular spasms which cause stridor of the larynx in infants, paraesthesias, cramps and carpopedal spasm. The ST segment of the e.c.g. is prolonged.

Table 23 Laboratory findings in hypocalcaemia states

	Phosphate	Blood Alkaline Phosphatase	Urine calcium
Hypoparathyroidism	H	N	L
Pseudohypoparathyroidism	H	N	L
Malabsorption	L	N	L
Rickets* (simple and vitamin D-resistant)	L	H, N	L
Renal failure	H	N, H	L
Hypoproteinaemia	N	N	N
Pancreatitis	L	N, H	

N = normal, H = high, L = low.
*See page 133 for earlier changes.

Treatment

The underlying cause of the calcium deficiency and hypocalcaemia will determine the detailed management. Blood calcium may be restored towards normal and neuromuscular symptoms controlled by supplementary oral calcium and vitamin D. Urinary and blood calcium should be determined at regular intervals. Crystalline dihydrotachysterol may be more suitable for prolonged use than vitamin D_2 or D_3. A daily dose of 1 mg is probably sufficient. Blood calcium concentration cannot be maintained without some form of vitamin D which causes not only enhanced gastrointestinal absorption but also resorption of bone. Dietary supplements of calcium are also necessary to make the calcium available for enhanced absorption.

Vitamin D is usually given as ergocalciferol (D_2) 1000 to 2500 μg daily together with several grams of additional calcium as lactate or gluconate for chronic hypoparathyroidism. Acute hypocalcaemia following thyroid or parathyroid surgery needs intravenous calcium 15 to 20 mg/kg over several hours.

When chronic hypoparathyroidism following thyroid surgery seems likely vitamin D 5000 μg units should be given daily, tapering to maintenance levels as the extent of deficiency becomes apparent. $1\alpha(OH)D_3$ is active in very small doses (p. 134).

PHOSPHORUS

Deficiency does not occur spontaneously in man because of the widespread distribution in foodstuffs. The prolonged and excessive use of non-absorbed antacids containing magnesium or aluminium hydroxide limits the absorption of phosphate and produces symptoms and X-ray changes indistinguishable from osteomalacia. Phosphate depletion may occur in renal disease, alcoholism and with parenteral nutrition (p. 238). Symptoms and signs include confusion, dysarthria, paraesthesias, peripheral neuropathy, muscle weakness, anorexia, nausea and vomiting. Liver function tests are abnormal and oxygen release from red cells is impaired by 2, 3-DPG deficiency. Hypophosphataemic rickets is discussed on page 134.

MAGNESIUM

The serum magnesium level is the simplest and quickest approach to the evaluation of magnesium status. If the level is normal (around $2 \cdot 0$ mEq/1) and the clinical state is suggestive of deficiency the erythrocyte content and 24-hour urinary excretion should be measured.

Symptoms of deficiency are neuromuscular dysfunction, especially tetany and behavioural disturbances, ataxia, vertigo, tremors, depression, irritability and psychotic behaviour. The tetany is distinguished from that of hypocalcaemia by serum determinations and differences in the e.c.g. Significant hypocalcaemia and hypomagnesaemia may coexist especially from excessive loss of gastrointestinal fluids.

In symptomatic deficiency the serum level is usually less than 1 mEq/1 but not all with such low levels develop symptoms. Dietary inadequacy alone is not a cause; renal conservation is marked on a low intake and conditioning factors have to be present, such as PEM (p. 107), malabsorption or abnormal loss of fluids. Some cases are familial.

Treatment

In tetany, seizures or eclampsia, magnesium sulphate may safely be given parenterally if the calculated extracellular deficit is given over a 48-hour period. In other conditions where the need for replacement is less urgent, the oral route should be used because of the danger of magnesium intoxication (p. 159).

IRON

Few would contest the statement that this is the most widespread deficiency state of all. Even so satisfactory evidence upon which to base such a statement is not easy to assemble. Iron deficiency is depletion of body iron and anaemia is not essential for its presence. Most data in the literature relate to iron deficiency anaemia. There have been differences of opinion as to what level of haemoglobin signifies the presence of anaemia in various groups.

Definitions and diagnosis

Iron deficiency exists in varying degrees, from mild depletion of iron stores to severe anaemia.

Three stages in the process of increasing deficiency may be identified: (1) iron depletion; decrease in storage iron alone. Identified by decreased or absent haemosiderin granules within reticulo-endothelial cells of the marrow and with serum ferritin < 12 ng/ml; (2) iron deficiency without anaemia; absent iron stores and a saturation of transferrin (plasma iron/total iron binding capacity) of 15 per cent or less (normal 20 to 40 per cent). (3) iron deficiency with anaemia. In addition to the above findings a haemoglobin less than the levels shown in Table 24.

Table 24 Lower limits of normal haemoglobin (sea level)

Years	Sex	Haemoglobin (g/100ml)	Packed cell vol. (per cent)
0.6-4	Both	11	33
5-9	Both	11.5	34.5
10-14	Both	12	36
Adults	Men	14	42
	Women	12	36
	Pregnant women	11	33

Table 25 Laboratory tests for anaemias with defects in haemoglobin synthesis

	Iron deficiency	Infection	Porphyrin or globin block
Plasma ferritin	Decreased	Unchanged	Unchanged
Sideroblasts	Decreased	Decreased	Increased
Marrow reticulo-endothelial iron	Decreased	Increased	Increased
Morphologic type of anaemia	Normocytic or microcytic hypochromic	Normocytic or microcytic normochromic	Microcytic hypochromic

Iron deficiency is only one cause of anaemia in which there is a defect in haemoglobin synthesis. Appropriate laboratory tests as indicated in Table 25 will distinguish the various conditions.

Symptoms and signs

After acute blood loss symptoms relate to volume depletion and shock. Anaemia of insidious onset manifests as increasing fatigue and slight pallor of the mucous membranes. Later on cardiorespiratory signs of oxygen lack include dyspnoe, tachycardia, palpitations, angina and cardiac enlargement. Headache, tinnitus, anorexia, constipation and low grade fever also occur. Glossitis and angular stomatitis may be present. Iron-deficiency anaemia has some features not shared by other causes of anaemia, i.e. koilonychia (spoon-shaped nails), dysphagia (see Paterson-Kelly syndrome, p.000) and achlor-hydria.

Deficiency of iron even short of causing anaemia has been shown to impair work performance and, in young children especially, has an adverse effect on brain function.

Prevalence

Data in the literature are virtually confined to anaemia, with varying criteria for diagnosis, and do not deal with iron deficiency as such. Several studies suggest that the prevalance of iron deficiency anaemia is about 10 per cent in non-pregnant women, 10–60 per cent during pregnancy and 10–60 per cent in infancy. Contributory factors in early life include (1) low stores at birth, especially in prematures, (2) low iron content of milk, (3) high requirements for rapid growth, and (4) gastrointestinal loss due to sensitivity to cow's milk. Many young women have iron intakes well below the RDA, especially if they are 'on a diet' or 'watching their weight'. It is not clear whether they are truly deficient or whether the RDAs are unnecessarily high.

Treatment

If infancy and pregnancy are excluded, the cause of iron deficiency anaemia is usually blood loss, and appropriate measures must first be taken concerning the underlying cause. Repletion of stores takes months of therapy when iron is given orally, even when the haemoglobin has been restored to normal. With appropriate doses therapeutic response in haemoglobin synthesis is equal with oral or parenteral iron. The latter is necessary in malabsorption and may be preferable in serious gastrointestinal diseases or intolerance. Transfusion is reserved for rapid blood loss and chronic deficiency with Hb $<$ 4 g/100ml.

Oral therapy is usually 200 mg/day of elemental iron as ferrous sulphate, gluconate or fumarate. Intolerance to iron is rare with 100 mg/day and present in about 15 per cent at 200 mg/day.

The parenteral iron preparation of choice is iron dextran, i.m. or i.v. The daily dose should be limited to 100 mg. Sterile abscess and allergic reactions are rare. Indications are malabsorption, unchecked recurrent blood loss and the rare patient who cannot tolerate oral iron.

In severe anaemias the Hb concentration should begin to increase one week after treatment at the rate of 0·2 g/day or more.

The high incidence of iron deficiency anaemia in pregnancy and infancy warrants routine prophylaxis; 5 to 15 mg/day in infancy through fortification of food and 30 mg/day in the latter half of pregnancy medicinally.

It is well known that frank anaemia is associated with impaired muscular performance and intellectual activity. There is some evidence that iron deficiency without anaemia may cause irritability, lassitude and inability to concentrate.

The role of iron in resistance to infection is discussed on page 224.

Fortification of certain staple items of food is commonly practised and is considered to be necessary to meet the requirements of the vulnerable groups. Some authorities feel that the levels of fortification have been set too high and migh be conducive to iron overload in those who have the familial trait (see p. 160). Some foods consumed with the fortified item enhance iron absorption (e.g. fruit juice) but others impair it (e.g. boiled eggs). Some forms or iron are better absorbed than others; ferrous sulphate more readily than powdered elemental iron.

IODINE

Mild iodine deficiency manifests itself primarily by non-toxic enlargement of the thyroid gland or goitre ('simple', 'colloid', 'endemic', and 'nodular'). While the major factor in the production of non-toxic goitre is deficient intake of iodine, other factors are clearly involved, as the incidence is not uniform among people living together and exposed to the same environmental conditions.

In general the goitrous areas of the world have been found to be those where the iodine intake is low.

Goitre occurs in every continent. It has been estimated that 200 million people are affected. The problem has substantially declined in such countries as the United States, Switzerland and New Zealand, due to better living conditions and iodized salt programmes.

In recent years attention has been drawn to the serious consequences for the fetus of marked maternal iodine deficiency during pregnancy. Endemic cretinism is the consequence and takes one of two distinct clinical forms; the myxoedematous or the neurological (Table 000). In most areas the latter is much the more common. The Andes regions of South America, parts of Central America and of central and eastern Africa, the Himalayan region of Asia and Papua New Guinea are highly endemic areas.

People who are resident in goitrous areas can only obtain enough iodine by (a) consuming a substantial proportion of their food in the form of marine foods, (b) eating foods imported from iodine-rich regions or (c) by the use of iodized salt.

Various methods have been tried for the prevention of goitre. Iodization of domestic salt is universally recognized as the most satisfactory method. Iodide is unstable and has largely been replaced by iodate. The optimum level of iodization depends upon the per capita consumption of salt and the requirement to prevent goitre. In temperate climates the daily intake of salt is about 6 g but may be as high as 30 g in humid countries. A supplement of at least 100 μg daily should be supplied. Salt is usually iodized at a level of 1:10 000 to 1:40 000 parts per million.

Many of the endemic areas are remote and lack permanent health facilities. A single intramuscular injection of 4 ml of iodized oil, providing 2.15 g of iodine, has been found to be protective against severe deficiency for up to 4½ years and is there the prophylaxis of choice.

FLUORINE

Epidemiological studies have revealed an inverse relationship between the fluoride content of drinking water and the incidence of dental caries. Levels of 1·0 to 1·5 p.p.m. are associated with minimum caries and no mottling (see p. 219). The 'level of maximum health with the maximum of safety' is 1 p.p.m.

Fluoridation of water supplies using usually sodium fluoride, to maintain a level of 1·0 to 1·2 p.p.m. is carried out by public health authorities in many parts of the world. Evidence has shown that there are no harmful effects and that an average reduction of 60 to 65 per cent in prevalence of caries in permanent teeth of children has been produced. The caries rate has also been reduced by the topical application of fluoride in toothpaste. This latter measure gets around the objection frequently raised by 'action groups' that fluoridation of the water supply is a violation of the rights of the individual.

Bone density was studied in two areas of the United States: one of low fluoride intake and the other of high. In the area of high intake there was found to be less osteoporosis, fewer collapsed vertebrae and, as a surprise finding, less calcification of the aorta.

ZINC

Conditioned deficiency of zinc has been reported in cirrhosis, nephrotic syndrome, orthostatic albuminuria, porphyria, several neurological and psychiatric diseases, malabsorptive states, and protein-losing enteropathy. It is not clear what clinical manifestations can be attributed to the zinc deficiency *per se* although night blindness in some patients with cirrhosis has responded to zinc and not to vitamin A. In some of these states increased urinary excretion of zinc seems to be at least in part responsible.

From Egypt and Iran descriptions have come of hypogonadism and iron deficiency anaemia in males with very low zinc status and diminished faecal and urinary excretion. Zinc supplements to some patients resulted in growth of genitalia, appearance of pubic, axillary and facial hair and significant height increase. The specific role of zinc deficiency in the growth deficit and testicular aspects of this syndrome is not clear as these patients had been consuming a generally deficient diet. Excess of phytate or fibre, parasites and geophagia may all play a part. Most bread consumed in rural Iran is unleavened. Leavening of bread has been shown to increase the solubility of zinc.

Short stature and impaired taste (hypogeusia) have been shown to respond to zinc in apparently well-nourished children in parts of North America and Europe with low zinc hair concentration and a history of a predominantly milk diet.

A previously lethal autosomal recessive disease, *acrodermatitis enteropathica* has been shown to be due to malabsorption of zinc. Zinc sulphate 30 to 150 mg/day cures the skin lesions, diarrhoea and promotes growth.

Zinc appears to act beneficially in wound healing in man as well as in animals.

OTHER TRACE ELEMENTS

Copper

Deficiency in man is very rare because of the abundance of this trace element. The normal diet contains about one-third as much as it does of iron but the needs for iron are 50 times greater.

Hypocupraemia has occurred in malnourished infants, especially if fed exclusively on milk, and in the presence of diarrhoea. Anaemia, neutropoenia anorexia, growth failure, hair and skin changes, psychomotor retardation and bone lesions have been reported. A defect in copper absorption has been described in *Menkes' steely hair disease,* a sex-linked inherited disorder. Copper treatment has so far proved ineffective.

Cobalt

Cobalt is required as part of the vitamin B_{12} molecule. All ordinary diets supply much more than can be accounted for as the vitamin and there is no good evidence that human deficiency occurs. It causes polycythaemia and has been advocated in the treatment of the anaemias of chronic renal failure but toxicity is common.

Chromium

Trivalent chromium is the active ingredient of the glucose tolerance factor (G-TF)—a factor needed by rats to maintain normal glucose tolerance. Trivalent chromium has been shown to improve glucose tolerance in some diabetics, some elderly subjects and in PEM. A single patient on home parenteral nutrition after $3\frac{1}{2}$ years developed weight loss, peripheral neuropathy and glucose intolerance; all responding to chromium.

Selenium

Selenium is essential for many animal species, deficiency causing liver necrosis, myopathy and infertility. Its function, although not clearly understood, seems to be associated with that of vitamin E (p. 135). Deficiency has been reported in prolonged parenteral nutrition and endemic cardiomyopathy in the Keshan region of China is being brought under control by prophylactic selenium.

Manganese

Deficiency occurred when this trace element was inadvertently omitted from an experimental diet. Weight loss, nausea and vomiting, dermatitis and hair changes resulted.

Molybdenum

Deficiency resulting in mental disturbance has been reported in a single infant on prolonged parenteral nutrition.

14. OBESITY

Adipose tissue is the repository of excess ingested energy and is an ideal form for its storage. Under the conditions of life in the human race's infancy, adipose tissue was more frequently called upon at a moment's notice to supply energy than for massive fat storage. This may be why the mechanisms favouring fat mobilization are many and diversified while fat synthesis depends almost entirely on a single hormone, insulin. In contrast, the adipose tissue of modern man is more often called upon to store fat than to mobilize it. The consequence is one of the most common and disabling disorders of civilization: obesity.

Definition and diagnosis

Obesity may be defined as adiposity in excess of that consistent with health.

At present the most popular practical assessment of adiposity is by use of the body mass index (BMI) derived from weight/height^2 which is largely independent of height. Table 26 shows a proposed grading system:

Table 26 Grading of obesity by weight W (kg) and height (H)

	W/H^2
Grade III	> 40
Grade II	30-40
Grade I	25–29. 9
Not obese	< 25

However, this method ignores differences in body composition and frame size.

At age 25 the normal amount of fat at what is termed 'desirable' weight is about 14 per cent of body weight for males and 25 per cent for females. These figures tend to rise in later years, even when the weight remains constant, but that this is not physiological is suggested by the absence of this trend among some primitive peoples.

In recent years the measurement of skinfold thickness has been introduced as a relatively simple method for estimating the body fat (see p. 6). A triceps skinfold thickness equal to or greater than 23 mm in man and 30 mm in women between the ages of 30 and 50 is indicative of obesity.

Magnitude of the problem

Using one or other of the definitions of obesity described above it has been estimated that in the United States about 15 per cent of men and 20 per cent of women are obese. Figures for Europe are about half of these, but everywhere in the west obesity is increasing by about 1 per cent per decade.

Consequences to health

Obese patients are poorer surgical risks than the non-obese. They tend to be clumsy and more accident-prone. While obesity is not responsible for initiating certain disease processes it does tend to unmask or enhance these and, conversely, if treated contributes to amelioration of the underlying conditions. Among these may be included diabetes, hypertension and bone, joint and muscle diseases. Extreme obesity increases the work of breathing, decreases respiratory reserve and maximum capacity, and causes changes in the circulation contributing to dyspnoea.

The major evidence for the increased mortality carried by obesity comes from the data of life insurance companies. One study indicated that the mortality for men and women who were 20 per cent or more above average weight, was about 150 per cent of that of those with average weight. It also showed that for those who were this much overweight and who reduced weight and were then rerated for insurance purposes, the aggregate mortality fell to about 110 per cent. In old age, however, this association does not apply and heroic efforts to slim should be avoided and careful attention paid to any sustained weight loss.

Aetiology

Obesity results from an imbalance between energy intake, energy output and the energy stores. It would be surprising if such a fundamental and complex process of metabolism had a single aetiology or that there was a single disorder. The term obesity probably covers a variety of disorders which we are unable to separate at present and many factors are involved.

Studies of energy expenditure for the same task in individuals matched for age, sex, weight and body form have shown differences up to 600 Kcal (2·5 MJ)/day; indicating that 'personal' factors play a major part in the control of energy balance.

Heredity. The tendency of obesity to occur in families is well recognized, but this might be because members of the same family tend to have similar customs and preferences. Strong evidence for genetic predisposition to obesity comes from studies of identical twins reared separately in which the weight of the pairs was highly correlated. One study showed that the weights of monozygotic twins brought up apart was closer than those of dizygotic twins reared together. While the weights of adopted children show no correlation with those of their adopting parents, those of natural children do. Body build, or somatotype, appears to be inherited and among the three main somatotypes, ectomorph (tall and thin), mesomorph (average height and muscular), and endomorph (short and fat) it is the latter that is prone to obesity.

In several recent studies large numbers of people have been observed from infancy into middle age. The results provide overall strong evidence for the influence of both genetic and environmental factors (such as social class) in the development of obesity, or more correctly, the obesities.

Psychological factors

The obese react differently to external and internal stimuli related to food as compared with the way non-obese people react. Experiments have shown that obese and normal people do not refer to the same bodily state when they use the term 'hunger'. This was explored further by manipulating gastric motility in patients and by inducing fear in some and not in others. While in normal subjects there was a high degree of correspondence between the state of the gut and eating behaviour, for obese subjects there was no correspondence and nothing that was done could influence the amounts eaten by the obese.

The circumstances of eating seem to have a profound effect on the eating behaviour of the obese, but not on that of the normal. When food is dull and the surroundings uninteresting, the obese eat very little, whereas the normal person's behaviour is directly linked to his physical state, whether or not he is hungry, and little affected by external circumstances.

Gastric contractions stop after a small amount of food has been placed in the stomach. An individual whose eating is mainly under internal control should eat only enough to stop the contractions. Eating beyond this point is under external control: taste, sight, smell of food. The obese, whose eating is mainly externally controlled, find it difficult to stop eating. If the external cues were absent or ignored then a person under external control could almost starve. This seems to be the case sometimes in patients with *anorexia nervosa* (see p. 213), many of whom at some time in their lives have been obese. Another state in which the psychological changes border on the pathological is the *night eating syndrome*. Patients suffer from insomnia and voracious appetite at night, with marked anorexia in the morning. The obesity can be extreme.

Cultural influences

Obesity correlates well with social class, particularly in women. In western societies, mild to moderate obesity is due to the combined effect of overnutrition and underactivity. The economically deprived classes are particularly prone to obesity in highly developed societies, whereas in developing countries it is the ruling class which becomes overweight and develops associated degenerative diseases. Habits with regard to size and frequency of meals have been shown to be important in relation to the occurrence of obesity. The consumption of large infrequent meals, rather than frequent nibbling, is especially likely to contribute to the development of obesity. However, it appears that the frequency of feeding does not influence the rate of weight loss of obese patients on a reducing diet.

Eating is one of the most important social activities, both within the family circle and with friends. The generally accepted norm of body shape and size will largely influence the individual's ideas on the subject. In Arabic the word for health and wellbeing 'saha' also denotes plumpness. Such deeply rooted cultural concepts raise formidable barriers to the combat of obesity.

Obesity is more common in women than in men; even allowing for the fact that they usually have about twice as much fat. They are usually under much more constraint to overeat, being concerned with preparation of the family food and the meal times of the children. Many women attribute the onset of obesity to their pregnancies. Those already obese tend to put on even more weight after a pregnancy.

Physical activity

The view, commonly held, that all obese people overeat has not been substantiated by several surveys. It was found that obese school children actually ate less than their normal weight controls but spent very much less of their time in activities involving exercise. Excessive weight gain began especially in winter, when the opportunities for exercise are less.

Several studies of large groups of people who admit to an overweight problem have shown that most of them do not engage in any additional exercise and may be on the move for as little as one hour in the average day. In addition to helping to combat obesity, physical training has a beneficial effect on the risk of CHD, decreases absenteeism and accidents at work and promotes a feeling of wellbeing.

Cell size and number

Adipose tissue, like any other tissue, grows by increase in number and/or increase in size of cells. It is now no longer accepted that there is a critical period in early infancy when overfeeding can cause a permanent increase in the number of adipose tissue cells. More precise animal experiments, in which earlier methodological problems have been overcome, have failed to show that organs grow first by hyperplasia and then by hypertrophy (p. 7).

About 80 per cent of all overweight children remain so as adults and retrospective studies of obese adults indicate that 30 per cent of them were heavy as children. Birth weights do not correlate with adult weights but those at about age 5 do. From this it would seem that only a proportion of adult obesity arises in early life and most of this is genetic rather than influenced by diet.

Thermogenesis

It is common experience that some individuals maintain normal weight while consuming a diet that appears to provide energy in excess of their requirement while others readily put on weight despite restricted food intake. This clearly calls for an explanation other than in terms simply of energy intake and output. Variations in heat production (thermogenesis) may provide a clue and may be related to the presence of brown fat (p. 53).

Thermogenesis may be measured as changes in oxygen consumption and is known to be induced by eating. Following a meal, oxygen consumption rises by 10 to 20 per cent depending on the size and composition of the meal (p. 46). Several experiments in which subjects have consumed an excess of several thousand calories per day for many weeks or even months have been carried out. Some subjects gained weight but most maintained their normal weight and showed an increase in oxygen consumption, reflecting an increase in metabolic rate.

Nicotine and caffeine are known to increase the metabolic rate, but cigarette smoking and coffee and tea drinking are not to be recommended as means of reducing weight.

Metabolic rate

The BMR, expressed in terms of surface area, is usually reported to be normal in obesity. However, it is raised in absolute terms and appears to be related to an increase of about one-third in lean body mass. It falls during weight loss and this points to the need for a permanent reduction in food intake if a reduced body weight is to be maintained. Along with the fall in resting metabolic rate in energy restriction there is a fall in the calorigenic hormones, T_3 and noradrenaline. Evidence has been obtained for the importance of catecholamines in determining adaptive changes in metabolic rate by giving levodopa, a precursor of catecholamines (of which noradrenaline is one) and preventing the fall in metabolic rate consequent upon energy restriction in obese subjects.

Hormones

Some uncommon endocrine disorders result in obesity but other manifestations of hormonal imbalance assist in their differentiation from simple obesity.

In the fed state insulin promotes fat synthesis and plasma levels are raised in obesity. Levels return to normal when weight is reduced and the hyperinsulinism of obesity is probably due to insensitivity of the tissues. In some patients excess insulin initiates obesity, as in hypoglycaemia, because of the high carbohydrate feeding necessary to combat the symptoms. Loss of insulin secretory function, as in diabetes, is associated with weight loss.

Adrenocortical hyperactivity, as in Cushing's syndrome, produces obesity that is rarely extreme and involves the trunk and neck but spares the limbs and buttocks. Growth hormone is energy producing, promotes fat mobilization between meals, and favours muscle growth.

There is increased adiposity in eunuchs who lack testosterone and in the presence of oestrogens as in normal women. In both sexes a prepubertal increase in fat occurs, disappearing after puberty. Fat increase often recurs in pregnancy and at the menopause.

Distribution of body fat

Typically this is different in the two sexes; the android distribution in the male favours deposition on the trunk (chest and abdomen), while the female gynecoid form favours it on the periphery (upper arms, hips and thighs). Numerous studies have shown that both men and women with the android distribution have a significantly higher prevalence of coronary heart disease, cerebrovascular disease, hypertension and diabetes mellitus (type II). This state is also associated with a high incidence of metabolic abnormalities including higher blood pressure, glucose, insulin, C-peptide, cholesterol and triglycerides. The metabolic bases for these important changes are still being researched but it is probable that the sex hormones are primarily involved. Female sex hormones regulate lipoprotein lipase and stimulate the differentiation of adipocyte precursor cells into mature fat cells.

Prevention

In affluent communities everywhere, the desires of consumers are created by persuasion rather than need. This persuasion frequently has the effect of promoting excessive consumption of food and the purchase of labour-saving devices. Just as the occurrence of obesity is the result of gradual and imperceptible weight gain over the years, so is weight restriction a matter of daily resistance to small excesses in energy intake and regular exercise.

Nutrition education as part of health education, at various levels, in clinics and hospitals, schools, colleges, and through mass media should concentrate on weight control at certain times when it is most likely to occur, i.e. in pregnancy, menopause, reduction in physical activity for any cause, giving up smoking, etc. Prevention cannot begin too early and the pregnant woman should be taught how to prevent excessive weight gain herself but should also learn how to guard against inducing in early childhood lifelong obesity in her offspring.

The family doctor is in a key position to prevent obesity and it is the claim of one general practitioner with a special interest in the subject that no case of obesity has developed among the children brought up in his long-established practice.

Treatment

As research into the nature of obesity has greatly intensified in recent years an ever increasing number of factors have been implicated. This means that some will be more amenable to treatment than others and also that in any particular case there is at present no means of knowing what factor(s) are involved or when treatment is appropriate. Even so, considerable success has been obtained through behaviour modification.

The various methods of treatment based on behaviour modification depend on the ideas that overeating and underactivity are (1) to some extent learned behaviours and what is learned can be relearned, and (2) regardless of the aetiology of obesity its symptomatic expression is through overeating and underactivity and treatment should therefore be directed at these.

It involves an analysis of the circumstances in which eating occurs. Efforts are made to prevent excess eating in response to various social or psychological stimuli that previously have brought it about. Very often such programmes are administered by psychologists, social workers or nutritionists. Community self-help groups of various kinds—TOPS (Take Off Pounds Sensibly), OA (Overeaters Anonymous) and best known of all perhaps, Weight Watchers, have developed in recent years and more and more people are finding them of great help.

Before discussing dietary management which, in its various forms has to be the sheet anchor of therapy, it may be as well to mention ancillary treatment.

Exercise

Exercise within the limits of ability of the obese is always beneficial. Because of the inate inability of most obese people to take regular exercise, due no doubt in part to the extreme discomfort they experience in intense activity, rather little can be expected of this measure. However, an effort should be made to encourage the extremely obese to keep on the move, for it is at the extremes of under- and overactivity that there are really significant effects on weight.

Drugs

Weight loss does result, but there is regain when they are stopped and there is often the risk of drug dependence.

Thyroxine increases metabolic rate but also stimulates appetite and is not recommended routinely as only large doses result in weight loss. Diethylproprion and phentermine are anorectic drugs, but are also sympathomimetic stimulants. Fenfluramine increases satiety resulting in reduced meal size, rate of eating and weight loss, but when stopped after one year of treatment weight was regained. Hydroxycitrate interfers with lipogenesis and is under experimental trial. Ephedrine is also under clinical trial. It raises oxygen consumption and reduces body fat without affecting protein and is relatively safe. It may prove to be the first of a series of thermogenic drugs.

Principles of weight loss

Loss of weight is not a yard-stick of progress in the treatment of obesity. Negative energy balance is the objective of treatment and this depends on the relative amounts of fat and protein that are lost. The energy density of adipose tissue is 10 times that of lean tissue (8·0 kcal (33·5 kJ)/g versus 0·8 kcal (3·35 kJ)/g). Thus the same energy loss coming mainly from breakdown of lean tissue, or mainly from adipose tissue, gives rise to very different amounts of weight loss—much more in the case of lean tissue. During the first few days of energy restriction, while endogenous nitrogen loss is in its early phase of exponential decrease, weight loss is dramatic as it is occurring largely by loss of lean tissue. For every protein kJ spent about $\frac{1}{3}$g lean tissue is lost while for every fat kJ only about $\frac{1}{33}$ g of adipose tissue is lost.

Nutriment

Protein. Quantity and quality of the protein intake should be such that the body is maintained in nitrogen balance. Fifty grams of protein per day is adequate for a standard adult. *Protein-sparing Modified Fast*, providing 1·5 g/kg/day has received considerable attention recently. The claim that it differs from other low energy diets in lowering serum insulin, thus facilitating fat breakdown, has not been confirmed. It produces a number of side effects and in any case cannot form the basis for life-long weight control.

Fat. A diet very low in fat content is unpalatable and generally not acceptable. Linoleic acid must be provided. Some slimming regimes indicate that fat need not be restricted. The apparent success of these diets is limited to considerable weight loss achieved early on and this is not maintained for long. A palatable diet will usually have to include about 40 g fat/day.

Carbohydrate. Excessive consumption of sugars and starches is the usual basis for the occurrence of obesity and these have to be drastically reduced. Restriction of carbohydrate does not lead to the development of ketosis. In fact obese subjects are especially resistant to ketosis. Restriction of carbohydrate-rich items of diet is frequently the basis for popular suggestions for slimming. When carbohydrate is the main fuel, the body may require 2 to 4 kg more water in the tissues than when fat is being utilized. Loss of this extra water probably accounts for the rapid, but small, weight loss.

Vitamins. Multivitamin tablets will not be necessary under ordinary circumstances as the requirements can be provided by judicious use of dietary items. They are indicated during total starvation treatment. Fruits and green vegetables will meet requirements for vitamins A and C and also provide bulk to relieve hunger and prevent constipation.

Minerals. The iron intake may be low on a reducing diet, signs of anaemia have to be watched for, and prophylactic iron is justified. Inclusion of half a pint of milk will ordinarily prevent negative calcium balance.

Water and salt. These should not be restricted in any way unless abnormal retention of water and sodium exist due to heart failure or other cause.

Alcohol. If alcohol is consumed the energy value (7 kcal or 29·3 kJ/g) must be remembered and due allowance made in the diet.

Dietary management of moderate obesity

Energy expenditure of a subject is the sum of that necessary for basal metabolism (related most closely to the lean body mass) and the expenditure for various activities beyond the resting state (see p. 46). A clerical worker might require only about half of the energy intake of a heavy manual labourer (2000 versus 4000 kcal or 8·38 versus 16·76 MJ). A correctly devised diet providing about 1000 kcal (4·19 MJ)/day should result in a weekly loss of weight of about 1 kg in a moderately obese housewife. This calculation assumes a figure of 7·5 kcal (31·4 kJ)/g as the energy value of adipose tissue and a daily energy expenditure of the patient of 2200 kcal (9·21 MJ). The weekly negative energy balance is equivalent to $[7 \times (2200 - 1000)/7·5]$g or $[7 \times (9·21 - 4·19)/0·0314]$ or 1·12 kg. For an obese man performing hard physical work this would have to be augmented to about 1500 kcal (6·29 MJ) by suitable protein, fat or carbohydrate exchanges.

The best results with such a diet will be obtained if the food items are weighed. However, this may not be practicable for those with poor vision or physical or mental handicaps, and indeed is not necessary for the moderately overweight.

Treatment of the grossly obese

For patients who are very fat the 1 kg of weight loss/week achieved on the 1000 kcal (4·19 MJ)/day regime is usually dishearteningly little, and, providing there are no medical contraindications, a more drastic programme can be employed.

In recent years total starvation for days or weeks has been used by many to treat extreme obesity. Jaw-wiring is often instituted to ensure this. There is an initial dramatic loss of weight, much of which is due to extracellular water and sodium. Upon refeeding, even with minimal energy intake, water and sodium are markedly retained, together with nitrogen, and in the absence of fat deposition there may be regain of weight by about 25 per cent. However, this occurs to only a minor extent if a non-extendable nylon cord is worn like a belt around the waist.

Several metabolic complications of starvation in obesity may have serious consequences. Hyperuricaemia may result from competition of ketone bodies with uric acid for tubular excretion. Clinical gout may be precipitated during treatment, and on termination of a fast the rapid excretion of uric acid may cause crystalluria and nephropathy. Lactic acidosis has been reported in mildly diabetic obese persons. Porphyria, cardiac irregularities, postural hypotension and hypoglycaemia may occur. Renal lack of sodium and potassium may lead to hypovolaemic shock. Such treatment is contraindicated in the elderly and in those with cardiac complications in whom fatal results have occasionally been reported.

Surgery should be a last resort after all other treatment has really failed. Various intestinal bypass operations have largely been abandoned because of serious morbidity and mortality. Gastroplasty appears relatively safe and free from complications and in the long term less weight is regained than with diet alone.

15. VITAMIN TOXICITIES

HYPERVITAMINOSIS A AND HYPERCAROTENOSIS

Acute toxicity

There are many reports of sudden rise of intracranial pressure with bulging of the anterior fontanelle and vomiting in infants and young children given several hundred thousand units of vitamin A. Spontaneous recovery occurs, with no residual damage, when the vitamin is stopped and fatalities have not been reported.

In adults the few instances of acute poisoning have been confined to reports of the ingestion by Arctic explorers at a single meal of several million units of vitamin A in polar bear or bearded seal liver. Several hours after the meal, drowsiness, irritability, severe headache and vomiting have resulted, and after 24 to 48 hours the skin around the mouth, on the face and sometimes over large areas of the body has peeled off.

Chronic poisoning

This is characterized in children by anorexia, painful extremities, dry skin, sparse hair, hepatosplenomegaly, hypoplastic anaemia, leucopoenia and headache due to raised intracranial pressure and brain tumour may be suspected. Symptoms develop more rapidly in babies than in older children. Evidence of periosteal thickening of the long bones, as revealed by X-ray, is helpful in diagnosis.

The established condition in adults may present an unusual clinical picture consisting of headaches, blurring of vision and diplopia, pruritus, generalized pains, skeletal deformities, and liver enlargement.

Plasma vitamin A $> 100 \ \mu g/100$ ml is diagnostic and gradual recovery follows cessation of excessive intake.

Hypercarotenosis

This usually arises as the result of prolonged ingestion of large quantities of green and yellow leafy vegetables, or of carrots (often as carrot juice by food fadists), citrus fruits and tomatoes. In some cases of hypothyroidism, diabetes and various hyperlipaemic states, hypercarotenaemia may occur as a result of disturbed carotenoid metabolism. Yellow or orange discolouration of the skin (xanthosis cutis, carotenodermia) is usually not present until the concentration in plasma rises above 250 μg/100 ml. Carotenoids are secreted in sweat and sebum and reabsorbed by the stratum corneum. The staining is, therefore, especially prominent on the nasolabial folds, forehead, axillae and groins, and on the palms and soles where the horny layers of the skin are thick. The sclerae and buccal mucous membranes are unaffected, a distinguishing feature from jaundice.

Hypercarotenosis *per se* appears to be usually compatible with health. Hypervitaminosis A does not result. Any underlying metabolic disturbances require appropriate treatment.

HYPERVITAMINOSIS D AND IDIOPATHIC HYPERCALCAEMIA

Hypercalcaemia, from whatever cause, may be asymptomatic in early stages but sooner or later general fatigue, weight loss, constipation, anorexia, muscular weakness and renal colic may develop. Besides being caused by hyperparathyroidism it may result from a variety of malignancies in which a 'pseudohyper-parathyroidism' is produced. So-called idopathic hypercalcaemia has to be distinguished from all of these conditions. There are probably two different diseases. In the mild form there is usually a history of the ingestion of large doses, 500 to 1000 μg or more, of vitamin D daily for a period of several months although toxicity has been reported in very young children with a daily intake as low as 25 μg. The age of onset of symptoms is usually between 5 and 8 months. In contrast to uncomplicated hyperparathyroidism serum phosphorus levels tend to be increased rather than low. Alkaline phosphatase is often increased in hyperparathyroidism but low in idiopathic hypercalcaemia. On X-ray there is increased density of calcified cartilage at the ends of the tubular bones, with a broad zone of rarefaction proximal to the metaphysis. The condition was not infrequently reported in Great Britain following World War II. This may have been due to overfortification of milk and other foods with vitamin D. Since legislation was passed in Britain reducing the level of fortification, there has been a substantial reduction in the number of cases.

The rare severe form has a poor prognosis and constitutes a syndrome which includes osteosclerosis, hypercalcuria, nephrocalcinosis, mental retardation, 'elfin' facies, and anomalies of the great vessels.

Treatment consists in providing a diet as low as possible in calcium and vitamin D. A commercial product Locasel (Trufood Ltd), is an excellent substitute for milk in the treatment of these cases, as it has about one-tenth of the calcium content and contains no vitamin D. The urine should be kept acid.

VITAMIN K TOXICITY

Excessive dosing with menadione and its water soluble analogues (but not with phytonadione) in infants, especially prematures, led in the past to hyperbilirubinaemia with deposition of bile, called kernicterus, in parts of the central nervous system. Menadione is now banned. There may be increased haemolysis, especially in G-6PD deficiency, and hepatocellular damage. The mechanism is not understood.

16. WATER AND ELEMENT TOXICITIES

WATER EXCESS (HYPO-OSMOLAR SYNDROMES) AND SODIUM EXCESS

The impairment of water diuresis accounts for most of the hypoosmolar or hypernatraemic syndromes observed. Leaving aside those patients with chronic renal failure in whom the impaired water excretion results from a marked reduction in renal mass, there are three main groups of patients left. In these the failure is due to (1) alteration of renal function which prevents the delivery of an adequate volume of water to the diluting segments of nephron; (2) abnormal permeability of these segments to water despite the absence of antidiuretic hormone and (3) sustained level of circulating antidiuretic hormone.

There may or may not be oedema and the syndrome may be asymptomatic or there may be symptoms of water intoxication: confusion, lethargy, headache, anorexia, nausea, vomiting, weakness and rarely, convulsions. Unless there is some associated disorder the circulation is usually well maintained. Treatment consists of (1) removal or correction of the underlying cause; (2) rigid water restriction. An osmotic diuretic such as urea, glucose or mannitol will cause excretion of water in excess of salt and is useful in oedematous patients. If symptoms of water intoxication are marked, hypertonic saline may be used to correct the profound overhydration of the cells.

Sodium excess

The accumulation of salt in the body is usually mainly in the extracellular fluids. Hypernatraemia may be due to (1) dehydration (as in diabetes insipidus), or (2) normal hydration (certain brain conditions with a 'reset' osmoregulatory centre), or even (3) overhydration (primary aldosteronism, Cushing's syndrome, etc.). In the latter the fluid retention frequently results in oedema.

Experimental rats fed for several generations on a high salt intake eventually give rise to offspring that have a generic predisposition to hypertension. The disease in humans appears to occur more readily in some families and life-long high salt intake may play a part (p.000). The salt intake of the average artificially fed infant is considerably greater than its requirements. Half of this comes from milk up to the age of 6 months, but only a quarter from milk at a year. Then most is provided by processed vegetables, meat and eggs, added by the manufacturer. It is advisable that no infant foods have more than 0.25 per cent salt added. Introduction of semisolids and overconcentrated milk feeds in the first few months of life may cause hypernatraemia.

Hypertonic dehydration with hypernatraemia is a dangerous condition which poses great difficulties in management. Rehydration must be slow. Hypotonic solutions which might seem to be rational, must not be used as rapid expansion of brain cells occurs. Solutions containing Na, Ca and K are indicated.

Potassium excess (hyperkalaemia)

This may arise from excess ingestion or infusion of potassium salts, or in acute renal failure or adrenal insufficiency. The serum level is > 4.7 mEq/l and there are no obvious signs or symptoms but e.c.g. changes (shortening of Q–T intervals, tall T waves) assist in the detection of this dangerous state. Emergency treatment consists of intravenous glucose, insulin, calcium gluconate and hypertonic sodium bicarbonate.

Magnesium excess

It often occurs following ingestion of Mg-containing antacids or purgatives in the presence of renal failure. Neuromuscular transmission is impaired throughout the body with hypotension, respiratory depression and cardiac abnormalities. Treatment consists of general support, diuretics and intravenous calcium.

Calcium excess

Adverse effects of excessive intake of calcium seem to be limited to the influence of calcium upon the utilization of other nutrients, especially magnesium, iron, iodine and manganese.

Hypercalcaemia has developed in patients with poor renal function who consume large amounts of calcium-containing alkalis and milk as treatment for peptic ulcer, the so-called 'milk-alkali syndrome'. Most commonly it occurs secondary to malignant disease invading bone. Hyperparathyroidism and vitamin D toxicity are less common causes. Manifestations include calcium deposition in the kidneys, lung and elsewhere; gastrointestinal, urinary and muscular symptoms, leading eventually to psychosis, coma and even death. The underlying condition requires treatment and oral phosphate administration is useful in the long-term management.

Iron overload (haemochromatosis)

A habitually high dietary intake is responsible in some Bantu and Ethiopian people in Africa. Heavy consumption of fermented alcohol drinks in South Africa and wines in Europe and North America is also held responsible. Habitual iron medication over several decades, repeated blood transfusions and even iron-rich drinking water may be the cause. When pathological changes have been produced by excessive parenchymal deposits the process may be potentiated by other factors such as malnutrition, alcoholism, toxins and viral hepatitis. Only about 1 to 2 per cent of all cases are what is termed 'familial haemochromatosis', due to an inborn error of metabolism leading to increased absorption of iron.

The pathology appears to differ in the dietary and the idiopathic forms. In the former there is maximal involvement of Kupffer cells, portal tract phagocytes and spleen, whereas in the idiopathic form most of the iron is in the parenchymal cells of the liver. Increased absorption of iron has been shown to occur in relatives of patients with the idiopathic form, who may show isolated signs of the disease, such as skin pigmentation, hepatomegaly, raised serum iron, or excessive free iron on liver biopsy. This provides some evidence in favour of a genetic defect with an intermediate form of inheritance with the mildly affected siblings representing the heterozygous state.

Treatment of iron overload entails reducing the intake. Venesection may be necessary in severe cases. Deferoxamine chelates iron and reduces stores. In patients with the idiopathic form and near relatives these measures are still indicated, even though the intake is not excessive.

Acute poisoning

This usually occurs in children swallowing iron tablets and causes vomiting, upper abdominal pain, cyanosis, diarrhoea, drowsiness and shock. Fatalities are not infrequent.

Fluorosis

Drinking water provides the principal source of fluorine. The concentration of fluorine in bone is proportional to the amount in drinking water. There is no final answer to the question of the critical toxic level of fluorine in skeletal tissues and the level of intake to produce it. At least in temperate climates a level of 1.0 p.p.m. in drinking water will result in skeletal and dental fluoride retention, but without cumulative harmful effects.

Mottled enamel is a defect almost confined to the permanent teeth, and develops during their period of formation. Deciduous teeth are only affected by extremely high levels. Mottled teeth have chalky, white patches distributed irregularly over their surface with secondary infiltration of dark brown staining. In severe cases the weak enamel is lost, resulting in 'pitting'. However, in some parts of the world, notably the Arabian Gulf, parts of India and Africa where the drinking water concentration exceeds 10 p.p.m skeletal fluorosis has been reported. After constant exposure for about 30 years pain and stiffness of the spine and joints develop and on X-ray the spine appears to be one continuous column of bone with numerous exostoses and calcification of tendons and ligaments. Genu valgum with localized osteoporosis has been reported as a common feature of fluorosis in central India.

There is no effective treatment, but prevention is possible by boiling water for a few minutes, and ensuring that it is separated from the precipitate formed.

Zinc

Ingestion of the metal in large amounts is usually associated with the intake of an acid food or drink from a galvanized container, and causes vomiting and diarrhoea. Metal fume fever is caused by the inhalation of zinc oxide. It is also known as 'brass founder's ague', and 'zinc shakes'. Cure results in a few days on removal from the environment.

Copper

Acute poisoning results from the ingestion of grams of copper, usually in the form of the sulphate.

Chronic toxicity exists as Wilson's disease or hepatolenticular degeneration inherited as an autosomal recessive. The first evidences of the abnormality are persistently low concentration of caeruloplasmin (<20mg/100 ml) and high level of hepatic copper (>250 μg/g). Urinary copper excretion is increased. Liver parenchymal cells are eventually destroyed and replaced by fibrous tissue. Copper also deposits in other tissues, especially the central nervous system, kidney and cornea. Heterozygous carriers have moderate decrease of caeruloplasmin and increase of liver copper and although they are symptom-free they require therapy.

Treatment consists of 1 to 3 g D-penicillamine daily, which chelates copper and increases urinary excretion. Foods rich in copper should be avoided and 25 mg vitamin B_6 daily should be prescribed as penicillamine complexes with the aldehyde groups of pyridoxal to form a thiazolidine compound. Life-long treatment with penicillamine is probably indicated.

Recent evidence suggests that Indian childhood cirrhosis may be due to excessive ingestion as a result of preparation of food in copper vessels.

Cobalt

Cobaltous chloride (20–30 mg/day) has been advocated in the treatment of the anaemia of chronic renal failure for its polychyhaemic effect. Toxicity may result in hypothyroidism and cardiomyopathy.

Selenium

The discovery of widespread occurrence of chronic selenosis in animals in the United States led to community surveys in seleniferous areas. No conclusive evidence of a human public health problem has been obtained there, but in several regions of China loss of hair, dermatosis and neuropathy have been related to high selenium intake. Some 'health' store preparations contain toxic amounts.

Manganese

Toxicity has been seen in man following chronic inhalation of manganese dusts by miners. After months or years of exposure a neurological condition resembling Parkinsonism or Wilson's disease occurs. The appearance of manganese in the urine may be of diagnostic value.

Treatment is to stop exposure and neurological improvement may be hastened with ethylenediaminetetraacetic acid (EDTA). The condition does not appear to be fatal.

Molybdenum

Areas of very high intake in the United States are associated with a high incidence of gout and, in India, with bone changes related to fluorine toxicity.

Strontium

^{90}Sr is one of the most abundant and potentially hazardous radioactive by-products of nuclear fission. Radiostrontium is retained, especially in the bones, and is readily transmitted to the milk and to the fetus. Because there is preferential absorption of calcium from the intestinal tract, and preferential excretion of strontium in the urine, high dietary calcium is protective against strontium retention.

Aluminium

Aluminium-containing antacids given to uraemic patients on long-term dialysis have been reported to cause neurological damage. Brain damage has been produced in animals dosed with aluminium and a high aluminium content has been found in parts of the brain affected in patients with some forms of dementia. Dialysates with a high aluminium content have been associated with osteomalacia in renal patients.

MULTIPLE CHOICE QUESTIONS

Answer each question true *or* false .

1. In starvation:
    i) tachycardia and raised venous pressure are common
   ii) urea/total nitrogen ratio in urine falls progressively
  iii) BMR is reduced only late on
   iv) Anaemia is usually microcytic hypochromic
    v) during recovery diarrhoea may be due to lactase deficiency.

2. Xerophthalmia:
    i) is the name given to all stages of vitamin A deficiency eye disease
   ii) is almost always accompanied by PEM
  iii) is almost always present in PEM
   iv) is likely to be present in a child with plasma retinol of 30 μg/dl
    v) accounts for about 250 000 cases of blindness each year.

3. Kwashiorkor is characterized by:
    i) marked hunger
   ii) skin lesions on areas exposed to ultraviolet light
  iii) accumulation of triglyceride in the liver
   iv) a raised plasma ratio of non essential/essential amino acids
    v) prolonged breast feeding supplemented by starchy foods.

4. Iron:
    i) status is best assessed by transferrin in plasma
   ii) deficiency impairs the growth of bacteria
  iii) deficiency in infants is related to prolonged breast feeding
   iv) deficiency is the most widespread deficiency state
    v) overload is most commonly of genetic origin.

5. Obesity:
    i) is frequently associated with hypertension and diabetes mellitus
   ii) of gynecoid distribution is a risk factor for several diseases
  iii) is 'morbid' when weight/height is > 200 per cent standard
   iv) has a strong genetic component in its aetiology
    v) does not correlate strongly with social class.

Explanation and answers and page 286

FURTHER READING

10. Starvation
Bistrian B R 1977 Interaction of nutrition and infection in the hospital setting. American Journal of Clinical Nutrition 30: 1228–1232

Cahill G F 1970 Starvation in man. New England Journal of Medicine 282: 668–675.
Keys A, Brozek J, Hanschel A, Mickelson O, Taylor H L 1950 The biology of human
    starvation, vols 1, 2. University of Minnesota Press, Minneapolis

11. Protein-energy malnutrition
Alleyne G A O, Hay R W, Picou D I, Stanfield J P, Whitehead R G 1977 Protein-energy
    malnutrition. Arnold, London
Coward W A, Lunn P G 1981 The biochemistry and physiology of kwashiorkor and
    marasmus. British Medical Bulletin 37, No 1, 19–24
Cravioto J, Hambraeus L, Vahlquist B (eds) 1974 Early malnutrition and mental
    development. Swedish Nutrition Foundation, Stockholm
Golden M H N 1982 Protein deficiency, energy deficiency, and the oedema of
    malnutrition, Lancet i: 1261–1265
Hansen J D L, Buchanan N, Pettifor J M 1982 Protein energy malnutrition: signs,
    symptoms, pathology, diagnostic tests and treatment. In: McLaren D S, Burman D (eds)
    Textbook of paediatric nutrition 2nd edn. 1982 Churchill Livingstone, London
McLaren D S 1982 Protein energy malnutrition: classification, pathogenesis, prevalence
    and prevention In: McLaren D S, Burman D (eds) Textbook of paediatric nutrition, 2nd
    edn. Churchill Livingstone, London

12. Vitamin deficiency and dependency
De Luca H F 1979 Vitamin D: metabolism and function. Springer, Berlin
Marks J 1985 The vitamins, their role in medical practice. M T Press, Lancaster
McLaren D S 1982 Vitamin deficiency, toxicity and dependency In: McLaren D S,
    Burman D (eds) Textbook of paediatric nutrition, 2nd edn. Churchill Livingstone, London
WHO Expert Committee 1982 The control of vitamin A deficiency and xerophthalmia.
    Technical Report Series no 672. WHO, Geneva

13. Water, electrolyte and element deficiencies
Addy D P 1986 Happiness is: iron. British Medical Journal 292: 969–970
Fairbanks VF, Fahey JL, Beutler E 1971 Clinical disorders of iron metabolism, 2nd edn. Grune
    and Stratton, New York
Rose B D 1977 Clinical physiology of acid-base and electrolyte disorders. McGraw Hill,
    New York
Stanbury J B, Hetzel B S (eds) 1980 Endemic goiter and endemic cretinism. Wiley, New
    York
Underwood E J 1977 Trace elements in human and animal nutrition. 4th edn. Academic
    Press, New York

14. Obesity
Andersen T, Backer O G, Stockholm K H, Quaade F 1984 Randomised trial of diet and
    gastroplasty compared with diet alone in morbid obesity. New England Journal of
    Medicine 310: 352–356
Anon 1984 The shape of fatness. Lancet i: 889–890
Bray G A 1982 Regulation of energy balance. Proceedings of the Nutrition Society 41:
    95–108
Craddock D 1978 Obesity and its management 3rd edn. Churchill Livingstone, Edinburgh
Garrow J S 1978 Energy balance and obesity in man 2nd edn. Elsevier, Amsterdam
Hirsch J 1978 What's new in the treatment of obesity? In: Freinkel N (ed) The year in
    metabolism 1977. Plenum, New York, p 169
Rothwell N J, Stock M J 1983 Luxuskonsumpstion, diet-induced thermogenesis and brown
    fat: the case in favour: Clinical Science 64: 19–23

III

Nutrition and diet in systemic disease

'Where sciences meet, their growth occurs. In scientific borderlands not only are facts gathered that are often new in kind, but it is in these regions that wholly new concepts arise.'
F. GOWLAND HOPKINS, 1938

17. INTRODUCTION

Nutritional disorders may arise secondary to various disease processes in the body as shown in Table 27. Besides actually producing nutritional disease there are several ways in which food and nutriment interact with the body in a harmful or a helpful way. Examples are shown in Figure 18 and detailed consideration of many such subjects is given in other parts of the book.

1. Many diseases interfere with a number of essential functions and lead to secondary malnutrition. Table 27 lists these functions and gives examples of diseases in which they are deranged.

Table 27 Secondary malnutrition

Defect in	Examples
Digestion	Pancreatic disease, intestinal surgery
Absorption	Malabsorption syndromes (coeliac, sprue etc.)
Transport	a-β-Lipoproteinaemia
Storage	Cirrhosis, haemochromatosis
Metabolism	Inborn errors, (phenylketonuria, galactosaemia, etc.), vitamin dependency (B_6/B_{12}), obesity?
Elimination	Trauma, renal failure, protein-losing enteropathy
Requirements (increased)	Pyrexia, injury, thyrotoxicosis

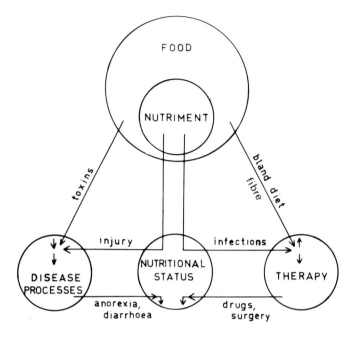

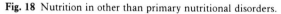

Fig. 18 Nutrition in other than primary nutritional disorders.

2. Treatment of disease may, as a side-effect, interfere with the body's nutrition. Examples of this include resection of the gastro-intestinal tract, destruction of vitamin-producing gut flora by antibiotics, treatment with antifolate drugs, isoniazid and the like.

3. Nutritional status may influence the response of the body to a disease process as seen in the synergistic effect of malnutrition and infection, impairment of the immune response, wound healing and metabolism of some drugs.

4. The effects of treatment may be diminished by poor nutritional status in infectious diseases, e.g. tuberculosis.

5. The dietary treatment and management of non-nutritional disease forms a major part of this section and is gaining in importance all the time. The harmful effects of many inborn errors of metabolism can be largely overcome by appropriate dietary measures to eliminate or reduce the harmful matabolites in these patients. Dietary management of gastrointestinal, renal, liver and metabolic diseases is becoming increasingly rational as it is related to newer knowledge of the aetiology of these conditions.

6. Of rather different nature are the many conditions which result from the presence of toxic substances in the diet, be they food additives or contaminants, or pathogenic organisms. The nutrition of the patient is often not affected and the management consists of identifying the toxin, preventing its further ingestion and treating symptoms.

7. Epidemiological and human experimental evidence suggests that a number of diseases result directly (diverticulitis, appendicitis) or indirectly (haemorrhoids, varicose veins) from intestinal stasis and their high incidence in affluent societies might be due to the low fibre content of the diet. Likewise it has been suggested that cancer of the colon may be related to the intestinal stasis and more prolonged action of any carcinogen. Low-fibre diet has been postulated by some, with little evidence at present, to play a role in coronary thrombosis (decreasing reabsorption of bile salts and lowering cholesterol), cholelithiasis (absorption of actor that facilitates precipitation of cholesterol) obesity (excess energy absorption) and diabetes mellitus (excess sugar consumption).

Principles of diet therapy

A knowledge of the patient's background is important with regard to planning a diet if it is to be long term. Socioeconomic circumstances, work patterns and meal habits, cultural and religious practices and the adequacy of the previous diet should all be enquired about.

Dietary modifications may be of the following kinds:

1. Quality or consistency, e.g. tube feedings, restricted fibre diets, gluten-free diet.

2. Quantity: modifications of total energy, or individual nutrient, e.g. Na, Ca, phenylalanine.

3. Combinations: modifications of interrelated nutriment, e.g. protein, Na, K.

The normal dietary requirements and appropriate foodstuffs for the individual should always be carefully considered before adaptation is advised for special cases. This is especially important for children.

For acute, short-term diseases the diet may be unbalanced and very restrictive for the patient, e.g. postoperative, during test procedures and acute kidney disease. In chronic conditions, such as diabetes, peptic ulcer, chronic renal failure, etc. all nutritional requirements must be met and due attention paid to all practical details. In this connection the motivation of the patient to follow the diet has to be taken into account. The relationships between the patient and all responsible for his treatment and the members of the patient's family, especially those concerned with preparation of the food, are very important. Follow-up should include explanations before leaving hospital, and the use of outpatient departments, clinics and home visits.

In addition to having an adequate knowledge of her subject, the dietitian must have the ability to communicate her knowledge to the patient and to work with the physician; gaining his invaluable support in her work, advising him on dietary aspects of treatment as well as interpreting his dietary orders and prescriptions.

18. NUTRITIONAL ASSESSMENT OF HOSPITALIZED PATIENTS

A series of steps can be recognized in the development of any deficiency state, beginning with depletion of stores, progressing to deterioration in normal cell function, then to the clinical symptoms of deficiency of the acutely malnourished patient and ending eventually with morbidity and mortality. Although the most precise way to quantify nutritional depletion remains unsettled, a variety of somatic measurements and laboratory tests exist (Table 28). These measurements and tests should follow a complete dietary history and physical examination, carefully investigating symptoms and signs suggesting malnutrition or specific nutrient deficiencies (Table 29).

Table 28 Data base used for evaluating nutritional depletion

Data	Comment
Clinical data	
Medical history	
Current illness	Nutritional state particularly affected if disease impairs appetite, taste sensations, chewing, swallowing, absorption
Nutrient intake	Inquire about change in eating pattern and weight change. A food diary, 24-hour diet recall, or hospital calorie count can confirm the intake deficit
Energy expenditure	This may be subtle, such as dyspnoea (increased work of breathing) or the increased metabolic cost of fever, trauma, or surgical stress
Treatment modality	Medications, chemotherapy, and radiation therapy can alter appetite, taste, nutrient absorption, and metabolism
Social factors	Excessive alcohol, drugs, poverty, or 'shut-in' situations
Physical examination	
Routine physical evaluation	Note signs suggesting a nutrient deficiency
Anthropometric measurements	
Body weight	Best measured in underwear, at the same point in the day and on the same scale. May be expressed as percent weight change: $$= \frac{\text{usual weight} - \text{actual weight}}{\text{usual weight}} \times 100$$ Rate of weight lost and circumstances (deliberate dieting versus loss due to illness) are most important
Height	Must be verified because loss of height after age 20 is universal (± 1 cm every decade) and accelerated by bone diseases
Triceps skin fold (TSF)	Measured with calipers (Lange, Harpenden) midway between acromium and olecranon
Arm muscle circumference (AMC)	Measured with a centimeter tape at same midpoint of humerus in the non-dominant arm. Arm muscle mass is calculated from: idealized equation: arm circumference ($0.314 \times$ TSF)
Creatinine-height index	Validity of single measurement is uncertain

Immune function
  Skin tests for *Candida*,
  mumps
  Trichophyton, SK/SD, and PPD

Response is graded after 48 hours:
0, no response (anergic)
1, less than 1 cm wheal (impaired)
2, greater than 1 cm wheal (reactive)

Laboratory tests
Routinely available
  Complete blood count and
  blood smear examination,
  reticulocyte count

Diagnoses: microcytic (Fe, Cu, vitamin B_6), macrocytic (folic acid, B_{12}, vitamin C), normocytic (PCM, chronic disease), haemolytic anaemia (vitamin E in newborn, P)

  Total lymphocyte count

Normal 1500–4000 cells per cm; <1500 suggests PCM

  Blood glucose

May indicate diabetic state, often aggravated by stress

  Serum albumin

Less than 507 μmol per liter (3.5 g per dl) suggests PCM but also falls with hepatic disease, renal and gut protein leak

  Total iron-binding capacity

Indirect measurement of transferrin

  Na, K, Cl, HCO_3, Ca, P, Mg, Fe

Interpretation of these mineral changes is outlined in text

  Blood urea nitrogen (BUN)

End-product of protein catabolism, decreased with protein depletion but also liver disease; increased by renal dysfunction

  Creatinine

Reflects muscle breakdown. In normal men 1.5 g excreted per day, in women 1.0 per day

  Triglycerides and cholesterol

Usually decreased in PCM, may be increased by hyperlipidaemic states (including i.v. fat solutions) or liver disease

Less commonly available
  Transferrin
  Retinol-binding protein
  Fibronectin protein
  Plasma ferritin
  Vitamin
  Trace elements
  Essential fatty acids

Half-life 8 days ⎫
Half-life 12 hours ⎬ More sensitive indices than albumin of change in protein status
Half-life 4 hours ⎭
Reflects iron stores

See text

* SK/SD, streptokinase/streptodornase; PPD, tuberculin purified protein derivative; PCM, protein-calorie malnutrition.
(Howard LL, Meguid MM 1981 Nutritional assessment in total parenteral nutrition. Clinical and Laboratory Medicine 1 : 611.

Anthropomorphic measurements

The principal concept of anthropometry is that the metabolic physiological changes that occur in the human body reflect some morphological variations (Table 30). The two changes have a constant relation that can be followed by appropriate measurements. Height and weight expressed together are measures of gross morphology and reflect nutritional status (Table 31). For measurements of individual components of the whole body, skin fold calipers (e.g. fat and protein, muscle) the limb circumference and diameters of

Table 29 Metabolic function and clinical assessment of micronutrients

Nutrient	Metabolic function	Deficiency
Essential fatty acid	Components of all lipid membranes, precursors of prostaglandins	Scaly dermatitis
Calcium	Body content 600 g, bone crystal (99%), blood clotting, nerve and muscle excitability	Osteomalacia, tetany
Phosphorus	Body content 600 g, bone crystal (85%), ~P bonds, chief intracellular anion	Osteomalacia, haemolytic anaemia, $\downarrow$ HbO$_2$ dissociation, $\downarrow$ phagocytosis
Sulphur	Body content 175 g, occurs in methionine, cysteine, thiamin, insulin, chondroitin, sulphate, etc.	Unknown
Potassium	Body content 160 g, main intracellular cation	Muscular weakness, cardiac irritability, metabolic alkalosis
Sodium	Body content 100 g, main extracellular cation	$\downarrow$ Circulating blood volume, $\downarrow$ blood pressure $\downarrow$ urine output
Chloride	Body content 79 g, main extracellular anion	Metabolic alkalosis
Magnesium	Body content 25 g, cofactor for many enzymes including phosphorylases, phosphotransferases (Na-K ATPase, vitamin D hydroxylases)	Tetany, muscle weakness secondary to hypokalaemia and hypocalcaemia
Iron	Body content 4 g, haem compounds, cytochrome enzymes, iron stores	Microcytic, hypochromic anaemia; $\downarrow$ immunocompetence
Zinc	Body content 2 g, cofactor for many enzymes including carbonic anhydrase, alcohol dehydrogenase, carboxypeptidase	Growth retardation and hypogonadism; impaired wound healing and immunocompetence
Copper	Body content 100 mg, cofactor for lysil oxidase (collagen synthesis), cytochrome oxidase, tyrosinase	Anaemia and neutropenia, scurvy like osteopenia in children
Iodine	Body content 30 mg, component of thyroid hormones	Cretinism/myxoedema
Manganese	Body content 20 mg, cofactor for lipid, cholesterol, mucopolysaccharide synthesis	Abnormal clotting not corrected by vitamin K
Chromium	Body content 6 mg, part of insulin receptor mechanism	Glucose intolerance
Molybdenum	Body content 5 mg, cofactor for xanthine oxidase	Confusional state secondary to increased methionione
Selenium	Cofactor for glutathione preoxidase (GP)	Muscle weakness, haemolytic anaemia
Cobalt	Body content 80 μg, metallo-cofactor for cobalamin (B$_{12}$)	Unknown in humans
Ascorbic acid (vitamin C)	Microsomal electron transport, tryosine, trptophan, and dopamine synthesis, steroid synthesis, hydroxylation of collagen proline and lysine residues; folic acid metabolism	Scurvy, perifollicular haemorrhages, bleeding gums, osteopenia, and subperisteal haemorrhages; defective wound healing
Thiamin (vitamin B$_1$)	Cofactor (TPP) for transketolase pyruvate and ketogluterate decarboxylase, oxidation of branched-chain keto-acids	High-output cardiac failure, polyneuritis
Riboflavin (vitamin B$_2$)	Converted to electron acceptors and donators, flavin mononucleotide (FMN) and flavin adenine dinucleotide (FAD)	Cheilosis, glossitis, seborrhoeic dermatitis

Niacin (vitamin B_5)	Converted to electron acceptors and donators, nicotinamide dinucleotides (NAD, NADP)	Pellagra: pigmented dermatitis, ulceration of mucous membranes, central nervous system depression.
Biotin (vitamin B_7)	Cofactor for carboxylation enzymes where CO_2 is added, such as, pyruvate $\longrightarrow$ oxaloacetate, acetyl-coA $\longrightarrow$ malonyl-CoA	Alopecia, seborrhoeic dermatitis, neuritis
Pantothenic acid (vitamin B_3)	Converted to coenzyme A	Irritability, burning paraesthesias
Pyridoxine (vitamin B_6)	Cofactor (PLP) for many enzymes including transaminases, phosphorylases, amino oxidases	Glossitis, polyneuritis, seizures, microcytic hypochromic anaemia
Folic acid (vitamin B_9)	Cofactor for purine and pyrimidine synthesis and metabolism of serine, histidine, homocysteine, and ethanolamine	Megaloblastic defect of red blood cells and mucous membranes
Cobalamin vitamin B_{12})	Methyl B_{12} involved in methyl donor reaction, 5'deoxyadenosyl B_{12} involved in carboxylation reactions	Megaloblastic defect of red blood cells and mucous membranes, central and peripheral neuropathy
Vitamin A	Light-sensitive pigment in retina, epithelial maintenance	Night blindness and xerophthalmia, testicular atrophy, keratosis of skin
Vitamin D	Calcium, phosphorus, and possibly magnesium absorption from intestine, calcium deposition and mobilization from bone	Osteomalacia (rickets in growing children), muscle weakness
Vitamin E	Prevents peroxidation of polyunsaturated lipids	Haemolytic-anaemia of newborn, dystrophic changes of retina and posterior column nuclei
Vitamin K	Involved in synthesis of clotting factors II, VII, IX, and X	Bleeding tendency presenting as epistaxis, ecchymosis, gastrointestinal, urinary or central nervous system haemorrhage

various body parts are used. Most commonly used are the head, limb, and trunk circumference; less commonly used are lower limb length, biacromial and bi-iliac-crest diameters. Many formulas and standard tables have been developed and published in an attempt to overcome the biological variations of body fat distribution, muscle development, and skeletal form — until now with little success. The most commonly used measurements are height/weight index, triceps skin fold (TSF) and upper arm circumference.

19. GASTROINTESTINAL SYSTEM

This system has perhaps resisted investigation and understanding more than most. The intake and output, food and stools, have been little investigated compared with blood and urine. X-ray appearances are often non-specific or difficult to interpret as are various tests of organ function. Many conditions affecting the gastrointestinal tract are poorly understood and this naturally makes treatment unsatisfactory.

Table 30 Anthropometric criteria for assessing malnutrition in adults

Weight for height (Wt/Ht)
Men: 106 lb for 5 ft plus 6 lb for every inch over 5 ft (+ 10% over age 50)
Women: 100 lb for 5 ft plus 5 lb for every inch over 5 ft (+ 10% over age 50)

Triceps skin fold (TSF, mm)

	Standard	*90%*	*80%*	*70%*	*60%*
Men:	12.5	11.3	10.0	8.8	7.5
Women:	16.5	14.9	132	11.6	9.9

Mid-arm circumference (MAC, cm)

Men:	29.3	26.3	23.4	20.5	17.6
Women:	28.5	25.7	22.8	20.0	17.1

Mid-arm muscle circumference (MAMC, cm)

Men:	25.3	22.8	20.2	17.7	15.2
Women:	23.2	20.9	18.6	16.2	13.2

Tentative anthropometric criteria of protein-calorie malnutrition §

Degree of PCM	Wt/Ht	TSF	MAMC
Mild	>90%	>70%	>90%
Moderate	80–90%	50–70%	70–90%
Severe	<80%	<50%	<70%

§ % = % of standard.

(Howard LJ. Meguid MM 1981 Clinical and Laboratory Medicine 1:611)

Mouth

Buccal lesions of nutritional origin include angular stomatitis, cheilosis (p. 118), certain appearances of the tongue (magenta in riboflavin deficiency, 'raw beef' in pellagra and atrophic in pernicious anaemia) and gums (spongy and bleeding in scurvy, p. 129) and teeth (p. 218).

Salivary glands

Bilateral painless enlargement of the parotid glands is common in school-age children in poor communities in Africa and Asia. Although it is usually associated with mild to moderate forms of PEM, it is not a feature of acute kwashiorkor or marasmus. In undernourished populations acute and painful enlargement of the parotids has been reported to occur on refeeding.

Oesophagus

Dysphagia, or difficulty in swallowing, is the main symptom of any disease affecting the oesophagus. It becomes extreme in stricture from any cause and parenteral nutrition may be necessary (p. 238).

Table 31 Ideal weight and creatinine — height index

Height		Medium frame ideal weight		Total mg Creatinine/ 24 hours*	mg Creatinine/ cm body weight/24 hours
Men					
5' 2"	157.5 cm	124 lb	56.0 kg	1288	8.17
5' 3"	160.0 cm	127 lb	57.6 kg	1325	8.28
5' 4"	162.6 cm	130 lb	59.1 kg	1359	8.36
5' 5"	165.1 cm	133 lb	60.3 kg	1386	8.40
5' 6"	167.6 cm	137 lb	62.0 kg	1426	8.51
5' 7"	170.2 cm	141 lb	63.8 kg	1467	8.62
5' 8"	172.7 cm	145 lb	65.8 kg	1513	8.76
5' 9"	175.3 cm	149 lb	67.6 kg	1555	8.86
5'10"	177.8 cm	153 lb	69.4 kg	1596	8.98
5'11"	180.3 cm	158 lb	71.4 kg	1642	9.11
6' 0"	182.9 cm	162 lb	73.5 kg	1691	9.24
6' 1"	185.4 cm	167 lb	75.6 kg	1739	9.38
6' 2"	188.0 cm	171 lb	77.6 kg	1785	9.49
6' 3"	190.5 cm	176 lb	79.6 kg	1831	9.61
6' 4"	193.0 cm	181 lb	82.2 kg	1891	9.80
Women					
4'10"	147.3 cm	101.5 lb	46.1 kg	830	5.63
4'11"	149.9 cm	104.0 lb	47.3 kg	851	5.68
5' 0"	152.4 cm	107.0 lb	48.6 kg	875	5.74
5' 1"	154.9 cm	110.0 lb	50.0 kg	900	5.81
5' 2"	157.5 cm	113.0 lb	51.4 kg	925	5.87
5' 3"	160.0 cm	116.0 lb	52.7 kg	949	5.93
5' 4"	162.6 cm	119.5 lb	54.3 kg	977	6.01
5' 5"	165.1 cm	123.0 lb	55.9 kg	1006	6.09
5' 6"	167.6 cm	127.5 lb	58.0 kg	1044	6.23
5' 7"	170.2 cm	131.5 lb	59.8 kg	1076	6.32
5' 8"	172.7 cm	135.5 lb	61.6 kg	1109	6.42
5' 9"	175.3 cm	139.5 lb	63.4 kg	1141	6.51
5'10"	177.8 cm	143.5 lb	65.2 kg	1174	6.60
5'11"	180.3 cm	147.5 lb	67.0 kg	1206	6.69
6' 0"	182.9 cm	151.5 lb	68.9 kg	1240	6.78

* Creatinine coefficient = 23mg/kg body weight in men, in women.

Paterson–Kelly (Plummer–Vinson) syndrome

This is the association of iron deficiency anaemia, glossitis, dysphagia and achlorhydria, usually in middle-aged women. In severe cases postcricoid webs and even carcinoma may develop. B group vitamin deficiency is also present and treatment should consist of iron and multivitamin therapy.

Stomach and duodenum

Dyspepsia, or difficulty with digestion, may take many forms such as nausea, heartburn, epigastric discomfort, distension and pain, and has many causes.

Persistent dyspepsia should be thoroughly investigated as it may be an indication of serious underlying disease.

One form, flatulent dyspepsia, is common with or without evidence of cholelithiasis. It consists of epigastric discomfort after meals, a feeling of fullness, eructation with temporary relief, and regurgitation of sour fluid to the mouth with heartburn. It is possibly associated with abnormal gastrointestinal motility, leading to regurgutation of duodenal juice into the stomach and delayed gastric emptying. Meals should be small and chewed well.

Peptic ulcer

The aetiology of ulceration in the stomach, duodenum and other parts exposed to gastric juice remains obscure. The term 'peptic' implies autodigestion of the mucous membrane by gastric secretions, but whether this is the way ulceration occurs is not known. Peptic ulcers do not occur in the absence of gastric acid. The anatomical situation makes considerable difference to the behaviour of the ulcer.

Gastric ulcer does not appear to be directly related to nutritional deficiency and it is rare in developing countries. In contrast to duodenal ulcer it is not associated with increased acid secretion and occurs later in life. These ulcers heal under treatment but they often relapse and as they have a tendency to undergo malignant transformation, follow-up is essential.

In Britain and North America duodenal ulcer is about ten times commoner than gastric ulcer and is more common in men than women, smokers than non-smokers, related than non-related subjects, and those with blood group O than those with groups A, B or AB. Nutritional factors do not seem to play a part. Emotional stress and responsibility may predispose.

In India and some other parts of Asia and Africa it is very common among peasants. Diet does seem to play an important role but how it does so is not clear. In India cases are almost entirely confined to the rice- and cassava-eating south. The very highly spiced curries of south India have often been blamed but these are also eaten by the well-to-do classes who do not suffer from a high incidence of ulcer. Here cases often present at hospital in a very advanced state, with a large cicatrized mass palpable in the epigastrium and causing pyloric stenosis. As a consequence treatment almost always has to be surgical.

Treatment The management of peptic ulceration has been revolutionized by the introduction of drugs, such as cimetidine, that act as antagonists to histamine receptors in the gastric mucosa and inhibit H^+ secretion. Use of these drugs has almost entirely replaced surgical management and greatly reduced the need for alkalis. Dietary management is still directed at diminishing H^+ ion secretion and facilitating healing by:

1. Preventing the stimulation of acid by avoiding alcohol, coffee, meat extracts, etc.

2. Suppressing motility by frequent feeding.

3. Protecting the mucosa by the use of 'bland' foods.

There is, however, very little evidence that any of these processes actually takes place during healing. Patients with severe ulcer symptoms often experience rapid relief when admitted to hospital and given frequent milk feeds. Psychological factors might be largely responsible for the improvement. The antacid effect of alkalis and food seems to be short-lived and it has never been demonstrated that spicy or coarse foods actually damage the gastric mucosa. Dietary invalidism, if induced, can be worse than the disease itself. Healing of the ulcer occurs as rapidly on a liberal diet as on the traditional bland diet. The patient should be encouraged to take a fully nutritious diet divided into frequent small meals. Any particular type of food that seems to cause discomfort regularly, the potent stimulants, coffee and alcohol and ulcerogenic drugs, such as aspirin, steroids and the non-steroidal anti-inflammatory agents should be avoided.

Gastritis

The lesion may be either acute and erosive or chronic and atrophic. It may be due to blood-borne toxins, bacterial or metabolic; ingestion of food or drugs which act as irritants, or foods to which the patient is allergic (p. 226). Gastroscopy has shown that a considerable degree of gastritis can exist without producing symptoms.

In acute gastritis the cause should be identified if possible and then withdrawn or neutralized. Solid food should be withheld for 24 to 48 hours and alkalis, bismuth and opium prescribed. Dehydration and electrolyte imbalance due to vomiting should be corrected (p. 137).

Chronic gastritis in which there are often atrophic changes in the mucosa, requires removal of the cause which may often involve a deep-rooted habit such as smoking, drinking or prolonged consumption of some food item. Alkalis and a bland diet may help.

Dumping syndrome

After gastric resection, partially digested food with a high osmotic pressure enters the proximal small bowel more rapidly and in large amounts. Small molecules, especially sugars, attract water from the plasma into the small bowel lumen. The rapid fall in plasma volume causes faintness, weakness and sweating. Hypoglycaemia occurs but does not usually coincide with symptoms. Simple sugars should be eliminated from the diet and starch restricted. Fluids should be taken one half hour after a meal.

INTESTINES

Symptomatology referable to disorders of the intestines may result from diarrhoea, constipation, obstruction and malabsorption. Treatment will naturally depend upon diagnosis.

Diarrhoea

This may be acute, intermittent or chronic. The causes are legion, but among the most important are various types of bacterial 'food poisoning', 'traveller's diarrhoea', and 'weanling' diarrhoea associated with protein energy malnutrition (p. 101). Diet plays no special role but is part of general management.

Abstention from food may prove necessary, especially if vomiting is also present, but should not be persisted in for longer that 48 hours. A decarbonated mineral solution containing glucose (e.g. flat Coca Cola) should be sipped in small amounts. Drug therapy consists of antibiotics if sensitive organisms are responsible, and bismuth carbonate, kaolin, opium or atropine for symptomatic relief. In persistent cases water and electrolyte replacement may necessitate parenteral therapy (p. 238).

Constipation

Most people have a daily bowel movement, but defaecation only once every 2 to 3 days is compatible with perfect health. Diet plays an auxiliary part in treatment, along with the encouragement of sound bowel habits, especially important in the young, and the taking of adequate and regular exercise.

Cellulose is not digested, but by its bulk and consistency stimulates peristalsis. Sources of roughage are whole-meal cereals, leafy vegetables, roots and fresh and cooked fruits. Quantities should be increased slowly to permit tolerance. An adequate fluid intake helps to keep faeces soft.

Malabsorption

Malabsorption should be distinguished from maldigestion. The former is a defect in the intestinal mucosa leading to a defect in the uptake of nutrients or bile, or the proper secretion of digestive enzymes. Maldigestion is due to an intraluminal defect of digestive enzymes, e.g. lipase.

Many disease processes result in malabsorption and, therefore, one form of secondary malnutrition (see Table 27) by interfering with nutrition and metabolism in: (1) the intestinal lumen, (2) the passage of digestion products across the intestinal mucosa, and (3) the transport of the products in the intestinal lympatics. Table 32 lists some common causes of malabsorption.

Clinically, malabsorption and maldigestion have similar outcomes: weight loss, steatorrhoea with a greater that 20 g fat loss in the stool, diarrhoea due to hydroxylated fatty acids and bloating, usually due to gas. One practically never sees a patient who has malabsorption without some weight loss. Persistent chronic diarrhoea without weight loss may be spastic colitis, due to food

Table 32 Common causes of malaborption

Abnormalities within the intestinal lumen
1. Inadequate digestion
   Pancreatic exocrine insufficiency (chronic pancreatitis, cystic fibrosis, pancreatic atrophy or ductal obstruction)
   Gastric hypersection (Zollinger-Ellison syndrome)
   Postgastrectomy malabsorption

2. Altered bile salt metabolism
   Hepatobiliary disease
   Bacterial overgrowth
   Blind loop syndrome
   Short gut syndrome
   Extensive ileal resection

Abnormal function of intestinal mucosa
Disaccharidase deficiency
Coeliac disease; gluten enteropathy
Lipophagia granulomatosis
Dyslipoproteinaemias
Diabetes mellitus with steatorrhoea
Tropical sprue
Intestinal lymphoma
Radiation enteritis

Obstruction of intestinal lympatics
Congenital lymphangiectasia
Constrictive pericarditis and congestive heart failure
Lymphoma
Tuberculosis
Retroperitoneal fibrosis

---

allergy. Other more severe symptoms include anaemia due to malabsorption of water-soluble vitamins and copper; hypoproteinaemic oedema due to loss of protein secondary to a defect of the mucosal lymphatics; tetany due to malabsorption of calcium in the duodenum and magnesium in the duodenum and jejunum and frequent bruising due to malabsorption of the fat-soluble vitamin K.

Specific treatment varies with the cause, but general management in all cases consists of treatment of the underlying cause including surgery and antibiotics and diet therapy with nutrient supplements to maintain normal nutrition as far as possible. Special dietary restriction is indicated in disaccharidase deficiency (p. 185) and coeliac disease (p. 188). The introduction of diets rich in medium-chain triglycerides (MCT) has revolutionized the management of many of these conditions (p. 187) by permitting absorption of fat and consequently much-needed energy. Iron, calcium, fat-soluble vitamins and folic acid and vitamin B_{12} most commonly need to be given as supplements. In severe cases with inanition, total parenteral alimentation therapy at home is currently recommended.

Bacterial contamination of the gut

This occurs most commonly in the long afferent loop (blind loop) of duodenum following gastric surgery, strictures, or fistulae of the bowel and diverticulae of the small intestine. The intraluminal bacteria compete with the host for vitamin B_{12}. Antibiotic treatment prevents this.

The steatorrhoea that sometimes occurs is probably due to bacterial hydrolysis of conjugated bile salts which normally aid emulsification of fat by activating pancreatic lipase, incorporating products of lipolysis into micelles and stimulating re-esterification within epithelial cells.

Frequent small feeds are recommended of a high energy, high protein and low fat diet. Iron and vitamin B_{12} supplemens are usually necessary.

Protein-losing enteropathy

There are a number of conditions in which the rate of loss of protein into the intestine exceeds the reabsorption of the constituent amino acids. They result in obstruction of the gastrointestinal lymphatics, exudation through damaged mucosa, and excessive secretion of mucus. There is usually also loss of minerals and lipid. Some cases may have an allergic basis. Treatment must be directed at the cause but a high protein diet is always indicated.

Obstruction

There are many causes and several types of intestinal obstruction, all of which are life-threatening conditions requiring surgical management. Nutritional aspects are confined to parenteral feeding (see p. 238).

Crohn's disease (regional enteritis)

This is a chronic inflammatory disease of unknown aetiology with a high familial incidence and may persist a lifetime. It is usually progressive, with exacerbations and remissions and tends to recur following surgery, which is indicated for its complications: obstruction, perforation and bleeding.

The diet should be high in protein, energy and of low residue. Meals should be unhurried and the food chewed thoroughly. Severe cases with fever, loss of blood and mucus, and tissue destruction readily become protein energy malnourished. Lean meat and liver are included as much as possible. Milk is permitted unless there is lactose intolerance. Supplemental feeding with MCT and amino acid preparations may be necessary. Known irritants—alcohol, coffee, tea—should be avoided. Multivitamin tablets are indicated. Vitamin B_{12} should be given parenterally (1 mg intramuscularly once a month) as its normal site of absorption, the terminal ileum, is usually involved. Most iron preparations are poorly tolerated by the gastrointestinal tract but ferrous gluconate—polysorbate 20 (1 to 2 capsules 3 times a day) appears to be well absorbed.

Ulcerative colitis

This is one of the most difficult diseases to treat and there are no specific preventive or curative measures. These patients are usually tense, unduly sensitive and easily depressed and psychotherapy may be of considerable help if started early. In some the disease may have an allergic basis to cow's milk or other foreign protein.

A low residue diet is usually prescribed on the principle of reducing physical stimulation to a minimum. Low residue foods that are more completely absorbed include meat, fish, chicken, rice, white bread, noodles and macaroni, dextrose, gelatin and hard-boiled eggs. High residue foods to be avoided are apples, oranges, celery, cabbage, tomatoes, berries and raw egg albumin. Such a liberal, smooth, non-irritant regime tends to be vitamin deficient and a polyvitamin preparation should be given. A small number of cases has been shown to benefit from withdrawal of milk and milk-containing products.

If abdominal pain, defaecatory urgency and pronounced diarrhoea are not controlled by such a dietary regime, total parenteral alimentation (p. 238) with intramuscular vitamins for up to 2 weeks may provide sufficient rest to the alimentary tract to allow it to recover.

Fulminating cases require hospitalization for nasogastric suction, antibiotics and adrenococorticosteroids parenterally. If adequate response has not been obtained in 2 or 3 weeks, or if severe haemorrhage or perforation occurs, surgical intervention is indicated.

Diverticulosis and diverticulitis

Symptomless diverticulae, affecting mainly the distal colon, are found on X-ray with great frequency in adult western populations. It is now recognized that the main factor in their causation is prolonged consumption of a diet low in fibre, especially cereal fibre. Use of wholemeal bread and about 5 to 20g of unprocessed bran per day may prevent symptoms developing. These consist of alternating diarrhoea and constipation, colonic pain and tenderness and flatulence and indicate the presence of diverticulitis. The diet should be high in fibre, but in severe recurrent cases antibiotics or even surgical treatment may prove necessary (see also p. 167).

Irritable bowel syndrome (IBS)

This is an intermittent disease of the gastrointestinal tract exacerbated by stress, due to a motor disorder which usually begins in the sigmoid colon with increasing intraluminal pressures and hypermotility. Symptoms include crampy abdominal pain, bloating, gas, belching and explosive diarrhoea starting 20 to 30 minutes after a meal. Fibre with its bulking properties is the current treatment of choice.

LIVER

Nutritional deficiency commonly affects the liver. The most notable instances in man are the fatty liver in kwashiorkor (p. 106) and the alcoholic fatty liver leading to cirrhosis if the cause is not removed (p. 242). There is no evidence for a human counterpart to the fatty infiltration due to methionine or choline deficiency, or the massive necrosis resulting from deficiency of cystine, vitamin E or selenium in experimental animals.

Veno-occlusive disease results in serious damage to the liver in young children and is especially common in Jamaica. It is probably due to alkaloids in *Senecio* herbs found in bush teas (p. 26).

Infantile biliary cirrhosis occurs in Indian children. Recent evidence suggests in may be due to excess copper accumulation (p. 161).

Aflatoxin contamination of food has been suspected of causing primary liver cancer (p. 24) and resulting in liver necrosis in some cases of Reye's syndrome (p. 24).

Acute viral hepatitis

Three immunologically distinct but clinically similiar forms, hepatitis A hepatitis B and non-A non-B hepatitis exist. They may be transmitted by the exchange of body fluids (orally and sexually) or via the parenteral route. Hepatitis A has a shorter incubation period and extensive outbreaks have been traced to contaminated water or milk and ingestion of foods including uncooked clams and oysters. Contamination of needles and syringes is an important source of spread of hepatitis B and less so of hepatitis A. Transfusion-associated hepatitis may be of either type. Australian antigen is a specific marker for hepatitis B. It is found in a small percentage of normal people and in some diseases.

A high carbohydrate, low fat and low protein intake has usually been recommended. In the early stages anorexia is marked and craving for certain foods is not unusual. There is no evidence that any particular foods are unsuitable for these patients, and frequent small feedings of attractive food should be provided.

Every effort should be made to provide the energy and protein requirements of the patient within the limits of tolerance. Intravenous feeding will occasionally have to be resorted to. Especially in the first few days nausea may be extreme and meals should be small, easy to masticate and attractively served.

Cirrhosis

Diffuse fibrotic changes in the liver are the end result of a number of diseases affecting the liver, including chronic alcoholism (p. 242). Considerable improvement however may be obtained if the nutritional state has been especially poor prior to starting treatment. There is often wasting, hypoalbuminaemia, sodium retention, oedema, ascites, obstruction to hepatic and portal veins and anaemia. There is no specific diet to recommend but a normal energy, normal protein intake (about 0·8g/kg/day) should be aimed at as long as liver function is not grossly impaired.

Sodium restriction (1 to 2 g per day) is a valuable measure in combating fluid retention manifested as ascites or oedema. A salt-poor diet is difficult to consume over a prolonged period, imposes a burden on the dietitian, and is expensive. The use of modern diuretics makes rigorous salt restriction less important. However, the 'low salt syndrome' is a hazard of sodium restriction. It may arise in cirrhosis patients as a result of depletion of body stores from repeated paracenteses, the use of diuretics, or in renal failure.

Hepatic coma

Advancing liver failure leads to symptoms of precoma and then coma. The first change may be a vacant stare and lack of personal tidiness. The patient is distant, confused, performs acts clumsily and follows directions with difficulty. The characteristic 'flapping tremor' consists of coarse irregular flexion — extension movements at the metacarpophalangeal and wrist joints. The e.e.g. is abnormal.

Hepatic coma may be primary, when it is due to progressive disease, or precipitated by (1) paracentesis, (2) portacaval shunt, (3) barbiturates or morphine, and (4) nitrogenous substances such as protein, amino acid mixtures, ammonium salts or in gastrointestinal haemorrhage.

Nutrition has to be maintained by nasogastric tube or intravenously (p. 238). Special problems include hypernatraemia (less commonly hyponatraemia), hypokalaemia, hypocalcaemia and alkalosis. Severe anaemia may require blood transfusion and salt-poor albumin may be given in daily doses of 25 to 50 g to combat hypovolaemic shock.

The oral administration of broad-spectrum antibiotics, such as neomycin or paromomycin, (0.5 to 1g 6 hourly of either) has been shown to bring about improvement, together with restriction of intake of protein to 20 g/day. This comes about by the destruction of the normal flora in the caecum and elsewhere which is capable of splitting urea into ammonia. The hyperammonaemia appears to be harmful but exactly how is not clear. In some patients the catabolic state leads to release of aromatic amino acids which penetrate the blood–brain barrier as a result of the coincident fall in branched-chain amino acids. Treatment consists of supplementing the diet with the latter acids with a high energy intake.

Gall stones and cholecystitis

The aetiology of this disease complex remains ill-understood. It has been shown that the liver secretes an abnormal bile that is supersaturated with cholesterol. The bile has a low phospholipid: cholesterol ratio in comparison with normal. The bile salt pool is contracted, facilitating precipitation of cholesterol.

Predisposing factors include familial occurrence, female sex, tendency to obesity, pregnancy leading to stasis of bile in the gall bladder and accompanying diabetes mellitus, cardiovascular disease and familial hypercholesterolaemia. The habitual diet is often high in energy and fat.

Dietary treatment is in no way prophylactic or curative and at best can only be palliative. These patients have intolerance to greasy or fried foods and onions, cabbage, radishes, cucumbers and spiced foods. Dietary fat should be limited and, much of this should be vegetable oils, such as corn oil, which are unsaturated and stimulate bile flow. Chenic (chenodeoxycholic) acid which comprises about 40 per cent of the bile acids of normal human bile has been shown to reduce cholesterol secretion into bile, probably by inhibiting liver synthesis. Patients with cholesterol stones and a functioning gall bladder have responded to 15mg/kg.day at meal times. A diet low in cholesterol enhances the effect of chenic acid.

Chronic obstructive jaundice

Acholia results from a number of congenital, postoperative or other conditions affecting the bile ducts. Steatorrhoea leads to malnutrition affecting energy, proteins, minerals and vitamins. Lack of bile salts prevents micelle formation with fat and poor absorption. Vitamin K is not absorbed and prothrombin deficiency results (p. 135). A regime high in energy and protein should be provided. Fat is poorly tolerated and should be limited to 40 g per day.

Pancreatic insufficiency

Lack of enzymes, particularly lipase, causes failure in splitting triglycerides to monoglycerides with diarrhoea, steatorrhoea and inadequate absorption of all nutrients. The main diseases are acute or chronic pancreatitis, carcinoma, and cystic fibrosis. The most common cause is chronic alcoholic pancreatitis.

Substitute pancreatic preparations of varying potency are available commercially. They should be given before and with the meal. The enzyme deficiency can rarely be entirely met in this way. Fat consumption is modified and medium chain triglycerides are a valuable means of increasing the energy intake (p. 187). Protein intake must be adequate and in a readily absorbed form. Long-term nocturnal elemental diet (p. 238) has promoted catch-up growth in a teenage child with cystic fibrosis. In the latter, long-term treatment with intravenous fat has ameliorated the clinical cause.

20. METABOLIC DISORDERS

DISORDERS OF CARBOHYDRATE METABOLISM

Diabetes mellitus

The availability of insulin therapy in no way lessens the importance of providing the diabetic patient with a nutrionally adequate diet.

The degree of glucose wastage by excretion in the urine is the primary cause of the metabolic symptomatology. The energy deficit due to the glycosuria gives rise to hunger and polyphagia. This and the water loss lead to thirst, polydypsia and weight loss. Protein ingested is largely made into sugar and therefore used inefficiently. Loss of both exogenous and endogenous carbohydrate results in rapid mobilization of fat leading eventually in severe cases to ketosis and coma. There are broadly two forms of diabetes mellitus.

Insulin-dependent diabetes mellitus (type I, juvenile). The ketotic severe form is found more commonly among the young. There is an absolute insulin deficiency. Nutritional adjustments are only of secondary importance to insulin therapy. Animal fat should be limited but it is now recognized that a reasonable amount of sugar is well tolerated and fibre intake should be normal. Meals should be frequent and small to spread the energy intake over the day. It is very important to strike an energy balance through the use of insulin. Restriction may lead to fat mobilization and ketosis, and excess to either weight gain or glycosuria with polyuria, demineralization and ketosis.

Non-insulin dependent diabetes mellitus (maturity onset, type II). This milder form of the disease, manifesting itself in middle life, is also characterized by insulin deficiency but of lesser degree and of a different kind. Insulin release is delayed and does not coincide with the glucose peak during a glucose tolerance test. High inappropriate insulin levels occur late on, giveing rise to the impression of hyperinsulinism, but overall there is deficiency. About 20 per cent of the healthy population, often relatives of diabetics have what has been termed prediabetes. These are subjects who show diminished insulin secretion despite normal glucose tolerance. It is believed that the occurrence of some stress factor, especially increasing obesity, may covert them into true diabetics.

Diet and exercise alone used judiciously can give excellent results in this form. Every effort should be made to achieve a weight about 5 per cent below that recommended in life insurance tables. At the present time emphasis is given to a diet adequate in all nutrients and prudent in relation to fat and refined carbohydrate as recommended generally (p. 281).

The proneness of diabetics to atheroma necessitates the reduction of fat to 20 to 25 per cent of total energy and most of it in unsaturated form.

Although many patients with the 'carbohydrate-induced' form of hyperlipidaemia (Frederickson type IV, see p. 190) have abnormal glucose tolerance there is no evidence yet that this is related to diabetes mellitus.

Long-term complications. A prudent diet should be followed to avoid excess intake of energy, saturated fat and refined sugars.

The microangiopathy of diabetes is a specific lesion consisting of the deposition of collagenous glycoprotein in capillary basement membranes. It has especially serious results in the kidney as glomerulosclerosis producing uraemia. Protein restriction has proved helpful in this and other forms of renal failure (see p. 209).

In the retina the microangiopathy often leads to blindness. No specific dietary measures are of value for this process.

Hypoglycaemia

This is usually considered to occur when the blood glucose falls below 50 mg/100 ml, due to either excessive removal of glucose from the blood, or decreased secretion into the blood. Each of these states may be caused by a variety of pathological conditions. Several of these may be alleviated by dietary means.

In functional hypoglycaemia there is normal fasting blood glucose, but mild hypoglycaemia develops 2 to 4 hours after a meal, perphaps as a result of excess insulin response to the glucose load. Symptoms can usually be controlled by avoiding refined sugar and taking a diet generally low in carbohydrate.

The *dumping syndrome* following partial gastrectomy sometimes results in hypoglycaemia (p. 175).

Several amino acids stimulate the release of insulin but only leucine has so far been found to produce symptomatic hypoglycaemia. Many infants have responded in an exaggerated way to this amino acid and it is now thought that leucine sensitivity is an important cause of spontaneous hypoglycaemia in children. Treatment consists in limiting the intake of protein but not sufficiently to interfere with normal growth.

Fructose intolerance is a disorder inherited as an autosomal recessive in which after fructose ingestion blood fructose rises steeply and severe hypoglycaemia is produced. Aldolase activity in the liver is greatly depressed, fructose-1-phosphate accumulates and inhibits action of fructokinase, and so fructose rises in the blood. Fructose prevents the release of glucose from the liver. These patients have to omit sucrose and sweet fruits from their diet, the main dietary sources of fructose.

Jamaican vomiting sickness, due to consumption of *akee nut* is characterized by severe hypoglycaemia; from hypoglycin in the nut.

Glycogen storage diseases

At present eight types of this rare group of inherited disorders of glycogen metabolism have been identified. Dietary management is indicated in only two. The most common is *type 1 glycogen storage disease* (glucose-6-phosphatase deficiency, von Gierke's disease). Features are stunting, hepatomegaly, and fasting hypoglycaemia unresponsive to adrenaline or glucagon. Small frequent meals containing glucose or starch should be given to control blood glucose level. Sugars other than glucose should be avoided. *Type III glycogen storage disease* (Debrancher enzyme deficiency) is a rare disorder of glycogenolysis producing milder degrees of stunting, hepatomegaly and hypoglycaemia than type I. Frequent small meals are indicated, high in protein, in contrast to type I, as the gluconeogenic pathways from amino acids to glucose-6-phosphate and thence glucose are functional.

Galactosaemia

This congenital disorder leads to impairment of galactose metabolism due to the absence of the enzyme, galactose-1-phosphate uridyltransferase, necessary to catalyse the reaction together of galactose-1-phosphate and uridine diphosphoglucose. In its absence galactose-1-phosphate acccumulates in erythrocytes, liver, kidney and cerebral cortex. In severe cases, shortly after birth there are hypoglycaemic attacks, jaundice, cataracts, and mental deficiency. Later in life alternative pathways may develop permitting prolonged survival.

Treatment consists in removing milk from the diet, both human and bovine, and milk sugars. Galactose intake should be avoided by the mildly galactosaemic mother during pregnancy. Control of the adequacy of dietary restriction may be obtained by estimating the concentration of galactose or galactose-1-phosphate in red cells.

Galactokinase deficiency

This is a much rarer and milder disorder than galactosaemia, manifest mainly by cataracts. These usually appear late in infancy, but if diagnois is made early a galactose-free diet promotes normal development.

Abnormalities of sugar absorption

Several sugars may be affected and the abnormality may be either inherited when enzymes are deficient from birth or acquired. Disaccharides are usually affected but a few instances of monosaccharide malabsorption, involving glucose and galactose, have been reported. Symptoms consist of abdominal pain,flatulence and diarrhoea. A classification of the syndrome is given in Table 33 and the criteria for diagnosis in Table 34.

True congenital lactose intolerance in infants is rare. Of 25 cases reported about half had lactosuria with aminoaciduria and renal acidosis.

More than 60 cases of sucrose-isomaltose intolerance have been reported, nearly all children. Symptoms occur when the child is weaned onto a diet containing sucrose, and dextrin or starch which contain isomaltose residues.

Table 33 Disaccharide malabsorption syndromes

Congenital
1. Lactose intolerance (with or without lactosuria)
2. Sucrose-isomaltose intolerance
Acquired (primary) lactase deficiency
Secondary deficiency in other diseases
1. Tropical and non-tropical sprue
2. Other diseases with malabsorption (e.g. infectious diarrhoea, lipophagia granulomatosis lymphoma, ulcerative colitis, cystic fibrosis)
3. Protein-energy malnutrition (kwashiorkor and marasmus)
Disaccharide malabsorption with normal disaccharidases
1. Bowel resection or bypass
2. Physiological diarrhoea of the newborn

Table 34 Criteria for the diagnosis of disaccharidase deficiency

Major criteria
1. Symptoms produced by the offending disaccharide (by history or during tolerance test)
2. Symptoms improved by removal of disaccharide
3. Abnormal disaccharide tolerance test
4. Low level of enzyme in mucosal biopsy
Helpful additional features
1. Low faecal pH
2. Increased lactic acid in faeces
3. Small bowel X-ray (barium + offending disaccharide) — malabsorption pattern

In man lactase production is maintained at high levels until after weaning, but in later childhood and adult life most populations, who do not consume milk then, have a 70 to 95 per cent incidence of deficiency. Only those of northern European origin, who usually drink milk throughout life, maintain lactose secretion. Moderate amounts of milk can be tolerated by children and affected adults alike, best in the form of whole milk, with a meal, several times a day. Milk aid programmes should not be curtailed on this count.

Secondary disaccharidase deficiency may complicate malabsorption of any cause. Protein energy malnutrition is among these (p. 108) and the intolerance to milk may necessitate the substitution of a vegetable food mixture or lactose-free milk in recovery.

Breast-fed newborns, especially prematures, may be temporarily intolerant. Human milk contains about 7 per cent lactose.

DISORDERS OF LIPID METABOLISM

These are classified in Table 35 and common examples of each type are given. Some are considered in detail elsewhere.

Steatorrhoea

This term implies the presence in the stools of an excessive amount of fat,

Table 35 Main disorders of lipid metabolism

Intestinal lipid metabolism (steatorrhoeas)
  Pancreatic disease
  Coeliac disease
  Abetalipoproteinaemia
  lipophagia granulomatosis and the like
Lipid transportation in serum
  Inherited hyperlipoproteinaemias
  Secondary hyperlipoproteinaemias
Lipid metabolism by liver and other tissues
  Atherosclerosis (cholesterol)
  Diabetes mellitus (fatty acids)
  Biliary cirrhosis (phospholipids)
  Fatty livers (triglycerides)

usually greater than 20 g per day after a 100 g fat load. The gross appearance may be soft, greasy and pale. Microscopic examination may be necessary to reveal fat droplets by staining. Definite diagnosis requires that a fat balance be performed. Other tests will be necessary to reveal the underlying cause of the malabsorption and also what other nutrients are affected, especially calcium, potassium, magnesium, iron and water- and fat-soluble vitamins.

Treatment should first be directed to the underlying condition. If steatorrhoea cannot be controlled by this means it can be considerably reduced by cutting down the dietary fat to about 25 g per day. This decreases intestinal motility, distension and pain, but negative energy balance may occur. Medium-chain triglycerides (MCT) have proved of value in this regard. The metabolism of MCT differs in a number of ways from that of long-chain triglycerides (LCT) (Fig. 19). MCT can be absorbed without previous hy-

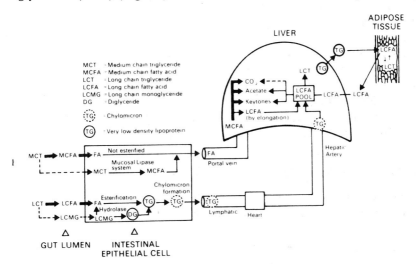

Fig. 19 Physiology of medium-chain triglycerides. (Greenberger 1969 New England Journal of Medicine 280: 1045)

drolysis, although absorption is better in the presence of pancreatic lipase and bile. Virtually complete hydrolysis of MCT takes place in the microsomal fraction of intestinal mucosa. The octanoic acid released is transported directly to the liver by the portal vein, where it is catabolized to carbon dioxide and water. Energy is thereby readily made available to the body, and this happens even where there is liver disease, as MCT are oxidized in many other sites.

A list of conditions in which they are indicated is given in Table 36.

MCT may be given either as oil in fruit juice or as a liquid formula diet; both commercially available. Side-effects may include abdominal pain, hyperketonaemia, and hypoglycaemia occasionally. Recipes are available for palatable diets (Beck p. 218).

Coeliac disease

Childhood and adult forms of the disease are probably the same. Other names for the adult disease are *gluten-induced enteropathy, ideopathic steatorrhoea* and *non-tropical sprue*. The condition is characterized by weight loss, crampy abdominal pain and malabsorption of fat, nitrogen, vitamins, minerals and water. It is of familial occurrence but the mode of inheritance is not clear. It is precipitated by part of the α gliadin fraction of gluten, a water-insoluble protein in wheat, barley, rye, buckwheat and malt. The primary abnormality is not known but is thought to be either due to peptidase deficiency or result from an immune defect.

Pathological changes in the villi visible by light microscopy and better revealed by electron microscopy are striking but not pathognomonic.

Complete clinical remission usually occurs within a few days or weeks of introducing a gluten-free diet. The mucosal changes may not revert to normal until after a year or more.

Food containing gluten must be excluded. Surprisingly, wheat products may occur in such items as hot-dogs, cold cuts, salad dressings, ice-cream and meat loaves. Flours from oats, maize, soy, rice and potato may be safely used. Some patients settle down only after milk is also excluded, probably due to associated lactase deficiency.

Lipoprotein disorders

In *a-β-lipoproteinaemia* (acanthocytosis) complete absence of circulating β-lipoprotein leads to failure of transport of lipids and other substances, failure to thrive, abnormal red cells, ataxia and retinal damage. MCT permit transport of fat since chylomicron formation is not necessary. Long term effects of this treatment on the red cells and nervous system are not yet known.

Two other rare lipid transport defects have been described. In *Tangier disease* there is lack of high density lipoproteins in serum and cholesterol

Table 36 Rationale for use of MCT

Physiochemical characteristics	Physiological considerations	Potential therapeutic applications
MCT present more interfacial surface for enzyme action/unit time	Intraluminal enzymatic hydrolysis of MCT is more rapid and more complete than LCT	Decreased intraluminal concentrations of pancreatic lipase (pancreatic insufficiency, cystic fibrosis) Decreased small-bowel absorptive surface (intestinal resection)
Greater water solubility of MCT hydrolysis products	Bile salts are not required for dispersion in water	Decreased intraluminal concentrations of bile salts (intrahepatic and extrahepatic bilary-tract obstruction, chronic parenchymal liver disease)
Smaller molecular size of MCT *vs* LCT	Small amounts of MCT may enter intestinal cell without prior hydrolysis	Pancreatic insufficiency
Shorter chain length of fatty acids derived from MCT	More efficient penetration of diseased mucosal surface	Non-tropical sprue, tropical sprue
Small molecular size and lower pK of fatty acids derived from MCT	*Intramucosal metabolism of MCFA different from LCFA:* decreased affinity for esterifying enzymes, decreased affinity for activation enzymes, minimal re-esterification of MCFA to MCT, no chylomicron formation	A-β-lipoproteinaemia Hypo-β-lipoproteinaemia
Greater water solubility of MCFA	*Different routes of transport of MCT vs LCT:* portal transport of MCT (as MCFA), lymphatic transport of LCT (as chylomicrons)	Lymphatic obstruction (lymphomas) Intestinal lymphangiectasia

(Greenberger 1969 New England Journal of Medicine 280: 1045) ester is deposited in the reticuloendothelial system. Lecithin:cholesterol acyltransferase (LCAT) is the enzyme in plasma that acounts for most of the esterification of cholesterol. It is considered necessary for normal lipoprotein formation and metabolism. Several cases of *LCAT deficiency* have been reported with abnormal plasma lipoproteins and renal failure. There is no treatment for either condition.

Hyperliproproteinaemias. In these conditions there is an excess of various lipoproteins in the serum (p. 52). They may be genetic or acquired in association with another disease.

Congenital hyperlipoproteinaemias have been classified into five types by Fredrickson on the basis of the particular lipoprotein abnormalities found by electrophoresis and preparative ultracentrifugation. Type I is characterized by excess of chylomicrons. Treatment consists of restricting fat intake to 15 to 30 g daily. On this diet patients tend to continue to have hyperlipaemia induced by the high carbohydrate diet they have to consume. The prognosis is reasonably good. Repeated attacks of pancreatitis are the most serious feature.

In type II familial hyperbetalipoproteinaemia or hypercholesterolaemia, there is deposition of cholesterol in skin (xanthomas), cornea (arcus senilis) and blood vessels (atheroma). Coronary artery disease is common at a young age. It is probably the most common type. It has been divided into IIa with an increase in LDL and IIb with raised LDL and VLDL. The hypercholesterolaemia is usually of severe degree (as high as 1000 mg/100 ml).

The objective of treatment is the lowering of serum cholesterol levels. Xanthomas regress but it is not clear whether the atheromatous process can be controlled. Dietary cholesterol should be as low as possible and saturated fat no more that 20 to 30 g daily. Polyunsaturated fats should be two to three times this level. In type IIb carbohydrate should be restricted to reduce triglyceride levels.

Type III is a rare form with an excess of β-lipoproteins which have acquired an abnormally low density because of increased amounts of triglycerides. Marked fall in circulating lipids has been produced by restriction of energy intake and substitution of polyunsaturated fats.

Type IV is also called hyperpre-β-lipoproteinaemia and carbohydrate-induced hyperlipaemia. The mainstay of treatment is energy restriction, and many patients are obese and the disorder is common in diabetics. These patients have an unusual tendency to develop hypertriglyceridaemia on ingestion of carbohydrate. Both alcohol and MCT predispose to this and should be excluded (p. 187).

Type V is a mixed form, and treatment consists in weight reduction and energy restriction.

Acquired hyperlipoproteinaemias are associated with such conditions as pregnancy, diabetes mellitus, pancreatitis, hypo- and hyper-thyroidism, nephrosis, liver disease, and multiple myeloma. Restrictive diets have only limited benefit and many patients find it difficult to adhere to them. If the hyperlipaemia is fat induced, fat intake should be limited to 20 to 30 g per day. Patients with hypertriglyceridaemia may achieve normal levels by using polyunsaturated oil or margarine for cooking. Some overweight patients respond to energy restriction.

Refsum's disease

In this rare recessively inherited defect phytanic acid accumulates in tissues due to the absence of phytanic acid *a* hydroxylase. Neurological damage, eye lesions and heart disease occur. Fat meat and fish and whole dairy products are rich in phytanic acid and exclusion of these foods from the diet has resulted in considerable improvement.

Disorders of purine and pyrimidine metabolism

Gout

This disease is characterized by hyperuricaemia resulting from a combination of a genetic predisposition and environmental factors. Free uric acid is precipitated in and about joints and tendons and in the kidney parenchyma. The high blood level of uric acid is probably due to biochemical abnormalities leading to excess uric acid formation and to diminished renal excretion. An effective armamentarium of drugs is now available for the control of blood uric acid and relief of acute inflamation of joints.

Dietary measures play a relatively minor but not negligible role. A diet low in purines, with no more than a quarter of a pound (113 g) of meat in a week, is recommended for gouty patients until there is evidence of effective control by drugs of acute attacks and the serum urate level. Most patients may then resume a normal diet. In those with severe renal disease dietary restriction may need to be continued. Liver, kidney, sweet bread, brain, fish roe, sardine, crab, anchovy, sprats, peas, and beans are rich in purines and can easily be avoided.

A high fat intake and alcohol consumption both tend to raise the serum urate and should be avoided. Starvation and low energy intake provoke acute attacks of gout through mobilization of endogenous lipid which leads to ketonaemia and renal retention of urate. Weight reduction in the obese gouty patient is therefore best postponed until acute attacks and serum urate level have been brought under control.

Hereditary orotic aciduria

This is a very rare condition in which affected children develop a severe megaloblastic anaemia during the first few months of life. Mental and physical development are retarded. Two enzymes of pyridopyrimidine metabolism are deficient. Large quantities of orotic acid are excreted in the urine.

Treatment with uridine has proved to be very effective. The dose appears to be of the order of 150 mg per kg body weight per day.

Hereditary xanthinuria

In this rare condition xanthine oxidase is grossly deficient, and as a result xanthine and hypoxanthine, precursors of uric acid, are in high concentration in plasma and urine. Xanthine calculi may form in the urinary tract. The condition is usually benign. A high fluid intake, alkali therapy and restriction of purine content of diet are indicated.

Disorders of porphyrin metabolism and porphyrias

The porphyrias are a large group of primary and usually hereditary disorders of porphyrin or porphyrin precursor metabolism, difficult to define and classify. The enzymatic defects have not all been identified yet. Nutrition has a limited place in management.

Acute intermittent porphyria is an inborn error characterized by overproduction of porphyrin precursors by the liver. The central and peripheral nervous system is severely affected. Photosensitivity is not a feature of this type of porphyria. A high carbohydrate intake, together with insulin therapy, may be beneficial. Starvation is known to precipitate attacks, and a high carbohydrate intake has been shown to increase secretion of porphyrin precursors. Such a regime may also benefit another form, *variegate porphyria*, which presents with skin sensitivity, or neurological manifestations, or both together.

DISORDERS OF AMINO ACID METABOLISM

This is a large and complex group of disorders the diagnosis and management of which form an interesting part of paediatric practice. Attention here will be confined to the better recognized examples of those conditions for which dietary management has proved effective. For greater detail the reference at the end of the chapter should be consulted.

There are three types of disorders of amino acid metabolism: (a) an inherited enzyme or membrane transport defect, (b) a defect secondary to other diseases affecting liver, bowel or kidney usually resulting in marked aminoaciduria, and (c) a transient defect of early infancy. Only the first of these types of disorder will be considered here. Some of these conditions are apoenzyme disorders in which the coenzyme is a vitamin and respond partially or completely to large doses of appropriate vitamin. The best substantiated instances of this state, vitamin dependency, involve pyridoxine, (p 121), cobalamin (p. 128) and biotin (p. 129).

Dietary management of these disorders, designed to provide an adequate intake of essential amino acids and total protein, as well as all other nutrients, to promote optimum growth and development in early life, demands expert medical, dietetic and biochemical supervision over a number of years. At the same time the amino acid(s) where metabolism is affected have to be restricted. Appropriate low amino acid diets and low amino acid protein substitutes have been devised and are commercially available for many of these disorders.

All of these conditions are rare; only a few instances of some have been reported. Phenylketonuria is the commonest, occurring in 1 of every 12 000–30 000 births in most Caucasian populations. With a few exceptions they are transmitted by Mendelian recessive inheritance.

Phenylalanine and tyrosine

Phenylketonuria and hyperphenylalaninaemia

During growth less than half of the dietary intake of phenylalanine is used for growth and the remainder is mostly oxidized to tyrosine but there are several alternative pathways. In classical *phenylketonuria* there is irreversible deficiency of liver phenylalanine hydroxylase, and phenylalanine accumulates throughout the body. The untreated homozygous case is severely mentally retarded (intelligence quotient < 20); half the patients die by the age of 20. There are various neurological manifestations, lack of pigment in hair, skin and irises and frequently eczema.

A diet low in phenylalanine gives favourable results if treatment is begun before 3 months of age with poorer prognosis after this time.

The diet is made up from natural foods low in phenylalanine and specially treated protein foods, such as milk and soya beans, to lower the phenylalanine content. The diets tend to be monotonous but have been consumed for years by children. The phenylalanine tolerance at all ages is between 200 and 500 mg/day. The results depend considerably upon the quality of the biochemical control that can be exerted. Overenthusiastic restriction can cause hypophenylalaninaemia with retarded growth. At present it seems wisest to advise continuation of treatment for as long as possible under reasonable circumstances, certainly well into mid-childhood. Return to a normal diet in children aged 5–15 years resulted in a fall in intellectual progress in many in a recent trial.

Phenylketonuric females, some of whom are mentally retarded, bear children. There appears to be an inverse relationship between maternal phenylalanine plasma level and final I.Q. of the offspring. It may prove necessary to resume dietary restriction during pregnancy to protect the fetus.

Besides classic phenylketonuria, several other disorders of phenylalanine metabolism have been described. *Phenylketonuria, mild variant I* is the same as the classical form but there is a high tolerance for dietary phenylalanine. *Phenylketonuria, 'transient' variant II* resembles the classical form but under treatment tolerance to phenylalanine increases. Care has to be exercised to prevent the symptoms of hypophenylalaninaemia in these sensitive cases.

Benign persistent hyperphenylalaninaemia and *neonatal hyperphenyl-alaninaemia* are important to distinguish from those forms that require treatment.

Disorders of tyrosine metabolism

Tyrosine is derived predominantly from dietary phenylalanine and from protein-bound tyrosine. The main catabolic pathway is conversion to acetoacetate. Several inherited disorders of tyrosine metabolism have been recognized. The commonest condition is *transient neonatal tyrosinaemia* or *tyrosyluria* in which there is a temporary deficiency of *p*-hydroxyphenyl-pyruvic acid oxidase which is vitamin C-dependent. The infant may be lethargic or fail to thrive. There is response to vitamin C (50 to 100 mg/day) or lowered protein intake.

Hereditary tyrosinaemia (Baber's syndrome, cirrhosis and the Fanconi syndrome) is due to deficiency of *p*-HPPA oxidase. In the acute form there is liver failure and death. A more chronic state is characterized by nodular cirrhosis and renal tubular dysfunction. In both forms of the disease restriction of dietary tyrosine and phenylalanine, as in the treatment of phenylketonuria (300 to 500 mg/day), is of distinct benefit. Methionine restriction in the acute stage is also beneficial. A defect in methionine-activity enzyme has been described, resulting in depletion of tissue ATP. Hypo-glycaemia and electrolyte imbalance have to be corrected.

Methionine and cystine

Homocystinuria (cystathionine synthetase deficiency)

Homocystine, an amino acid normally not detected in urine, appears there in large amounts. The plasma levels of both homocystine and methionine are elevated.

Homocystine condenses with serine to yield cystathionine, the reaction being catalysed by cystathionine synthase. Activity of this enzyme has been shown to be virtually absent in liver and brain of these patients.

Earlier reports suggested mental retardation, growth failure and light complexion as constant features but these are not always present. The skin tends to be coarse, the gait may be flat-footed, and there is hepatomegaly with normal function. Other clinical features such as skeletal changes (kyphosis, scoliosis and arachnodactyly) and ectopia lentis have caused confusion with Marfan's syndrome. Vascular thromboses are common and may lead to death in the second or third decade.

About half the patients respond to large doses of vitmin B$_6$ (250 to 500 mg daily). It is not clear yet whether pyridoxal phosphate is a coenzyme for cystathionine synthase (see Table 16, p. 122). Folic acid requirements are increased as methytetrahydrofolate is consumed by the disposal of excess homocysteine.

A low protein, low methionine diet will reduce elevated plasma methionine and homocystine levels. Cystine supplements have also been advocated in view of the block that prevents the formation of cystine. Possible long-term retarding effects of low protein, low methionine intake have to be guarded against.

Homocystinuria also occurs in two rare disorders of vitamin B_{12} and folic acid metabolism and these vitamin dependency states respond to large doses of the vitamins.

Cystathioninuria

This occurs in two forms: (1) acquired cases in association with vitamin B_6 deficiency , liver disease, certain tumours and following administration of thyroxine; (2) inherited cases which respond dramatically to large doses of vitamin B_6 and are considered to be a form of pyridoxine dependency (p. 122).

Cystathionine serves to transfer the sulphur atom of methionine to cystine under the action of cystathionase which is inactive without pyridoxal phosphate. It has been shown in liver homogenates of two patients that cystathionase activity is very low. The addition of pyridoxal phosphate in vitro restored activity to normal.

No consistent clinical pattern has emerged associated with cystathioninuria. It is probable that the various associated abnormalities, including mental retardation, are coincidental.

Daily administration of 200 to 400 mg of pyridoxine has suppressed the excretion of cystathionine.

Cystinuria

This is one of the longest recognized and most common inborn errors of metabolism. It is inherited as an autosomal recessive trait. Although, besides cystine, lysine, arginine and ornithine are excreted in great excess by the homozygous individual, cystine is the least soluble naturally occurring amino acid and is responsible for the formation of renal, ureteral and bladder calculi. These same four amino acids are poorly absorbed by the gut.

The most important single aspect of treatment is the maintenance of a high fluid intake. Alkalinization of the urine has the same effect. Encouraging results have been reported with 1 to 3 g D-penicillamine daily. Results from lowering cystine excretion by limiting dietary protein and methionine have not been encouraging.

Branched-chain amino acids

This is a complex group of organic acidaemias with a common symptomatology of vomiting, ketosis, hypoglycaemia, mental retardation, coma and death. Some are vitamin dependency states involving thiamin, biotin or vitamin B_{12}.

Maple syrup urine disease (branched-chain ketoaminoacidaemia BCKA)

BCKA affects the decarboxylation step in the degradation of all three of these amino acids. Classical BCKA is inherited as an autosomal recessive trait, but an intermittent form is probably the result of a mutant allele.

The disease is named after the odour which is detectable from the urine and the body of the patient. Feeding difficulties, vomiting, hypertonicity and a shrill cry are characteristic in the first week of life. Flaccidity and apnoea may supervene, followed by convulsions and death. Untreated children who have survived have suffered severe mental and motor retardation.

Effective treatment necessitates a semisynthetic diet, restricted in branched-chain amino acids but otherwise nutritionally adequate. One patient has been successfully maintained for over 5 years from 6 days of age on a gelatin-based diet to which were added other amino acids and nutrients. Therapy has to be begun within the first month of life if permanent neurological damage is to be avoided. The hypoglycaemia often encountered is reminiscent of leucine-sensitive hypoglycaemia and may result from impaired glucose absorption. It responds to the general treatment.

Isovalericacidaemia

In the three patients studied so far there was a pungent odour ('sweaty feet syndrome') due to the short-chain fatty acid, isovaleric acid, severe metabolic acidosis and neurological manifestations. The condition appears to be a disorder of leucine metabolism with deficiency of the enzyme which specifically oxidizes isovaleryl CoA.

Restriction of protein intake to the minimum requirement prevents isovalericacidaemia, but during infancy this may be especially difficult to achieve. Early diagnosis and treatment are very important. If acidosis and dehydration occur they have to be corrected as soon as possible.

Urea cycle

Many disorders of enzymes of this cycle that takes place in the liver have been described. All are rare and feature hyperammonaemia, and mental retardation. Early death is common.

Argininosuccinicaciduria

High concentrations of this urea cycle intermediate have usually been associated with mental retardation. It is thought that elevated blood ammonia may play a part in central nervous system dysfunction.

No successful treatment has so far been devised. A high protein diet or administration of ornithine and citrulline increases the excretion of the amino acid, and a low protein diet diminishes it. Arginine supplementation, together with just enough protein to sustain normal growth and control the hyperammonaemia, warrant further trials. Early diagnosis in the newborn period before brain injury has occurred is most important.

Familial protein intolerance

This has been described in 10 children of 7 Finnish and Lapp families. All patients tolerated breast milk well but diarrhoea and vomiting began after weaning and they failed to thrive. When old enough to select their food they rejected cow's milk, meat, fish, liver and eggs and symptoms subsided on grains, vegetables and juices. There was evidence of defective renal and intestinal transport of dibasic amino acids.

Treatment consists of avoidance of proteins of animal origin but vegetable proteins seem to be well tolerated. Arginine may be added in view of the apparent deficiency.

Tryptophan

Hartnup disease

This condition was first described in 1956 in 4 children of a single sibship. More than 20 other cases have been reported and the disease is named after the original family. It consists of a syndrome characterized by a pellagra-like dermatosis, temporary cerebellar ataxia and a constant renal aminoaciduria (p. 118).

There is a transport defect selective for monoamino-monocarboxylic amino acids with neutral or aromatic side chains. The defect is present in both kidney and intestine but the signs appear to be secondary to malabsorption of only one amino acid, tryptophan.

Nicotinamide, 40 to 250 mg daily, leads to striking improvement in the dermatosis and the neurological signs. Exposure to sunlight should be guarded against as the skin lesions are photosensitive. Temporary sterilization of the colon by neomycin has been suggested in order to reduce bacterial caboxylation of unabsorbed dietary amino acids and lessen absorption of indoles and other amines.

Other disorders

Defects in the transport or degradation of tryptophan have been described. None, surprisingly, cause pellagra. One, xanthurenic aciduria is pyridoxine-dependent (p. 122).

Histidine

Histidinaemia

This is an autosomal recessive trait which has been described in over 30 patients. There is diminished histidase (histidine α-deaminase) in tissues and the main degradative pathway to urocanic acid is blocked. By another pathway imidazole pyruvic acid is produced in excessive amounts.

The predominant clinical manifestations are mental retardation and disturbed speech although some untreated cases appeared unaffected on follow up.

Several groups have reported successful control of the biochemical abnormality by restriction of L-histidine intake to 25 mg/kg/day. Patients have tended to grow poorly on these restricted diets but it is not yet known whether this is due to the histidine restriction or to some other aspect of these artificial diets.

21. ENDOCRINE SYSTEM

A number of aspects of nutrient-endocrine interrelationships have been touched on in other sections. These include the hormonal control of metabolism (p. 69), endocrine changes in starvation and PEM (p. 106), obesity, (p. 152), diabetes mellitus (p. 183) and interrelationships of vitamin D, parathyroid hormone and calcitonin (p. 76). The nutritional effects or oral contraceptives are touched on later (p. 250).

In the present context it is intended to refer to the nutritional consequences of some of the major endocrine disorders.

PITUITARY AND HYPOTHALAMUS

Excessive secretion of growth hormone by the adenohypophysis (anterior pituitary) results in *gigantism* during development and *acromegaly* in the adult. The formation of lean body protein is favoured, with decreased levels of urea in blood and urine, and positive nitrogen balance.

Energy for protein anabolism comes largely from lipolysis in adipose tissue. Plasma NEFA and α- and β-lipoprotein levels rise.

Acromegalic patients often have diabetes mellitus and therefore need to be cared for from this point of view. Injections of growth hormone decrease glucose tolerance in normal subjects as well as in diabetic patients. While insulin and growth hormone appear to have divergent influences on intermediary metabolism, they are both required to prevent the nitrogen loss associated with diabetes.

Growth hormone influences mineral metabolism by causing retention of phosphorus, magnesium, potassium and sodium. Excessive amounts cause hypercalcaemia.

Hypopituitarism

Panhypopituitarism is associated with a low metabolic rate and anorexia. Fat stores are preserved due to the unopposed action of insulin and patients are susceptible to hypoglycaemia. When growth ceases, the requirements for hormones related to growth are reduced.

Diabetes insipidus

When antidiuretic hormone (ADH, vasopressin), secreted by the neuro-hypophysis (posterior pituitary), is deficient, a significant increase in water intake is necessary to offset polyuria. Diminished ADH output acts by decreasing the solute load and so causing energy deficiency dwarfism.

Hypothalmic and posterior pituitary disease

Abnormalities of these regions are rare causes of obesity. In *Froehlich's syndrome,* overeating and decreased activity are the most important factors in weight gain, but hypogonadotrophic hypogonadism plays a part in the characteristic distribution of fat.

Severe hunger results from destruction of the ventromedial nuclei of the hypothalamus. Tumours involving the lateral nucleus of the hypothalamus can cause cachexia and inanition.

THYROID

Hyperthyroidism (thyrotoxicosis)

Hyperthyroidism increases the need for all nutrients and energy. Intestinal absorption is stimulated and enzymatic reactions are accelerated. Excessive secretion catabolizes protein and fat. Decreased glucose tolerance is offset by an adequate insulin reserve in most hyperthyroid patients.

Hypothyroidism (myxoedema)

Iodine deficiency, if severe in infancy, may cause hypothyroidism and cretinism, but in the adult results only in simple goitre.

Metabolism is decreased and there is poor appetite, decreased intestinal absorption and constipation. There is fluid retention and mucopolysaccharide deposition in subcutaneous tissues.

Raised serum cholesterol results from a greater reduction in breakdown than in incorporation of acetate into cholesterol. Triglycerides are also elevated.

A mild anaemia often accompanies myxoedema. It usually responds to iron therapy together with thyroid hormone. Thyroid hormones facilitate the conversion of β-carotene and other pro-vitamin A carotenoids to vitamin A. In hypothyroidism, hypercarotenaemia may develop (p. 157).

ADRENAL

Cushing's syndrome results from excessive production of glucocorticoids. There is fluid retention, hypernatraemia and hypokalaemia. Gluconeogenesis is enhanced, resulting in catabolism of protein, amino acids are converted to glucose, nitrogen excretion is increased, and there is aminoaciduria. Hyperglycaemia results, and in time, with exhaustion of islet cell reserves, 'steroid diabetes' may be produced.

Hyperaldosteronism

This is an important, although rare, cause of hypertension. Aldosterone, secreted by the adrenal cortex, influences mainly mineral metabolism. It stimulates RNA synthesis of various enzymes that participate in sodium transport. Excessive secretion causes sodium retention and potassium loss. The hypokalaemia is associated with a metabolic acidosis.

Addison's disease

Deficiency of all adrenocortical steroids results in hyponatraemia, hyperkalaemia, and a defect in gluconeogenesis in the untreated patient. Weakness, weight loss, dehydration, anorexia, vomiting, diarrhoea and pigmentation of the skin are prominent features. Replacement therapy with cortisol and a mineralocorticoid corrects the deficits. Atrophy affecting both adrenals is the most common cause.

Phaeochromocytoma

This a rare tumour of the adrenal medulla.

Hypermetabolism results from the excessive secretion of catecholamines, producing increase in metabolic rate and in lipid breakdown and hyperglycaemia and usually presents as hypertension. Pellagra may result (p. 118).

GONADS

Hypogonadism in males

Testosterone is a powerful anabolic hormone and its absence depresses protein synthesis in muscle, bones and other organs. Androgens favour the development of lean body protein at the expense of fat breakdown.

Hypogonadism in females

Oestrogen deficiency elevates serum cholesterol and β-lipoproteins. It causes a mild catabolism of protein, especially in bone matrix, possibly related to osteoporosis (p. 217).

22. CARDIOVASCULAR SYSTEM

Atherosclerosis and its complications

Atherosclerosis derives its name from the combination of soft, lipid-rich material in the centre of typical intimal plaques (*athero:* porridge) combined with connective tissue and calcification (*sclerosis:* scarring). This process, commencing in the early years of life, appears to occur spontaneously only in the human species. It affects the medium and larger arteries of the body but clinical disease becomes manifest in those situations where marked narrowing of the lumen or thrombosis resulting in ischaemia or necrosis is especially likely to occur. In the coronary arteries this gives rise to three main syndromes of *coronary heart disease* (CHD): *myocardial infarction, angina pectoris* and *sudden unexpected death.* In the arteries of the neck and circle of Willis it results in *stroke* or *cerebrovascular accident;* either transient ischaemic attacks due to platelet microemboli or paralysis from infarction of brain tissue. In the leg arteries periphero-vascular disease causes *claudication* (pain on walking) or *gangrene.* In the renal arteries hypertension and renal failure may occur. Although the underlying pathological process appears to be common to all conditions the predisposing factors differ considerably and it will be necessary to deal with these separately in that connection.

The pathogenesis of the progression of atherosclerosis is complicated and ill-understood and a variety of hypotheses have been proposed that involve lipid infiltration (lipogenic), smooth muscle cell proliferation (myogenic), and mutagenic and thrombus formation (thrombogenic). It is probable that each of these factors is involved to some extent at various stages in the process.

The process of atherosclerosis has generally been regarded as inexorable, incapable of reversion, but experimental regression of atheromatous plaques with low cholesterol, high polyunsaturated fat intake provides some hope for similar improvement to be brought about in man.

Risk factors

These have been established on the basis of clinically manifest disease in longitudinal epidemiological studies and vary considerably according to the particular segment of the arterial system involved.

Age. Atherosclerosis is the majar cause of death in ageing populations and increasing age is the greatest risk factor although it is rarely listed as such.

Sex. CHD is about eight times more common in men than women but after the menopause the rate in women rises to equal that in men. However, sex steroid hormones are not protective; they actually cause excess mortality among men who have survived a heart attack.

Heredity. The concordance rate for CHD death is higher among monozygotic than dizygotic twins, as is serum cholesterol level. The heritability of serum cholesterol has been calculated to be 35 to 40 per cent. Body build, in which heredity plays an important role, is a relatively neglected factor. Mesomorphs are more vulnerable than other body types and android fat patterning predisposes (p. 152).

Hypertension. This is an important risk factor for both CHD and stroke, with its greatest effect on the cerebral arteries. It is associated especially with more severe atherosclerosis and increase in fibrous plaque formation. Obesity is frequently associated with high blood pressure and dietary management of overweight has been shown to be a most effective means of lowering blood pressure in such patients.

Obesity. From evidence provided by long-term epidemiological studies on a relatively fixed population such as that carried out in the town of Framingham, Massachussets it is considered that the effect of obesity on cardiovascular disease is mediated through its influence in raising blood lipids and blood pressure and impairing carbohydrate tolerance. In obese subjects who are 30 per cent over their ideal weight, the risk of developing cardiovascular disease CHD is 30 per cent greater.

Tobacco. Coronary heart disease is nearly three times greater in cigarette smokers than in non-smokers. Mortality in cigar, pipe and former cigarette smokers is about the same as in non-smokers. Cigarette smoking is also closely associated with peripheral vascular disease with intermittent claudication, and some studies have found greater incidence of stroke. Cigarette smoking seems to have an acute pharmacological action responsible for increase in sudden death and myocardial infarction by producing arrhythmias, myocardial ischaemia, decreased oxygen-carrying capacity of haemoglobin and possibly increased coagulability of the blood. Of all factors cigarette smoking alone will materially alter the risk of subsequent disease by a change at any age. This makes the cessation of cigarette smoking a very important element in the treatment of established coronary thrombosis and the discouragement of it in young people a key feature of prophylaxis. Recently even passive smokers have been noted to have an increased incidence of CHD.

Alcohol. There is evidence that CHD is less common in those who drink moderately. The postulated mechanism is that alcohol in mild to moderate doses stimulates hepatic VLDL clearance.

Diabetes mellitus. This disease confers an increased risk of the atherosclerotic diseases and there is increased severity of atherosclerosis in diabetics. Their serum lipids tend to be raised but this is not a sufficient explanation of the association. The dietary restriction of refined carbohydrate in the treatment of diabetes with an increased proportion of energy coming from complex carbohydrates and fat, especially if saturated, may play an important part.

Plasma lipids. The lipid in atheromatous arterial lesions is principally cholesterol and although the correlation between plasma and tissue concentrations of cholesterol is weak, determination in plasma is the only practical method. Even so, studies of populations in many countries and in individuals have shown a close correlation between plasma cholesterol levels and the occurrence of CHD. This is not true of stroke. Total body cholesterol has been shown to be proportional to body size and weight. The obese tend to have hypercholesterolaemia and levels can be lowered by weight reduction. Recent epidemiological evidence from the Framingham study, and confirmed elsewhere, shows that the negative correlation between HDL concentrations and CHD mortality are more important than positive correlations with plasma cholesterol or LDL. Even more recently some workers have suggested that apoproteins are more predictive than lipid fractions.

In a study of 500 3-month CHD survivors 31 per cent were found to be hyperlipidaemic as compared with healthy controls; 7.6 per cent had hypercholesterolaemia alone, 15.6 per cent hypertriglyceridaemia alone and 7.8 per cent both hypercholesterolaemia and hypertriglyceridaemia. In-depth family studies of these patients revealed that more than half had monogenic forms of hyperlipidaemia, thus emphasizing the importance of heredity. These hereditary forms contributed a disproportionate share of CHD in the young male.

Stress. A behaviour pattern has been described, characterized by an overwhelming sense of time urgency, aggressiveness, ambition and an excessive competetive drive, which seems to predispose to premature coronary heart disease. Association of this personality type with coronary heart disease has not invariably been found.

Exercise. Coronary heart disease has been shown to have a lower incidence and mortality among groups engaged in work with a moderate degree of physical activity than among those of sedentary occupation. In middle-aged men dying of causes other than coronary thrombosis it was found that myocardial fibrosis and occlusion of a main coronary artery were more common in those with the more sedentary occupations although the prevalence of coronary atherosclerosis was equally high in all groups. There is recent evidence that a programme of regular leisure time physical training helps to prevent coronary thrombosis. Mild physical exercise lowers the mortality rate in subjects who have had a heart attack, probably by improvement of myocardial function.

In certain Bantu tribes, the Samburu in Kenya and the Masai in Tanzania, physical activity appears to protect against the harmful effects of a diet of high fat content, for their serum lipid levels are low and they rarely develop coronary heart disease.

Although atherosclerosis is not uncommon, it is reported that their coronary arteries have wide lumens, perhaps as a consequence of high physical activity, and therefore less likely to be occluded by thrombus formation.

Drinking water. An inverse association has been found between drinking water hardness and cardiovascular death rates in several countries. The highest correlation is with the calcium and carbonate fraction.

Thrombogenesis. In recent years attention has again been paid to risk factors for abnormal clot formulation (thrombosis) in arteries. In particular, high levels of factor VII coagulant activity and plasma fibrinogen are strong indicators — according to some even more so than cholesterol — for coronary thrombosis. Cigarette smoking, probably, and diet, possibly, have their effects

The effects of all these risk factors are additive. Thus for the three major risk factors — blood cholesterol > 250 mg per cent, diastolic blood pressure > 90 mmHg and cigarette smoking (any number) — any one of these factors more than doubles the risk of a major coronary event. Two concurrent factors again doubled the risk, and the presence of all three factors doubled the risk yet again—to eight times the rate for those with none present. However, it must be realized that the survival rate over a 10-year period for the worst category, those with all three factors present, is 93 per cent, i.e. the risk of CHD for the high risk groups is not in absolute terms very high. Furthermore any measure, such as diet control which can only be expected to influence one of the factors, namely blood cholesterol, can have relatively little effect and cannot be expected to return the vascular tree to a pristine state.

For stroke, the four major aetiologically related diseases are diabetes mellitus, obesity, atherosclerosis and hypertension.

Diet and coronary heart disease

Diet composition

Data derived from WHO and FAO figures for food consumption and coronary heart disease deaths in men aged 55–59 years in 30 countries have shown significant positive correlations for the intake of animal protein, cholesterol, meat, total fat, eggs, sugar, total calories and animal fat. Significant negative correlations were found for intake of starch and vegetable protein.

Not all of the many intercountry and intercommunity studies that have been carried out agree with the evidence presented above. In general the closest relationship has been found with intake of saturated fat. Nevertheless when the intake of saturated fat within a given community of a developed country has been studied no such correlation has been demonstrated.

Small changes in dietary cholesterol intake, between 250 mg and 1.5 g per day, do not affect plasma cholesterol and larger intakes have only a temporary effect.

Sucrose intake has shown a high correlation in epidemiological studies, but if the calculations are made holding dietary fat consumption steady then the correlation disappears. There is also usually a correlation between sucrose consumed and cigarettes smoked.

It has been suggested that dietary fibre may reduce the reabsorption of cholesterol and there is epidemiological evidence for a negative correlation of dietary fibre content with CHD incidence. Human experiments over a few weeks have shown that lignin and pectin lower plasma cholesterol levels but that wheat fibre, cellulose and various gums fail to do so.

Intervention studies

These are extremely costly, very difficult to design and, if prospective, take many years to complete. Two of the larger have been MRFIT (Mulitple Risk Factor Intervention Trial) in the United States and the WHO European Collaborative Group Trial. Diet is only one of the risk factors taken account of and results have been difficult to interpret for various reasons, including the fact that compliance in the intervened group varies and the controls often change their life-style spontaneously. From studies such as these and the monitoring of blood cholesterol and other factors in large population groups it does appear that there are two, not necessarily mutually exclusive, approaches open for control measures. Most cases of CHD occur among the large numbers in whom risk factors are only moderately raised — only a mass (population) approach can help them. On the other hand, the 20 per cent or so who have very high risk factors can be dealt with more readily, although the yield will be much less. To some extent there is a debate as to which method should be adopted. In the case of diet the issue is further complicated by the conflicting opinions of the experts (p. 282).

A further factor has been introduced recently by the evidence that Greenland eskimos have an extremely low incidence of CHD. This seems to be attributable to their diet which is high in fish such as cod and mackerel rich in polyunsaturated oils containing ω 3 fatty acids (eicosapentaenoic, EPA, and docosahexaenoic, DHA, fatty acids). Experimentally it has been shown that these oils reduce platelet aggregation and may thus prevent thrombus formation.

Trends. Cardiovascular disease as discussed here is the major health problem in western societies today. It has been on the increase over the past 50 years or so to reach this position. However, there are signs, at least as far as CHD in the United States and some other countries, is concerned, that the peak has been passed. Mortality figures began to take a downward trend after 1968 and this has been maintained since then. The reasons are not known but several factors are probably involved. There is greater attention being paid to diet in relation to obesity, and hyperlipidaemia; smoking is declining among males, but not in young females, and more people are taking exercise. Even so there is evidence that improved child health has enhanced physiological age and contributed to the trend.

Cardiomyopathies

This term embraces a heterogeneous collection of heart conditions in which the heart muscle is affected and sometimes both pericardium and endo-cardium are also involved. Some instances are secondary to a serious infection or deficiency disease such as beriberi, but the primary form has no evident ae-tiology. *Endomyocardial fibrosis* has been reported from several parts of Africa, from Asia and Jamaica. The process predominantly affects the endocardium of the apices of the ventricles, extending into the posterior cusps of the atrioventricular valves.

Essential hypertension

Hypertension may be secondary to a known cause, such as kidney or endocrine disorder, but more frequently it is 'essential'. The blood pressure of healthy young adults is about 120 mmHg systolic and 80 mmHg diastolic. There is usually a slow rise with advancing age. However, this rise may be pathological and related to the occurrence of obesity and atherosclerosis for among some so-called 'primitive' communities it does not occur. Their salt intake has also been shown to be low (<10 mmol/day compared with the usual range of 100 to 250 mmol in the West).

Some individuals with mild hypertension respond to salt restriction and are thought to have a sensitivity to high salt intake, while others do not. Lowering of the blood pressure may be brought about by weight reduction. Although stress cannot be avoided, learning to cope with it through biofeedback has demonstrated beneficial effects. In severe hypertension salt restriction to 1 to 2g per day should be combined with drug treatment to assist sodium excretion.

Hypertension is defined as a diastolic pressure (PD) of over 90 mmHg. This number was determined by using life insurance tables indicating an increase in mortality and morbidity among those with PDs over 90. A systolic pressure (PS) greater than 140 is also associated with hypertension.

In the US, 25 per cent over 30 years of age are said to have hypertension. But one-third of them have PDs and PSs in the normal range if tested at home, when relaxed and at different times of the day. Usually BP peaks between 9 and 10 a.m. and falls off during the afternoon. The peak in BP is closely related to the daily peak incidence of myocardial infarction.

The treatment of hypertension is directed at controlling PD, although the Framingham study found that PS is more closely associated with morbidity. Before resorting to drug treatment it is best to fist advise exercise, weight reduction, relaxation, biofeedback and dietary modification. Not all patients respond to salt restriction.

The dietary requirement for Na^+ is 1 to 2 g/day, while the average salt intake in the US is 4 to 8 g/day (1 g salt = 43 mEq or 17.1 mmol Na^+). Thus, the average American consumes about 4 times the Na^+ intake needed. More than 50 per cent of dietary sodium comes from meat and grain. Dairy products are relatively high in Na^+, while breakfast cereals also contain about 300 mg Na^+ per ounce. Thus, a treatment of hypertension is the restriction of sodium intake to 2 g/day, which leads to BP control in 30 to 40 per cent of patients with mild hypertension and a decrease in the amount of medication needed by 50 per cent of patients with high BP.

Other elements have been linked to the cause and treatment of hypertension. Both calcium excess as well as calcium deficiency may exacerbate or alleviate hypertension. The ability of oral calcium supplements to lower blood pressure in some subjects with essential hypertension not only emphasizes the link between hypertensive disease and clinical aspects of calcium metabolism, but also suggests the possibility of increased calcium intake as a primary treatment for hypertension.

The circumstantial evidence supporting the association of Ca^{++} and hypertension are: (1) Ca^{++} is the primary ion responsible for making water 'hard'. The incidence of cardiovascular morbidity and mortality is decreased in areas with hard water. (2) Blacks in the US have a higher incidence of hypertension. They also often are lactase deficient and therefore consume less milk and other dairy products which contain a high Ca^{++} amount. (3) Pregnant women consuming less than 0.5 g Ca^{++} per day were found to have a 20-fold increase in the prevalence of gestational hypertension.

The average recommended Ca^{++} intake is 800 mg/day. There are no specific dietary recommendations concerning Ca^{++} and hypertension, but low renin hypertensives may respond to dietary Ca^{++} supplementation because Ca^{++} is linked to excitation-contraction coupling.

The evidence concerning K^+ is circumstantial. A high K^+ diet also often means a diet low in Na^+, so it is difficult to determine which factor helps keep BP low. The mechanism involving K^+ may include lowered renin and angiotensin receptor levels. There is no evidence that K^+ supplementation helps the majority of hypertensives.

There is no hard evidence concerning the effects of trace metals (e.g. Zn, Cu, Fe), fibre, or simple sugars. Coffee increases PS by 5 to 10 mmHg 1 to 2 hours after drinking a cup, but it is not known if it has long-term effects.

Excessive alcohol consumption is definitely linked to hypertension. The mechanism is unknown. A theory is that heavy drinkers often stop drinking for a day or two before a doctor's visit. This could produce a state of mild withdrawal, making them hyperadrenergic. The increase in BP is not related to excess calories or salt ingested; it may be linked to the effects of Ca^{++}. Alcohol may lead to structural changes in cell membranes. A change in the membrane of arteriolar smooth muscle may allow excessive amounts of Ca^{++} to enter the cells, increasing the excitation and thus contraction of the cells.

Congestive heart failure

In mild congestive heart failure there is breathlessness on effort and puffiness of the ankles noticed in the evening. At this stage considerable improvement can be expected from a reducing diet. When the cardiac decompensation is severe there is breathlessness on slightest exertion and oedema becomes generalized. Oedema is due to increased venous pressure and retention of sodium. If the intake of sodium is moderately restricted and a diuretic is used there is no need to reduce water intake below 1½ or 2 litres daily. With appropriate drug treatment a restricted salt regime providing 1 to 2 g sodium (40 to 80 mEq) daily may be persisted in for some months without life becoming unbearable. Almost all processed foods are rich in sodium, as are cereal products. Fresh unprocessed food such as meat, fish, eggs, milk and vegetables are moderate sources. Fruits and unprocessed cereals contain very little sodium. On a restricted regime table salt is not permitted and it should not be used in cooking. Rich sources must be avoided and moderate sources used in small amounts.

Varicose veins

Dilatation and tortuosity of the superficial leg veins occur when the deep saphenous system becomes thrombosed and occluded. The condition is much more common in developed than in developing countries and this may be related to constipation and pressure from an overloaded colon associated with the differences in fibre content of the diet (p. 50).

Pulmonary embolism and deep venous thrombosis

Thrombosis in the deep veins of the legs may be associated with the rise in intra-abdominal pressure in pregnancy and the enforced inactivity of patients undergoing surgery. Embolism to the lungs is a serious complication, frequently fatal if sufficiently massive to block the major vessels. These conditions are also more common in western countries and may be related to colonic stasis consequent upon a low-fibre diet.

23. RENAL SYSTEM

Through glomerular filtration and subsequent selective reabsorption and tubular secretion, the constituents of urine are finally obtained from the blood. In this way waste products of metabolism, such as urea, creatinine and toxic substances, are eliminated and water, electrolyte, and acid-base equilibrium is maintained.

Acute and chronic renal failure

This generally occurs as a secondary event to shock from acute blood loss, surgery or trauma. The increased metabolic requirements of stress and injury are dicussed on p. 231. Nutritional management should be directed to meet the increased energy requirement of the stress situation (35 to 45 kcal/kg body weight) by providing equal amounts of glucose and fat. In patients who are being dialysed protein requirements should be 0.8 g/kg/day to meet reparative needs of stress and injury. If these patients are unable to eat, energy is provided intravenously as total parenteral alimentation (p. 238).

Because of oliguria, fluid intake is restricted and, thus, the intravenous solutions need to by hyperconcentrated in order to provide the appropriate total calories as glucose and fat, and protein requirements as amino acids, in a smaller volume. All the electrolytes usually added to the solution are also needed in addition to vitamins. Phosphate is needed to avoid the risk of hypophosphataemia since this is more of a threat than mild hyperphosphataemia. Magnesium and other electrolytes are added to replace losses or deficits.

Under these cirumstances, acute renal failure generally lasts for 8 to 14 days following which a gradual return to normal renal function and urine output occurs. During the latter period fluid requirements are increased to replace fluid losses, and the hyperalimentation solution does not need to be hyperconcentrated.

For patients who develop chronic renal failure or who have chronic renal failure and develop an acute illness but do not require dialysis, energy requirements remain unchanged (cf. acute renal failure). Protein intake would need to be modified to provide 0.6 g/kg/day. In either acute or chronic renal failure 80 per cent of the protein intake should be of high biological value. If the patient's condition mandates dialysis the patient is generally encouraged to eat a balanced diet with the knowledge that extra fluid and by-products of metabolism will be removed during dialysis.

Acute glomerulonephritis

Protein should not be restricted unless oliguria or anuria develops. Sodium restriction is only necessary if urine output falls.

Chronic glomerulonephritis

In the absence of renal failure or other complications, no special dietary restriction is necessary. Salt should not be routinely restricted. If there is unrecognized salt-losing nephritis this can lead to hypovolaemia, with hypotension and aggravate renal failure.

Nephrosis

This syndrome, characterized by proteinuria, hypoalbuminaemia and hypercholesterolaemia may result from many causes of an infectious, toxic or allergic nature. These underlying conditions have to be treated. The diet should be high in protein, sufficient to maintain positive nitrogen balance. Calcium and potassium supplements are usually necessary. Salt restriction, to about 0. 5g daily, will prevent oedema and initiate diuresis.

Uraemia

Renal uraemia is most commonly due to disease affecting the kidney. In *prerenal uraemia* there is no primary disease of the kidney, but its functioning is affected by such states as water and salt depletion, shock, or haemorrhage. *Postrenal uraemia* results from obstruction in the renal tract, as in prostatic hypertrophy.

Acute uraemia is an emergency and the patient's life is always in danger. Initially, during the period of oliguria or anuria protein intake should be virtually nil. The daily intake of sugar should be at least 100 g to prevent weight loss due to catabolism of tissues. If the renal failure is mild and short lasting a limited intake of 20 g good quality protein should be given daily. If there is severe infection or excessive tissue damage the blood urea and potassium may rise and vomiting and mental confusion ensue. A blood urea of 250 mg/100ml or more and serum potassium of 7.5 mEq/1 or more are indications for haemodialysis.

The dietetic management of chronic uraemia is the same, whatever the underlying cause. If oedema is present, salt restriction is necessary. Generally fluid restriction is contraindicated because of the impaired concentrating power of the kidney. Occasionally in chronic nephritis there is an excessive loss of salt in the urine due to failure of tubular reabsorption, and additional salt up to 5 to 10 g/day is necessary.

In recent years attention has been focussed upon the management of patients with chronic uraemia by diets severely restricted in protein. This approach was pioneered in Italy with energy coming mainly from special low-protein biscuits and pasta manufactured in Italy and supplemented by items such as butter, jam, green leafy vegetables and fruit. The protein intake is about 20 g/day. Patients have been found not to tolerate well a very restricted protein intake. Important causes of the intolerance have been found to be the absence of meat and milk, the monotony of the foods, and the difficulty of preparing high energy—low protein foods.

Haemodialysis raises certain problems concerning dietary management, and the concept of low total protein diet high in essential amino acids has been developed to try to overcome these. The basic 20 g protein diet results in negative nitrogen balance due to dialysate nitrogen losses. Nitrogen balance is maintained by 0.75 g/kg body weight of high quality protein. This level of protein intake gives a lower urea level, higher serum albumin, fewer episodes of headache, nausea and vomiting during dialysis, and the need for briefer periods of dialysis. It is not yet clear whether the combination really prolongs life.

One diet formulation for uraemia consists of whey protein (lactalbumin) subjected to decaseination and electrodialysis to remove electrolytes. Neutralizing with calcium hydroxide increases the calcium content and the sodium and potassium contents can be made negligible.

On the basis that ammonium derived from urea breakdown in the gut could be utilized for protein synthesis by feeding the nitrogen-free ketoanalogues of some of the essential amino acids considerable nitrogen utilization has been achieved in uraemia.

Patients on regular dialysis become deficient in most vitamins and elements and regular supplements should be given. A group of bone disorders, referred to collectively as renal osteodystrophy, commonly occurs. Control of serum phosphate levels and maintenance of calcium balance are important measures. Impaired vitamin D metabolism is sometimes responsible (p. 140).

Other disturbances of metabolism in uraemia include glucose intolerance and hypertriglyceridaemia. The effect of insulin on glucose uptake appears to be blunted. The hypertriglyceridaemia in uraemia seems to result from both increased endogenous synthesis and impaired removal. The effect is exaggerated in haemodialysis patients.

Urinary lithiasis

This is not a single condition, but is divisible broadly on the basis of the chemical composition of the stones and on their location in the urinary tract. Urinary calculi are rarely 'pure' (e.g. cystine, see p. 195) but are usually composed of a number of chemical constituents. Most common among these are various urates and various calcium salts, especially oxalate, carbonate and phosphate.

All over the world urinary calculi form with considerable frequency, possibly more commonly in hot climates as a result of urine concentration, in kidneys, ureters, bladder and urethra. The urine of stone-formers has been found to be more saturated with respect to calcium oxalate than normal. Diet has not been shown to play a part in this form of stone disease. Hypercalciuria is frequently found and in some instances hyperparathyroidism is responsible.

Isolated bladder stone is quite a different problem, with stones composed largely of urates and calcium oxalate. Males are more affected than females, possible because of differences in the bladder outlet, and many cases occur in young boys. It seems to have been sufficiently common in the time of Hippocrates for lithotomy to have been a specialty with whose rights physicians promised not to interfere when they recited the Hippocratic oath.

Occurrence of bladder stone has changed greatly during the last century or so. Certain classic 'bladder stone areas', such as the fen district in England, the Netherlands, the New York area and Beirut, hardly see a case nowadays.

The aetiology of this condition remains obscure. Bladder stone patients do not exhibit any of the features of nutritional deficiency disease, and the bladder stone areas and the occurrence of nutritional deficiencies do not coincide. There does not appear to be any common dietary factor that links together all the foci of bladder stone. Wheat, millet, or rice may be the staple of such an area.

The aetiology of bladder stone has been intensively studied in recent years in Ubol, north Thailand, one of the most important foci of its occurrence. Oxalate crystaluria is common in urine of villagers but not of city inhabitants. High dietary phytate may cause phosphate depletion and supplementation has reduced oxalate crystalluria and clinical episodes.

At the present time the treatment of urinary calculi of all kinds is surgical. General measures include an adequate fluid intake, alkalinization of the urine, and restriction of foods of high purine content (liver, kidney and sweetbread) in the case of urate stones.

24. BLOOD

Iron, folic acid, vitamin B_{12}, vitamin B_6, ascorbic acid, vitamin E and copper and protein are of proven importance in haemopoietic disorders. The first three have been reviewed (pp. 141/124/126).

Protein

Anaemia is not a constant feature of even severe kwashiorkor or marasmus (p. 000). It is usually of the normocytic or slightly macrocytic type. The bone marrow is hypocellular and fatty. Granulocytes and platelets are not affected.

Protein deficiency may contribute to the macrocytosis commonly seen in chronic liver disease but folate deficiency is often responsible.

Vitamins

Niacin. The anaemia seen sometimes in pellagra is usually due to deficiency of iron or some other nutrient.

Riboflavin. Although dietary deficiency in man is not generally recognized to produce anaemia one claim has been made for its efficacy in the anaemia of kwashiorkor. Deficiency induced by the antagonist, galactoflavin has been reported to lead to erythrocytic hypoplasia (see p. 120).

Vitamin B_6. An increasing number of instances of microcytic hypochromic and of megaloblastic anaemia responsive to vitamin B_6 is being reported. Some are secondary to malabsorption, few seem to be purely dietary and some are familial and may be due to dependency (see p. 122).

Vitamin C. Anaemia in scurvy and the occasional relationship to folate deficiency have been referred to (see p. 130).

Fat-soluble vitamins. The evidence for a role for vitamin E in anaemia has been reviewed (see p. 135).

Hypervitaminosis A causes hepatosplenomegaly, anaemia and leuco-poenia. Vitamin D excess, by causing metastatic calcification in the kidneys, can lead to the anaemia of chronic renal disease. Vitamin K analogues induce haemolytic anaemia in infants with glucose-6 phosphate dehydrogenase (G-6PD) deficiency.

Elements

Other than iron, there is deficiency of only one element that has been definitely incriminated in anameia in man — copper (p. 146).

25. NERVOUS SYSTEM

Different parts of the nervous system tend to be affected by different nutrient deficiencies. The brain appears to be permanently affected in protein-energy malnutrition if the deficiency takes place in intra-uterine (p. 251) or very early postnatal life (p. 252). Mental changes, including alteration in the e.e.g. are commonly found in the acute state of kwashiorkor (p. 105).

Anorexia nervosa. This insidious disease is characterized by a complex psychiatric disturbance, usually in adolescent women (occasionally in young men), resulting in gradual weight loss due to chronic inadequate caloric intake leading to gross inanition.

The basis of the disorder appears to be phobia concerning the increase in weight at puberty and a consequent avoidance of food. There is a characteristic triad of disturbed attitudes which assists in the diagnosis and the management.

1. In spite of extreme emaciation the patient has such a disturbance of body image that she denies being excessively thin.

2. In spite of prolonged inanition she denies ever being hungry.

3. In spite of frantic and usually ritualized exercise she denies fatigue.

Other useful diagnostic criteria include secondary amenorrhoea, with low gonadotrophin levels but normal thyroid function.

In psychological terms the illness has been attributed to oral sadistic, cannibalistic and oral impregnation fantasies which are denied by refusal of food and by defeminization of the body through weight loss. In addition to food avoidance, laxatives, enemas, or self-induced vomiting may be resorted to. In the early stage foods that are high in carbohydrate are avoided. In some patients this avoidance breaks down periodically and they may pass through intermittent bulimia (increased appetite) to recovery. They may vomit in relation to the bulimic episodes and thus avoid weight gain. Amenorrhoea develops early in these patients and long precedes the state of panhypopituitarism which is generally considered to be secondary rather than primary in nature. A rather precise weight threshold of 44 kg has been found to be associated with lack of response of the pituitary.

Two forms have been indentified by some. In the *histrionic* type the patient should be isolated from the family and a good doctor-patient relationship established. The prognosis is favourable. The *obsessoid* type carries a higher mortality and prefrontal leucotomy may be necessary. Group and behavioural therapy should be tried.

This condition needs to be differentiated from chronic illnesses of adolescence including juvenile diabetes mellitus, Crohn's disease, hypopituitarism and neoplasms.

The early management consists of measures aimed at overcoming the aberrations in the attitude of the patient towards her own body. An injection of 5 units of soluble insulin before meals, causing mild hypoglycaemia, may stimulate the appetite. As emergency measures as much as 150 mg to 1 g chlorpromazine daily and 5 to 40 units of soluble insulin may be necessary. The dosage can be reduced once a daily intake of about 4000 kcal (16.76 MJ) has been reached. When all else fails these patients have been successfully supported by total parenteral hyperalimentation.

Vitamins

Cerebral symptoms are a prominent feature of acute and severe deficiency of thiamin (p. 115), niacin (p. 118) and pyridoxine (p. 121). Peripheral neuropathy charcterizes dry beriberi (p. 114), but other B vitamins are sometimes involved.

Vitamin B_{12} deficiency, whether dietary or due to lack of intrinsic factor, may involve the peripheral nerves as subacute combined degeneration of the cord or some cases of nutritional amblyopia (p. 126).

Hypervitaminosis A causes cerebral symptoms (p. 156) and hypervitaminosis D and K damage the brain (pp. 157, 158).

Elements

Iodine lack produces cretinism with mental retardation in severe deficiency (p. 144). Copper deficiency in Menkes' syndrome (p. 146) and toxicity in Wilson's disease (p. 161) are associated with brain damage. Lead causes encephalopathy in high doses and at lower levels may be responsible for some instances of hyperactivity in children (p. 26).

Metabolic disorders

Several aminoacidopathies, most notably phenylketonuria, may lead to brain damage (p. 193). Galactosaemia may cause mental retardation (p. 185) and cerebellar ataxia is a feature of a-β-lipoproteinaemia (p. 188) and Refsum's disease (p. 191).

Other conditions

Depression. Tryptophan has a key role in brain metabolism as precursor of the neurotransmitter 5-hydroxytryptamine (p. 36). Claims have been made for the relief of depression by oral tryptophan. The best substantiated evidence is for response to pyridoxine (involved in tryptophan metabolism, p. 56) of depression assoicated with pyridoxine deficiency in women taking oral contraceptives.

Schizophrenia appears to have a metabolic basis. Multivitamin therapy, based on the 'orthomolecular' concept of Pauling, awaits controlled evaluation. The increased incidence in patients with coeliac disease (p. 188) has led to claims of improvement on a gluten-free regime.

Multiple sclerosis is a progressive demyelinating disorder of the nervous system of uncertain aetiology. Serum linoleic acid levels have been reported to be low. Oral therapy with this essential fatty acid (p. 34) has generally lessened the duration and severity of relapses but not affected overall disability. Others have claimed improvement with a gluten-free diet.

26. SKIN

Starvation

Atrophic changes in skin and hair are characteristic signs in subjects of experimental stravation, victims of famine and prisoners of war (p. 98), marasmus in children (p. 101) and anorexia nervosa (p. 213).

Kwashiorkor

The 'crazy paving' dermatosis and hair changes are among the most characteristic clinical features of this disease (p. 102).

Vitamin deficiencies

Their role in dermatology has been referred to previously: vitamin A (p. 109), nicotinic acid (p. 121), riboflavin (p. 121), pyridoxine (p. 121), vitamin B_{12} (p. 127), pantothenic acid (p. 128), biotin (p. 129), vitamin C (p. 131), and essential fatty acids (p. 136).

Perifollicular hyperkeratosis (phrynoderma or toad skin)

The skin is generally dry and around the hair follicles on the affected parts there are small, hard, elevated papules, giving the skin a 'nutmeg grater' texture. The follicles may be filled with keratotic plugs. This appearance was originally described in patients who had xerophthalmia. The condition has been attributed to vitamin A deficiency. Others have claimed response to linoleic acid or to vitamins of the B complex. Like most nutritional signs, hyperfollicular keratosis is probably of multiple aetiology and many instances are not nutritional at all.

Acne vulgaris

A high carbohydrate intake and especially chocolate have been blamed. Double-blind studies have failed to incriminate any special dietary factor.

Retinoids (synthetic vitamin A-like compounds) are first choice treatement for severe acne and several other non-nutritional epidermal diseases, including some forms of skin cancer.

27. CONNECTIVE TISSUE

The chief members of the group of diseases affecting connective tissue are rheumatoid arthritis, rheumatic fever, systemic lupus erythematosus, sclerodema and polyarteritis nodosa. Although in none of them is a nutritional factor aetiologically involved, certain points of importance with regard to diet need to be emphasized.

Rheumatoid arthritis is a severe, crippling, generalized disease. It is often accompanied by marked weight loss and muscle wasting, fatigue and anorexia. Under these circumstances it is extremely difficult to maintain an adequate intake of protein and energy. These patients need small frequent meals with careful supervision. Community programmes to provide meals for those who are house-bound, and admission to long-term care institutions, have to be considered. About 5 per cent of patients with rheumatoid arthritis have involvement of the temporomandibular joints, and a soft or semiliquid diet may prove necessary. An uncommon complication, Sjögren's disease, with lacrimal and salivary gland atrophy, may make mastication especially difficult.

Scleroderma involving the oesophagus causes loss of extensibility and peristaltic movement. In the advanced stage a soft or semiliquid diet is necessary. The marked anorexia can lead to malnutrition and even death. Difficulty may even be experienced in opening the mouth because of the tight atrophic skin of the face. Retention of calcium in subcutaneous tissues. Restriction of intake of these minerals is indicated when calcification is widespread.

28. SKELETAL SYSTEM

The bones form about 15 per cent of the body weight or 10 kg in a 65 kg man. Of this about 2 kg is protein and 1.5 kg calcium. This amounts to 99 per cent of the total calcium in the body. The extracellular matrix of bone constitutes about 35 per cent of the tissue by weight and the inorganic mineral phase the remainder. Collagen accounts for 90 to 95 per cent of the bone matrix.

Hydroxyproline is an amino acid present almost exclusively and in high concentration in collagen in bone and connective tissue. It appears in the urine, mainly in peptide form, in proportion to the degree of collagen turnover and reflects growth in the child. The output is diminished in all forms of severe PEM and in failure to thrive (p. 106).

The bones show typical lesions in several nutritional disease. Deficiency of vitamin D results in a failure of the normal process of mineral deposition with the lack of calcification of performed bone matrix leading to rickets in the child and osteomalacia in the adult (p. 133)

In scurvy there is an impairment of synthesis of collagen in bone matrix and bone formation is greatly retarded (p. 131). The shafts of the long bones are thickened in hypervitaminosis A (p. 156). Bone growth is retarded in protein energy malnutrition (p. 102).

Osteoporosis

This denotes a diminished bone mass as compared with total bone volume. It is the most common metabolic bone disease, especially affecting the elderly. As determined by cortical thickness the process begins at about 35 years of age and among those who survive to 90 years of age the total loss amounts to 20 per cent in men and 30 per cent in women. It occasionally arises secondary to other diseases. Much more commonly it is idiopathic. There is no biochemical evidence of protein or calcium deficiency, or calcium/phosphorus imbalance in the elderly. Nevertheless there is evidence that calcium absorption diminishes with age and an intake of at least 1 g/day is now generally recommended. Osteoporosis is marked in ovarian agenesis and eunuchoid males and oestrogens stimulate osteoblast activity. Women receiving oestrogens postmenopausally have a reduced risk of fractures, although their long-term administration is not without its dangers. However, bone loss commences long before the menopause. Habitual inactivity in the aged may play a part as bone loss characterizes bed rest, immobilization of a limb and space travel. Some cases have been reported to respond to 1 a 25(OH)D. Fracture is the principal clinical manifestation and three syndromes have been described: lower forearm fracture mostly in women aged 50 to 65, fracture of the proximal femur in both sexes over the age of 70, and the relatively rare vertebral crush fracture syndrome presenting at any age but commonest in elderly women. All are associated with negative calcium balance, not from dietary deficiency but such causes as hypercalciuria in postmenopausal women or malabsorption in old age. There is no satisfactory treatment at present.

29. EYE

Various aspects of vitamin A deficiency have been fully covered elsewhere (p. 109).

B complex vitamins

Anterior segment. Vascularization of the cornea in man and certain other ocular signs were originally reported to respond to riboflavin. Subsequently many workers reported a high incidence of circumcorneal injection and corneal vascularization in groups receiving a reasonably adequate diet. This was due to misunderstanding of the normal variations in the vascular pattern of the limbic plexus. True vascularization of the cornea is an infrequent manifestation of hyporiboflavinosis in man.

A superficial keratitis in malnourished individuals, to which the name 'corneal epithelial dystrophy' was given, has also been attributed to deficiency of B vitamins, especially riboflavin.

Posterior segment. In nutritional amblyopia (nutritional retrobulbar neuropathy) the symptomatology is characterized by blurring of vision for both near and distant objects, often accompanied by photophobia and retrobulbar pain. Visual field examination reveals central or centrocaecal scotomas with little or no peripheral contraction. Many hundreds of cases occurred in the Far Eastern prisoner-of-war camps in World War II, leaving varying degrees of visual disability short of complete blindness. Under these conditions of special privation and also in several endemic foci, notably in Jamaica and Nigeria, the damage to the optic nerve was but part of a generalized neuropathy. Some cases have appeared to respond well to riboflavin, and others to vitamin B_{12} (p. 126). Tobacco-alcohol amblyopia is an identical syndrome in which cyanide from heavy pipe smoking may induce nutritional deficiency, especially of vitamin B_{12} which is effective as hydroxocobalamin.

Wernicke's encephalopathy, due to acute thiamin deficiency, occurs under prison camp conditions and in the terminal stages of chronic alcoholism. Ocular features include nystagmus, external rectus fatigue and paralysis, complete disconjugate wandering, loss of visual acuity and papilloedema (p. 116). A similar syndrome responds dramatically to niacin (p. 118).

Other eye conditions

Discrete colliquative keratapathy is the term applied by the writer to a mysterious disease of the cornea, first described in malnourished Bantu children in South Africa. The strictly localized area of corneal softening in an otherwise normal eye is distinct from the generalized keratinization and softening of keratomalacia.

Malnutrition and trachoma. The consensus of clinical opinion is that the corneal complications of trachoma progress more rapidly in the malnourished than the well-nourished subject, but cachectic children seem to be particularly immune to contracting infection. It may be that their conjunctivae lack certain enzyme systems essential for the virus.

Cataract has a higher incidence and earlier age of onset among the peoples of Asia and Africa than North America and Europe. Vitamin therapy has proved ineffective. It is possible that the cataract described in young malnourished adults in Indonesia is of nutritional origin.

Refractive errors. Whether environmental factors can influence refraction is not known; circumstantial evidence that they may do so is accumulating. A high incidence of myopia has been reported from a famine area in Tanzania, although the refraction of similar tribes in other parts of the country is normal. Both premature infants and marasmic infants are more myopic than normal controls. After infants recover from marasmus their eye refraction returns to normal, indicating a temporary disturbance in ocular dynamics rather than an effect on the growth of the eye.

30. TEETH

The enamel contains no capillary or lymph vessels for transport of nutrients.

When a tooth is improperly formed during development or when a portion is destroyed by decay or injury, it has no ability to repair the loss. When the tooth erupts, the blood supply to the enamel is cut and it comes into intimate contact with the environment of the oral cavity containing saliva, micro-organisms, food and epithelial debris. The tooth is in an especially vulnerable position with regard to adverse environmental, including nutritional, influences. Coronal caries has increased from the late 19th century coincident with the increased consumption of refined carbohydrate. *Streptococcus mutans* may play a part as it is more prevalent in carious lesions than in normal teeth and has been shown to cause caries in monkeys fed a high-sugar diet.

Vitamins. Vitamin A deficiency results in degeneration and atrophy of ameloblasts, as it does of other epithelial cells. Ameloblasts organize the epithelium which gives rise to odontoblasts, which consequently fail to differentiate and are arranged abnormally. Enamel hypoplasia is a consequence of these changes.

Gingival changes are a striking feature of scurvy and are described on page 131. Changes in the teeth in human scurvy, have been described. The dentine is resorbed and porotic, the pulp is atrophic and hyperaemic, and there is degeneration of osteoblasts, cyst formation, and foci of diverticulae of calcification.

Vitamin D deficiency and disturbance of the calcium/phosphorus ratio of the diet influence the development of teeth as well as of bones. First there is a line of disturbed calcification in the dentine. There is consequently retarded formation of predentine, and disturbance in calcification of dentine and cementum. The jaws undergo changes similar to those seen in other bones.

Elements. Among these the most important is fluorine, both in excess as the cause of the changes of fluorosis, and in deficiency in predisposing to caries (see pp. 145 and 160).

Selenium is reported to increase susceptibility to caries, while molybdenum and vanadium may have a beneficial effect.

Gingivitis and pyorrhoea. Although they may be associated with deficiency states there is no good evidence that they have a nutritional origin.

MULTIPLE CHOICE QUESTIONS

Answer each question true *or* false

1. In coronary heart disease:
   i) the major risk factors are cigarette smoking, high blood cholesterol and obesity
   ii) atherosclerosis can be reversed by a diet low in saturated fat
   iii) a low incidence is associated with a diet high in eicosapentaenoic acid
   iv) a high incidence is found in those with a high energy intake
   v) plasma HDL is usually raised.

2. Osteoporosis:
    i) is usually due to vitamin D deficiency
    ii) is more common after the age of 60 in women than in men
    iii) results in bending, rather than fracture, of bone
    iv) can be relieved after the menopause by female sex hormone therapy
    v) is accompanied by marked impairment of calcium absorption.

3. Hypertension:
    i) has a proven genetic component
    ii) is about 90 per cent of unknown aetiology
    iii) incidence in different countries correlates closely with salt intake
    iv) has close associations with cerebrovascular disease and diabetes mellitus
    v) is common in communities with a high potassuim intake.

4. Skin changes:
    i) are common in thiamin deficiency
    ii) are increasingly being treated with retinoids
    iii) of scurvy consist of petichiae and ecchymoses
    iv) do not occur in vitamin B_{12} deficiency
    v) of kwashiorkor may be due to zinc deficiency.

5. The following statements relate to nutrition and the nervous system:
    i) In anorexia nervosa gonadotrophin levels are low and thyroid function is normal
    ii) Multivitamin therapy of schizophrenia has proved to be beneficial
    iii) Excess vitamin A, D and K can all damage the brain
    iv) Copper deficiency causes neurological damage in Wilson's disease
    v) The e.e.g. is often abnormal in kwashiorkor.

Explanation and answers on page 286.

FURTHER READING

17. Introduction
Beck M E 1975 Nutrition and dietetics for nurses, 4th edn. Churchill Livingstone, Edinburgh
Dickerson J W T, Lee H A (eds) 1978 Nutrition in the clinical management of disease. Arnold, London
University of Iowa Hospitals and Clinics 1973 Recent advances in therapeutic diets, 2nd edn. Iowa State University Press, Ames, Iowa

18. Nutritional assessment
Jelliffe D B, Jelliffe E F P 1983 Assessment of nutritional states. Oxford University Press, Oxford

19. Gastrointestinal system
Royal College of Physicians of London 1980 Medical aspects of dietary fibre. Pitman Medical, Tunbridge Wells

20. Metabolic disorders
Jovanovic L, Peterson C M 1985 Nutrition and diabetes. Alan R Liss Inc, New York
McLaren D S, Burman D (eds) 1982 In: Textbook of paediatric nutrition, 2nd edn., ch 13–16. Churchill Livingstone, Edinburgh
Wood F C Jr, Bierman E L 1986 Is diet the cornerstone in management of diabetes? New England Journal of Medicine 315: 1224–1227

22. Cardiovascular system
COMA 1984 Diet and cardiovascular disease. HMSO, London
Denton D 1982 The hunger for salt: an anthropological, physiological and medical analysis. Springer, Berlin
Glomset J A 1985 Fish, fatty acids, and human health. New England Journal of Medicine 312 : 1253
Hazzard W R 1976 Aging and atherosclerosis: interactions with diet, heredity, and longevity and aging. Academic Press, New York

25. Nervous system
Bruch H 1978 The golden age, the enigma of anorexia nervosa. Open Books, London
Dickerson J W T 1978 Nutrition and disorders of the nervous system. In: Dickerson J W T, Lee H A (eds) Nutrition in the clinical management of disease. Arnold, London

28. Skeletal system
Schaafsma G, Van Beresteyn E C H, Raymakers J A, Duursma S A 1987 Nutritional aspects of osteoporosis. World Review of Nutrition and Dietetics 49: 121–159
Smith R 1987 Osteoporosis; cause and management. British Medical Journal 294: 329–332

IV

Nutritional
interrelationships

31. IMMUNITY AND INFECTION

Immunity is the ability of an individual to resist invasion by potentially harmful organisms. In a broader sense, immunity is the host's ability to react against antigens that are foreign to the body. The latter definition has resulted in the application of immunology to disciplines other than infections, including blood banking, autoimmunity, hypersensitivity, transplantation and tumour immunology.

The immune system comprises both humoral and cellular elements. Immunity is inborn or innate. A previous antigenic challenge is not necessary and such immunity is non-specific. It is acquired, as in infection, due to previous antigenic challenge and this immunity is specific as it is directed against a specific type of infectious agent. Acquired immunity may be obtained by either active immunization (use of an attenuated virus, e.g. polio) or by passive treatment (transfer of specific antiserum from one individual to the other).

The skin and mucosa act as physical barriers against the infectious organism. Factors such as pH, fatty acids, mucus, and normal flora may be harmful to infectious agents. When an organism breaks through the skin and mucosal barriers, systemic cellular and humoral immunity become critical to fight infection.

Cellular immunity consists of T lymphocytes and phagocytes. There are two major types of lymphocytes, the T and B cells. Although both types of lymphocytes originate in the bone marrow, the T lymphocytes are processed in the thymus (thymus-dependent). There are at least three subsets of T lymphocytes: (1) killer cells that kill cells by direct contact; they may also produce lymphokines that enhance the destruction of infectious organisms, (2) helper cells that aid in antibody responses, (3) suppressor cells that suppress antibody responses. The T lymphocyte response is generally specific. They are primarily involved in delayed hypersensitivity (skin test reactions), transplant rejections, and play a major role in body defence against viruses, fungi and certain intracellular bacteria. The B lymphocytes are thymus independent and are primarily involved in the production of the antibodies of humoral immunity. Phagocytes are cells that are capable of ingesting cells or micro-organisms into their cytoplasm. There are two types of phagocytes: (1) the macrophages or mononuclear cells, and (2) granulocytes or polymorpho-nuclear leukocytes. The phagocytic responses are generally non-specific.

Humoral immunity is mediated by antibodies or immunoglobulins, which are secreted by B cell derived plasma cells. There are five major types of anti-bodies: IgM, IgG, IgA, IgE and IgD. Ig is short for immunoglobulin. An antibody may neutralize an invading agent or lyse it with activation of complement. IgA is primarily a secretory antibody present on the mucous membrane of the gastrointestinal tract, the genitourinary tract and the pulmonary tree. Therefore, it is an important antibody in preventing the initial penetration of micro-organisms through the mucous membrane. When this barrier is broken, circulating IgM and IgG will come to bind with the invading agents. After an antigenic challenge, IgM is first formed and later followed by IgG. The latter is the predominant antibody in the blood and extracellular fluid. IgE is primarily involved in allergic reactions. The role of IgD has not been well defined.

Complement C3 is a set of proteins that may be activated by antibodies or endotoxins to lyse cell membranes. Opsonins are proteins that bind to cells or micro-organisms resulting in the facilitation of phagocytosis by macro-phages or granulocytes.

The importance of immunity is illustrated in immunodeficient diseases: T cell defects (DiGeorge syndrome) usually lead to serious infections with relatively innocuous organisms such as *Candida albicans* and *Pneumocystis carinii*, and is commonly found in AIDS (p. 224). In Bruton's agamma-globulinaemia, there is a high susceptibility to streptococcal, pneumococcal, meningococcal and haemophilus infections since specific antibodies are needed to combat these infections.

Impaired immune response and increased susceptibility to infection are of paramount importance in surgery. Many aspects of the immune process are affected by nutritional deprivation (Table 37). Whether these disturbances are

Table 37 Percentage change of immunological indices associated with varying degrees of protein-energy malnutrition

Immunological index	Malnutrition		
	Marginal	Moderate	Severe
Lymphocyte count	5%	10%	23%
T cells	30%	74%	98%
Delayed hypersensitivity	25%	70%	95%
Complement C3	26%	63%	87%
Opsonic function	37%	72%	90%
Bacterial capacity	27%	63%	87%
Secretory IgA	15%	48%	75%

(Meguid MM, Howard LJ 1983 Nutrition. In: Peters RM, Peacoc EE, Benfield JR (eds) Science applied to surgery. Boston, Little, Brown & Co, p 97-113).

the result of protein deficiencies or are consequent upon the depletion of specific factors such as iron or zinc is still controversial. A strong association exists between anergy (impaired cellular immunity), major sepsis and mortality in surgical patients. Anergy is associated with 7-fold increase in sepsis and an 18-fold increase in mortality.

Malnutrition not only may predispose to infection, but at the same time infection will tend to affect the nutrition of the host adversely. Rates of protein synthesis and gluconeogenesis are increased and the level of amino acids and some elements (e.g. zinc), fall in blood and are probably sequestered in the liver.

In niacin deficiency there are marked atrophic and inflammatory changes in the oral mucosa. Cheilotic lesions occur in riboflavin deficiency. Vitamin A deficiency results in metaplasia and keratinization of various epithelial tissues, most notably the conjunctiva and cornea of the eye, and the linings of the respiratory and urinary tracts and parts of the gastrointestinal tract. Secondary bacterial infection is an invariable accompaniment in the advanced state. The lesions seen in vitamin A-deficient germ-free animals are mild and take longer to produce.

Vitamin A controls the stability of the membrane surrounding the subcellular particles, lysosomes. Most of the evidence has been concerned with rupture of this membrane in the presence of excess vitamin A, but some work suggests that this also happens in the deficiency state. As a consequence the lysosomal contents are released. Included are several hydrolysing enzymes which could cause havoc to the body's defences.

One of the most potent weapons in natural defence of the body is phagocytosis by blood leycocytes and macrophages of the reticulo-endothelial system. In children with kwashiorkor and marasmus the activity of enzymes in leucocytes is depressed.

Most pathogenic organisms require considerable amounts of iron, almost all of which is either intracellularly in haemoglobuin, stored as the protein ferritin, or bound in the rapidly exchanging iron pool to transferrin in plasma. Iron deficiency often accompanies infection and may thus be to some extent protective, and dosing with iron may increase susceptibility to infection.

Acquired Immune Deficiency Syndrome (AIDS)

The virus causing AIDS was identified in late 1983 and early 1984. It is called HTLV-III (Human T-Lymphotropic Virus Type III) and is a blood-borne infectious agent. The emergence of AIDS among population groups already known to be at high risk for hepatitis B (male homosexuals, bisexual men, intravenous drug abusers and blood-product recipients, e.g. haemophiliacs) suggests a similar mode of transmission for the two diseases. AIDS has been reported in more than 40 countries on 5 continents. In the US about 50 per cent of risk group members have been infected. The prevalence of exposure in the general population is less than 1%. Heterosexual transmission from patients with AIDS due to bisexuality or haemophiliacs has been documented in the absence of anal intercourse. Also more than 250 cases in the US of AIDS in patients under 13 years of age have been identified since 1980. Sixty per cent have died. More than 70 per cent of such cases have involved children with one or both parents at risk for AIDS.

The spectrum of AIDS is very varied and summarized in Table 38. Common gastrointestinal manifestations of AIDS include oesophagitis (*Candida*, CMV, *Herpes*), hepatitis (MAI, CMV), and gastroenteritis (MAI, *Cryptosporidium, Isospora, Salmonella, Shigella, Campylobacter*, adenovirus). Investigators have also described a chronic malabsorption syndrome in AIDS patients characterized by weight loss, diarrhoea, and steatorrhoea, sometimes

Table 38 CDC classification of HTLV-III/LAV infection

Group I: acute infection	Mononucleosislike syndrome associated with seroconversion
Group II: asymptomatic infection	Positive HTLV-III/LAV antibody or viral culture. May be subclassified on basis of laboratory evaluation (CBC, platelet count, T-cell subset studies)
Group III: persistent generalized lymphadenopathy	Palpable lymphadenopathy (>1cm) at two or more extrainguinal sites for more than three months in the absence of a concurrent illness or infection to explain the findings. May be subclassified on the basis of laboratory evaluation
Group IV: other HTLV-III/LAV disease Subgroup A: Constitutional disease	One or more of the following: fever or diarrhoea persisting more than one month or involuntary weight loss greater than 10% of baseline; and absence of a concurrent illness or infection to explain the findings
Subgroup B: Neurological disease	One or more of the following: dementia, myelopathy, or peripheral neuropathy; and absence of a concurrent illness of condition
Subgroup C: Secondary infectious diseases	Infectious disease associated with HTLV-III/LAV infection and/or at least moderately indicative of a defect in cell-mediated immunity
Subgroup D: Secondary cancers	Diagnosis of one or more cancers known to be associated with HTLV-III/LAV infection as listed in the surveillance definition of AIDS and at least moderately indicative of a defect in cell-mediated immunity: Kaposi's sarcoma, non-Hodgkin's lymphoma (small, non-claved lymphoma or immunoblastic sarcoma), or primary lymphoma of the brain
Subgroup E: Other conditions in HTLV-III/LAV infection	Clinical findings or diseases, not classifiable above, that may be attributable to HTLV-III/LAV infection and are indicative of a defect in cell-mediated immunity; symptoms attributable to either HTLV-III/LAV infection or a coexisting disease not classified elsewhere; or clinical illnesses that may be complicated or altered by HTLV-III/LAV infection. These include chronic lymphoid interstitial pneumonitis and constitutional symptoms, secondary infectious diseases, and neoplasms not listed above

Adapted from CDC 1986 Classification system for human T-lymphotropic virus type III/lymphadenopathy-associated virus infections. Morbidity and Mortality Weekly Reference 35:334.

in the absence of specific bacterial or parasitic infection. Duodenal and jejunal biopsy samples have shown either a chronic inflammatory or atrophic pattern on histopthologic examination. The similarity between the onset of anorexia, the gradual loss of body weight, and cachexia during the course of AIDS and the clinical course with progressive disseminated cancer is striking. Isolated attempts at providing intense nutritional support in the form of total parenteral alimentation to ameliorate or reverse the clinical course have not been very successful. The rationale is that nutrition can improve the immune system (p. 224). Systematic study of the use of nutrients to support patients during this disease needs to be pursued and will become of prominence in the management of this syndrome once an effective vaccine has been developed.

Recent reports from central Africa showed much higher rates of HTLV-III/LAV antibody positivity in children with severe PEM and their mothers than in the healthy population. Thus AIDS may be considered to be one of the factors predisposing to childhood malnutrition.

Acquired immunity

In experimental animals, severe deficiency of protein, pyridoxine, pantothenic acid or folic acid consistently diminishes the level of circulating antibody in various infections. Cells of the lymphoid series produce antibodies and they have been shown to be grossly reduced in pyridoxine deficiency.

Several studies in human volunteers have provided some positive results. Antibody response to tetanus and typhoid vaccines was diminished on a low protein diet. Pantothenic acid deficiency depressed response to tetanus, but not to typhoid antigen. When pyridoxine deficiency was also combined there was marked depression of antibody response to tetanus and typhoid antigens. Vitamin supplementation restored normal response. Poliomyelitis antibody response was not affected by the combined deficiency.

The immune response has been studied intensively in PEM. There appears to be considerable reserve in the capabilities of the body and impairment has not been demonstrated in the mild and moderate degrees. Even in severe marasmus most evidence shows that both humoral and cell-mediated forms are adequate. In kwashiorkor there is atrophy of the cellular elements of the thymus gland and lymph nodes. Circulating immunoglobulin levels tend to be normal or increased, but circulating lymphocytes are reduced in number and functionally abnormal. Complement component levels are reduced except for CH. These changes revert to normal on recovery and there is no evidence of permanent impairment of immunity.

32. ADVERSE REACTIONS TO FOOD

These have been described as shown in Table 39.

Food intolerance may be defined as a reproducible adverse reaction to a

Table 39 Classification of adverse reactions to food

Food intolerance
1. Allergy
2. Enzyme defects (e.g. coeliac disease, hypolactasia)
3. Pharmacological effects (e.g. excess caffeine in tea or coffee)
4. Various unexplained effects (e.g. histamine release, fermentation of unabsorbed residues in the bowel)

Food aversion
1. Psychological avoidance (of particular foods)
2. Psychological intolerance (caused by emotions associated with a food and not the food itself)

specific food or food ingredient, which occurs even when the food is given in disguised form. *Food aversion*, on the other hand, does not occur if the food is given in disguised form. *Food allergies* involve a type I or III hypersensitivity reaction and are associated with raised serum IgE, circulating immune complexes and eosinophilia. The symptoms that can be securely ascribed to food allergy are given in Table 40.

True food allergy is rarely seen in adults and is much less common than other forms of food intolerance. Infants are most commonly affected and symptoms tend to decrease and disappear with advancing age. In them the condition frequently takes the form of an allergy to bovine protein. The main antigens seem to be beta-lactalbumin, casein, alpha-lactalbumin and bovine serum albumin. The condition is reported to occur in from 10 000 to 30 000 infants and young children in the United States every year, but seems to be much less common in the UK and other countries. Gastrointestinal, respiratory or skin problems or even catastrophic anaphylactic shock-type reactions have been reported. Such infants should be breast fed if possible, or

Table 40 Symptoms securely ascribed to allergy

General
Sudden death
Anaphylaxis

Alimentary
Vomiting
Abdominal pain and distension } in children
Diarrhoea

Skin
Urticaria
Angioneuritic oedema
Eczema

Respiratory
Rhinitis
Asthma

General (secondary to gut allergy)
Failure to thrive
Anaemia (iron loss)
Oedema (protein loss)

if not a suitable bottle mixture is Prosobee before 6 months and Nutramigen after 6 months of age.

A recent report has shown that while eczema in breast-fed infants has a high rate of spontaneous improvement, there are some cases that can be attributed to foods in their mothers' diets, especially egg and cow's milk.

Food intolerance not due to allergy

The symptoms due to most kinds of food intolerance arise at any time from 1 to 48 hours after ingestion of a food and mainly consist of abdominal pain and diarrhoea. Systemic symptoms are usually non-specific, i.e. general tiredness, muscle pains and headache. A high proportion of patients with the irritable bowel syndrome (p. 179) suffer from food intolerance.

Differential diagnosis

The possible causes of lower abdominal pain and diarrhoea are many, but the major diseases that have to be distinguished are summarized in Table 41.

The diarrhoea of food intolerance commonly occurs on waking in the morning with the rest of the day relatively free. There is no nocturnal diarrhoea or rectal bleeding. The pain is usually low and central or felt in one of both iliac fossae. It must be differentiated from that due to musculoskeletal disease, which often affects women of similar age. However, if the pain is associated with bowel actions, relieved by defaecation rather than by a night's sleep on a firm bed, and not aggravated by physical activity, it is reasonable to attribute it to the gut.

About half of patients in some series connect the onset of their symptoms with a gut infection, a course of antibiotics or gynaecological or abdominal surgery. Others observe that the gut symptoms vary with the menstrual cycle with a predictable pattern. These precipitants are worth enquiring for.

Investigations

Intolerance due to enzyme defects can be diagnosed by intestinal biopsy and challenge test; pharmacological effects can frequently be identified by

Table 41 Principal differential diagnoses to be excluded in patients suspected of having food intolerance

Symptoms of diarrhoea	Symptoms of lower abdominal pain
Infective	Cancer of the colon
Ulcerative colitis	Crohn's disease
Crohn's disease	Gynaecological problems
Cancer of the colon	Musculoskeletal problems
Malabsorption	

exclusion of the suspected substance. In true allergy there are signs of an abnormal immunological reaction to food (see above).

In the case of other instances of food intolerance investigations are aimed at excluding other diseases as at present there is no diagnostic test. Even if objective changes such as urticaria, asthma or vomiting occur, the diagnosis can be firmly established only if the symptoms disappear during an elimination diet and recur when a controlled challenge is given. Placebo responses are known to be very frequent. Among the tests in common use that are of no proven value are the pulse test, sublingual food tests, Rinkel's intradermal skin testing, cytotoxic food tests, and radioallergosorbent testing (RAST).

Management

Dietary manipulation. The most common foods usually found to provoke symptoms in patients with food intolerance are (in descending order): wheat, corn, dairy products, coffee, oats, rye, eggs, tea, barley, potatoes, citrus fruit, preservatives, chocolate and onions. Elimination dieting is a way of allowing the foods that cause symptoms in each individual to be identified. This should not be undertaken lightly as it may induce overt nutritional deficiency. In essence it consists of instructing the patient to limit the diet to one meat, one fruit and spring water for 5 to 8 days. When this leads to a complete remission of symptoms one food is reintroduced at a time, watching for those that provoke symptoms. Frequently this is too difficult and too unpleasant for patients. Supplements of iron, calcium and vitamin C are usually required. If a patient is not fully recovered after two weeks on an exclusion diet then it is not worth persisting further with a dietary approach. Those with multiple food intolerances are best treated symptomatically to avoid the development of an obsessional fixation on dietary manoeuvres. In many cases food intolerances tend to disappear after some months of dieting. Foods can be retested at yearly intervals and can be reintroduced when they no longer provoke symptoms.

Drug treatment. Some drugs may play a subsidiary role in management. Sodium cromoglycate can allow patients to stray from a diet when they have no control over what they eat. Four to six capsules opened and dissolved in a small quantity of very hot water with extra cold water added should be swilled around the mouth and swallowed 20 minutes before a meal and then again immediately before it. This technique should not be used more than once every 10 days. Ibuprofen 400 mg three times a day may be tried in patients who cannot adhere to a diet. It acts by blocking the production of 2-series prostaglandins from the large bowel. It is thought that prostaglandins from the large bowel may mediate food intolerance. Propranolol (40 mg tds) and amitryptyline (25 mg at night) block the peripheral effects of prostaglandins.

Food additives

Table 42 lists those additives for which there is evidence that they can cause reactions.

It should be emphasized that, in comparison with intolerance caused by natural food substances, that due to additives is very rare.

It seems that the mechanisms of adverse reactions to additives are varied. Additives are generally substances of low molecular weight, ingested irregularly, in very small doses. Available evidence suggests that immuno-allergic responses are much less commonly involved than pharmacological mechanisms.

Immunoallergic responses. A number of substances have the ability to bond covalently to macromolecules like proteins. They are called haptenes which are made immunogenic by this bonding. Some azo dyes can act as haptenes and in allergic patients IgE antibodies have been demonstrated against tartrazine, amaranth red, green S and sun yellow; and IgD antibodies specific to tartrazine. A delayed type of hypersensitivity, manifesting as eczema has occured after ingestion of such additives as azo dyes, BHT, BHA and quinine and after skin contact in the food, ointment and cosmetic industries.

Pharmacological mechanisms. There is evidence that tartrazine may provoke asthma by its inhibitory action on cyclo-oxygenase, leading to the inhibition of prostaglandin synthesis, particularly PGE_2 — a bronchodilator. Certain colouring agents — xanthenes and erythrosin — alter the membrane permeability of neurones in animals and it has been suggested that this could be responsible for behavioural disorders in humans. In animals, BHT and BHA cause a fall in serotonin, cholinesterase and cerebral noradrenalin associated with disorders of sleep, orientation and aggressiveness.

Table 42 Food additives that are capable of provoking reactions

Dyes
Tartrazine (E102)*
Amaranth (E123)
Sunset yellow (E110)

Antioxidants
Butylated hydroxyanisole (BHA) (E320)
Butylated hydroxytoluene (BHT) (E321)

Preservatives
Benzoates (E210–9)
Sodium nitrite (E250)
Sodium metabisulphite (E223)

Other
Flavourings — quinine, menthol
Enzymes — such as meat tenderizer (papain)

* E numbers are used in the EEC for identification on labels.

Hyperkinesis

Controversy has raged for more than a decade as to whether there is any scientific foundation to the claims of Feingold in California that hyperkinesis in children is caused by some foods and especially food additives, and that cure results from an additive-free diet. Most of the reports claiming dramatic benefit have been purely anecdotal and the few carefully controlled trials, which are very difficult to carry out, have produced largely negative results. Furthermore, the term 'hyperkinesis' and 'hyperactivity' commonly used to describe the disturbed state of the affected children are extremely vague and have included a widely heterogeneous collection of psychological and pathological states, making the proper study of response to diet manipulation virtually impossible. Nevertheless, there are suggestions that a very small group of children may have a true allergy to food additives such as those mentioned above.

33. INJURY

By injury is meant all kinds of trauma to the body, including, besides elective and emergency surgical intervention, radiation and burns.

Nutritional status and response to injury

A patient who sustains an injury may be suffering from any form of primary malnutrition, of either the under- or overnutrition type as described in Section II. On the other hand, many conditions requiring surgery affect nutrition by producing anorexia, vomiting, dysphagia or impairing digestion or absorption. The immediate needs should be met, parenterally if necessary (see p. 238), and operation should be proceeded with, as undue delay in an attempt to improve nutritional status does not meet with success.

Low peripheral concentrations of red blood cells, hypoproteinaemia, and ascorbic acid deficiency interfere with adequate would healing. Zinc has a key function in all protein synthesis, whereas copper is the metallocofactor for lysl oxidase, which is important in the formation of collagen crosslinkages and hence strong wounds. While primary wound healing has priority in even the malnourished patient and hence occurs even in severely cachectic patients; secondary wound healing, the healing of infected of dehisced wound, decubitus ulcers and skin graft takes are highly dependent on good nutrition.

Bone healing is delayed in protein deficiency. Fibroblastic repair and subsequent callus formation are depressed. Hypocalcaemia, secondary to hypoproteinaemia, may also play a part.

Acute injury phase

The metabolic 'set' of injury is initiated by the rise in catecholamines in response to anxiety, fear, pain and blood loss. This stimulates glucagon secretion, elevates cortisol levels and inhibits insulin secretion, leading to a catabolic hormonal mileau which facilitates release of gluconeogenic precursors (amino acids, lactate, glycerol, and ketone bodies) from the peripheral muscle and fat tissues and stimulates hepatic gluconeogenesis producing hyperglycaemia of trauma (pseudodiabetes of trauma), hyper-triglyceridaemia and elevated amino acid levels (branched chain and gluco-neogenic amino acids). Injured and repairing tissues are obligatory glucose utilizing. Other obligatory glucose utilizing tissues include the brain (140 g/day), the reticulo-endothelial system (25 g/day) and the renal medulla (35 g/day).

An increased metabolic rate occurs. It is associated with an elevated rate of oxygen consumption due to increased oxygen uptake by all major organ systems. An uncomplicated long-bone fracture increases the resting meta-bolic expenditure by 15 per cent to 30 per cent, multiple injuries and severe peritonitis increase it by 25 per cent to 50 per cent, and large thermal burns by 50 per cent to 100 per cent.

Following abdominal injury with peritonitis, the 24-hour nitrogen ex-cretion can reach 20 g or greater. This corresponds to a loss of about 120 g of protein or 0.5 kg of muscle tissue per day. It is worth noting that the increased nitrogen loss is due to generalized systemic proteolysis, particularly from skeletal muscle, and not just from the injured or infected tissue. As the magnitude of the stress subsides, the amino acid efflux from muscle decreases.

Since the systemic metabolic effects described can be blocked by anaes-thesia, their process seems to be initiated through the central nervous system. In patients with infections, these changes appear to stem from the release of endogenous pyrogens, leukocyte-endogenous mediation, and other sub-stances that are produced by infected tissues that stimulate metabolism directly and indirectly through the central nervous system and neuroendo-crine responses.

Anabolic chronic phase

This consists of an initial catabolic phase following on the acute phase that in turn is succeeded by one of anabolism of a duration depending on the degree of injury. By this process energy is primarily released from the depot fat to meet the additional demands for repair in the face of diminished food intake. Table 43 outlines the major changes characteristic of the two phases.

Long-term effects of injury

Among patients with operations on the stomach, anaemia may occur, usually iron deficiency. Megaloblastic anaemia is rare and then is due to vitamin B_{12} deficiency. Osteomalacia is not uncommon. Reference has been made elsewhere to the dumping syndrome (p.175) and blind loop syndrome (p.177). More serious malabsorption is likely to follow surgery of the intestine (p.178).

Table 43 Some major metabolic responses to injury

	Acute phase	Chronic phase
Metabolic rate	↑	↑
Body temperature	↑	↑
Cardiac output	↑	↑
Plasma insulin	↓	↑
Plasma glucagon	↑	slight↓ or normal
Plasma catecholamines	↑	slight↑ or normal
Blood glucose	↑	slight↑ or normal
Blood lactate	↑	slight↑ or normal
Plasma free fatty acids	↑	↓
Nitrogen balance	negative	negative becoming positive
Duration (days) (proportional to magnitude of injury)	1–5	6–10+ (depending on severity of injury)

Prolonged immobilization, espically during recovery from multiple injury involving fractures, repeated skin grafts, poliomyelitis, rheumatic fever, may lead to demineralization of bones. Physiotherapy and high calcium intake are indicated.

34. NUTRITIONAL SUPPORT OF THE HOSPITALIZED PATIENT

Indications for nutritional support

Nutritional support is indicated for those patients 'who cannot eat, should not eat, will not eat or cannot eat enough'. A patient's clinical course reflects the prognosis of his primary medical disorder, but concomitant malnutrition increases the risk of a complication and prejudices survival. Starvation studies have shown that physical performance begins to deteriorate when more than 10 per cent of body cell mass is lost, and malnourished patients succumb more readily to infection, to surgical stress and to the clinical crisis of major organ failure. If a prolonged period of gastrointestinal malfunction is inevitable, early initiation of nutritional support to prevent the onset of malnutrition is clinically indicated. If the patient is already malnourished, even if the prognosis is benign, starting nutritional support becomes imperative.

Nutritional support

The provision of adequate nutrients to hospitalized patients has three functions: (1) the supply of calories and amino acids needed for anabolism, and water, electrolytes, vitamins, and other micronutrients necessary for body functions; (2) to stimulate insulin and inhibit glucagon secretion, which reverses the catabolic hormonal picture of stress to one of anabolism (Injury,

p. 231); and (3) the requirements for protein are primarily the requirements for the indispensible amino acids used in the synthesis of body proteins. This process also requires about one-third of the daily energy consumption.

The provision of adequate nutrition involves a series of decisions to be made: these begin with the diagnosis of malnutrition and the selection of patients who need some form of nutritional support (see Table 44) as a part of their treatment. Other critical decisions are related to the choice of route for the provision of nutrients (oral/enteral, parenteral, or both) and the selection of the appropriate nutrient solutions.

The most physiological method of providing nutrition to a hospitalized patient is through voluntary eating. The average hospital diet is well-balanced and provides energy, nitrogen, vitamins and other micronutrients in accordance with recommended daily allowance (RDA) standards (p. 85). Unfortunately, the hospital setting does not always provide an environment conducive to eating; frequently patients are apprehensive, anxious, in discomfort or pain, and thus anorexic. Cancer patients may also suffer from anosmia and thus taste aversion.

In the absence of appropriate voluntary intake to meet the nutrient requirements of the non-stressed state or the increased requirements of stress, nutritional support must be provided.

Enteral alimentation

If a patient's gastrointestinal tract is functioning, it should be used. Its use maintains gastrointestinal mass and function. A variety of chemically formulated diets are available that can be given via an enteral route (see Table 45).

An elemental diet is indicated for patients with a malfunctioning gastrointestinal tract, including small bowel fistulas, short-bowel syndrome, oesophagogastric obstruction, radiation enteritis, pancreatitis, or inflammatory bowel disease in previously healthy patients who sustained acute trauma and are in a catabolic state with weight loss, failure to heal, and negative nitrogen balance.

Elemental diets are composed mainly of glucose, L-amino acids, and minimal quantities of fat in the form of short- and medium-chain triglycerides to supply essential fatty acid requirements and to provide a vehicle for the fat-soluble vitamins, minerals, and trace minerals.

Patients with dysphagia, oesophageal obstruction, or diversion, benefit from the use of enteral alimentation when ostomy tubes are placed. They require little or no active digestion and have minimal residue. When a portion of functional intestine is available for absorption this is a safer and cheaper alternative to total parenteral nutrition (see below) for the patient who cannot eat by mouth.

These diets are usually unsuitable for oral feeding; they are unpalatable, only small amounts (100 to 150 ml) can be tolerated at a time, and it is diffi-

Table 44 Clinical conditions indicating use
of nutritional support

Gastrointestinal tract obstruction
Pseudo-obstruction
Prolonged ileus
Wound dehiscence
Strictures
Gastroschisis
Neoplasia
Congenital atresia syndrome

Severe inflammation or loss of bowel surface
Regional enteritis/ulcerative colitis
Radiation enteritis
Intractable diarrhoea of infancy
Short bowel
Intestinal fistulas

Persistent vomiting or anorexia
Cancer chemotherapy
Anorexia nervosa
Severe depression
Chronic liver failure/dialysis

Increased demand of nutrients
Major trauma
Head injury
Burns
Sepsis
Heart failure
Cancer

Requirements for specific nutrients
Cystic fibrosis
Hepatic failure
Chronic renal failure
Heart failure

cult to monitor amounts given and prevent hyperosmolar dehydration.

Nasogastric feeding is preferred using a 16-gauge, 24-inch polyethylene catheter starting with 25 per cent weight/volume solution, 1 kcal/ml at a rate of 50 ml/h, increasing by 25 ml/h up to a total of 125 ml/h and 3000 kcal/24th. With jejunostomy feeding a 16-gauge, 36-inch polyethylene catheter is used starting with 10 per cent weight/volume solution at 50 ml/h and increasing by 25 ml/h each day up to daily fluid requirements. Concentration is thereafter by 5 per cent wt/vol/day until maximum tolerance is achieved (usually 20 per cent wt/vol concentration; 4/5 kcal/ml, at 125 ml/h for 2400 kcal/day).

A number of commercially formulated diets are available. Four generally basic groups of enteral products exist: blenderized formulas, milk-based formulas, elementally defined formulas, and disease-related formulas. More specific data on these choices are presented in Table 45.

As in other methods of enteral alimentation, hypertonic solutions should initially be administered at half strength and nutritional tolerance built up gradually. The maximum that can be given each day to any patient depends

Table 45 Commercial product comparison

Product/ Flavours	Manufacturer (Form)	Cal/ Ml	Cal/ Nitrogen Ratio	% Carbohydrate Source	g/l
Blenderized					
Compleat/ unflavoured	Doyle	1.07 B 1.00 B	156 : 1	8%	128.4 120
				Hydrolysed cereal solids, malto-dextrin, vegetables, fruits, orange juice	
Compleat modified formula/ unflavoured	Sandoz (liquid)	1.07	156 : 1	53% Cereal solids, vegetables, fruit, orange juice	141.8
Milk-based					
Instant breakfast/ vanilla strawberry eggnog chocolate chocolate malt	Carnation (powder)	1.06	113 : 1	51% Sucrose, corn syrup solids, lactose	135
Ensure/vanilla chocolate coffee strawberry eggnog black walnut	Ross	1.06	179 : 1	54.4% Corn syrup solids, sucrose	144.4
Lactose-free Isocal/ unflavoured	Mead Johnson (liquid)	1.06	195 : 1	50.2% Glucose	133
Osmolite/ unflavoured	Ross (liquid)	1.08	178 : 1	54% Hydrolysed corn starch	145
Defined-formula diets					
Vivonex High Nitrogen/ unflavoured	Norwich Eaton (powder)	1.0	141 : 1	81.5%	203.0
Special use					
Amin-Aid/ berry strawberry lemon-lime orange	McGaw (powder)	2.00	306 : 1	75% Maltodextrins, sucrose	375
Hepatic-Aid II/chocolate eggnog custard	McGaw (powder)	1.1	167 : 1	57% Maltodextrins, sucrose	169

Protein Source	g/l	% Fat Source	g/l	ml to meet RDA	Osmolality	Ch Lac	Per litre mEq Na$^+$	mEq K$^+$
5%	42.8 40	36%	42.8 40	1600/C 1500/B	390/C 405/B	24.6	52C 57B	33C 36B
eef, non-fat milk		Corn oil, mono-glycerides and diglycerides						
5%	42.8	31%	36.9	1500	300	None	29	36
eef, calcium aseinate		Corn oil, beef fat						
2%	58	27%	31	1400	NA	95.8	41	70
ilk, sodium aseinate, soy rotein isolate		Milk fat						
4%	37.1	31.5%	37.1	1887	450	None	37	40
odium & calcium aseinates, soy rotein isolate		Corn oil						
2.9%	34.2	36.9%	43.5	2000	300	None	23	34
Calcium & sodium aseinates, soy rotein isolate		Soy oil (80%), MCT oil (20%)						
4%	37	32%	39	1887	300	None	24	26
odium & calcium aseinates, soy rotein isolate		MCT oil (50%), corn oil (40%), soy oil (10%)						
7.7%	44.3	0.8%	0.9	3000	810	None	23	30
-amino acids		Safflower oil						
%	20	21.0%	46.7	Not Adequate	1095	None	<15	<6
Essential amino cids plus istidine		Soy oil, lecithin mono-glycerides and diglycerides						
5%	44	28%	36	Not Adequate	560	None	<15	<6
Amino acids increased branched-chain (decreased aromatic)		Soy oil, lecithin, mono-glycerides and diglycerides						

on the tolerance to a given fluid load or the development of diarrhoea or metabolic abnormalities. The complications of tube feedings are enumerated in Table 46.

PARENTERAL NUTRITION

Patients whose gastrointestinal tracts cannot support their nutrition must be fed parenterally. The various uses of parenteral nutrition are summarized in Table 47. A positive nitrogen balance can be achieved in a wide spectrum of diseases if a calorie/nitrogen ratio of 130 :1 to 200 :1 is provided; 35 to 45 kcal/kg/day and 0·2 to 0·3 g of nitrogen/kg/day. As might be expected, these ratios vary with different diseases and at different points during the course of the individual disease. Direct oxidation of infused glucose reaches a maximum level of approximately 55 per cent. At higher levels of glucose administration, carbon dioxide production is increased and fat synthesis is stimulated. Autopsy studies have shown that much of this tryglyceride remains in the liver. Thus, excessive exogenous glucose infusion would appear to embarrass both respiratory and hepatic functions in severely stressed patients.

In patients whose fat stores are markedly depleted, total calorie support is best provided by adding 10 kcal/kg/day as infused fat. Using exogenous fat rather than excess exogenous glucose circumvents the metabolic cost to the patient of converting glucose to fat. Over and above these caloric considerations, some intravenous fat is necessary in all patients on long-term TPN to supply essential fatty acid requirements (2 per cent of calories) (p. 34). Energy should be provided at 40–45 kcal/kg body weight and approximately 50 per cent from glucose and 50 per cent from fat.

Nitrogen is provided as synthetic crystalline amino acid solutions, which

Table 46 Complications of tube feeding

Type of complication	Frequency (percent)	Treatment
Gastrointestinal		
Bloating	15	Decrease flow rate
Diarrhoea and cramping	15	Decrease flow and/or concentration; consider different formula; add anti-diarrhoeal drug
Vomiting	<5	Decrease flow rate
Metabolic		
Hyperglycemia and glucosuria	5–10	Decrease glucose concentration or administer insulin
Oedema	5–10	Usually none, decrease sodium and fluid intake, use diuretics
Congestive heart failure	1–5	Decrease rate, administer diuretics and digoxin
Mechanical		
Dislodged tube	45	Secure meticulously
Clogged tube lumen	<10	Flush with water, replace tube
Pulmonary aspiration	<10	Discontinue tube feeding and start TPN
Tracheo-oesophageal fistula	<1	Discontinue tube feeding and start TPN

Reproduced with permission. Meguid MM, Gray GE, Debonis D 1984 The use of enteral nutrition in the patient with cancer. In: Rombeau JL, Caldwell MD (eds) Enteral Nutrition. WB Saunders, Philadelphia, pp. 303–337

Table 47 Summary of current usage and efficacy of TPN

Therapy	Efficacy	Disease	Outcome
Primary	Proven	Gastrointestinal fistula	Increases survival Reduces morbidity and mortality Increases incidence of spontaneous closure rate
		Short-bowel syndrome	Reduces morbidity and mortality
		Infants unable to eat	Reduces morbidity and mortality
		Myocardial infarction	Lower incidence of ventricular arrhythmias and lower vasopressor dependence
Supportive	Proven	Regional enteritis	Improves tolerance and response Increases temporary remission rates
		Gastrointestinal cancer	Decreases postoperative morbidity and mortality
		Chemotherapy/radiation therapy	Increases temporary remission rates
		Inflammatory bowel disease	Decreases complications
		Closed head injury	Earlier recovery and discharge
		Femoral fractures	Earlier ambulation and discharge
		Radical cystectomy	Earlier discharge
		Burns and trauma	Improves survival and shortens hospitalization
		Anorexia nervosa	Improves survival
Supportive	Suggestive	Cancer cachexia	Reduces postoperative complications
		Radiation enteritis	Augments survival
		Acute hepatic failure	Improves hepatic function and possibly survival
Supportive	Questionable	Acute renal failure	Reverses rise in BUN, potassium and PO_4 Possibly decreases length of anuric phase and possibly improves survival
		Acute pancreatitis	Decreases mortality but does not ameliorate respiratory or renal failure

have a well defined amino acid profile. They are especially indicated in special situations such as paediatric practice, renal failure and hepatic failure. Amino acid solutions should provide 30 per cent of their N as essential amino acid N for adults and about 40 per cent for infants.

Requirements for electrolytes and other elements and vitamins are met by addition to the intravenous solutions. Phosphate depletion (p. 141) has resulted when not specially added. Clinical folate, zinc and essential fatty acid deficiencies have also been reported. Toxicity of fat-soluble vitamins must be guarded against in prolonged administration.

Precautions. Preparation of solutions must be carried out aseptically under a laminar-flow, filtered-air hood. Catheter insertion and maintenance must be performed with strictest attention to surgical and aseptic techniques. The nutrient solution is generally delivered from a bottle or plastic bag to the patient by gravity or by a rate regulating infusion pump.

Monitoring. All patients on parenteral nutrition must be closely monitored clinically and biochemically. Fluid balance, metabolic balance, temperature, daily weight, electrolytes (daily initially), fat clearing capacity, serum P, Ca, Mg (every 3rd day), blood sugar (at least daily initially), liver function (twice weekly), haematology, urinary urea, electrolytes, urine and serum osmolality, acid–base balance; should all be monitored together with specific tests dictated by the presenting illness. Stringent monitoring is required because mechanical, metabolic, and infectious complications may develop rapidly and can be life-threatening. To pre-empt these complications it is useful to know when they most commonly develop. Catheter-related sepsis is rarely a cause of fever within the first 48 hours, whereas the acute extracellular–intracellular shifts of potassium and phosphate caused by glucose infusion occur rapidly, especially in malnourished fasting patients in whom significant total body depletion of potassium and phosphorus occurs. Table 48 lists the likely chronological sequence of complications of parenteral nutrition.

35. ALCOHOLISM

Alcoholism is a psychosomatic disease with both psychological and physiological determinants. People vary tremendously in their response to the ingestion of ethanol. Chronic alcoholism is a disease of multiple aetiology.

Table 48 Chronological occurrence of complications from total parenteral nutrition

	First 48 hours	First 2 weeks	Three months onward
Mechanical	Complications from catheter insertion: cephalad displacement pneumothorax haemothorax Detachment of catheter at catheter hub with blood loss or air embolism	Catheter coming out of vein Detachment of catheter at catheter hub with blood loss or air embolism	Detachment of catheter at catheter hub with blood loss or air embolism
Metabolic	Hyperglycaemia Hypophosphataemia Hypokalaemia	Hyperosmolar non-ketotic hyperglycaemic coma Hyponatraemia Hypomagnesaemia ($\downarrow$ K, $\downarrow$ Ca) Acid–base imbalance	Essential fatty acid deficiency Zinc, copper, chromium, selenium, molybdenum deficiency Iron deficiency Vitamin deficiency TPN metabolic bone disease TPN liver disease
Infectious		Catheter-induced sepsis Tunnel infections	Catheter-induced sepsis Tunnel infections

In the USA it is estimated that alcohol now supplies an important part of the daily energy intake, about 5 per cent for the average male if teetotallers are included and almost 10 per cent if they are excluded. This is an amount almost equivalent to that supplied by protein. These individuals are prone to develop obesity from excess energy consumption and are probably on a low-protein intake which may damage the liver over a long period of time.

Metabolism of alcohol

Ethanol on ingestion is distributed throughout the body water. Most persons are drunk when the blood level reaches 150 mg per cent and in danger of respiratory arrest at three times this level. The initial and rate-limiting step in alcohol oxidation is by alcohol dehydrogenase in the liver to acetaldehyde, which is then further oxidized to acetyl CoA and then to carbon dioxide and water via the tricarboxylic acid cycle. Niacin and riboflavin are directly involved in the metabolism of alcohol and most other B vitamins are affected, if less directly. The microsomal ethanol-oxidizing system (MEOS), containing cytochrome P-450, of the hepatocyte is equally important in oxidizing ethanol and is responsible for considerable metabolic adaptation in chronic high intake.

Changes in lipid metabolism include generation of reduced synthetic products of acetate, such as fatty acids and cholesterol, and increased reduction of dihydroxy-acetone phosphate to a-glycero-phosphate promoting triglyceride synthesis. These may partly account for the fatty infiltration of the liver.

Protein deficiency

This occurs in chronic alcoholism in association with severe dietary restriction in protein. The clinical manifestations are in most respects indistinguishable from those of kwashiorkor. Cirrhosis, so common a feature of chronic alcoholism, is not a sequel to kwashiorkor. The liver in relationship to alcoholism is considered separately (p. 242). A therapeutic trial, with a high-protein diet, will readily reveal the degree to which recovery may be expected. If liver function is essentially intact, response will be dramatic within a few days with disappearance of oedema, rise in serum albumin, recession of a large liver and reticulocytosis. In the absence of these changes liver damage must be suspected and recovery will be slow and partial, if occurring at all.

Vitamin deficiences

Among communities where food supplies are adequate alcoholism should be suspected as one of the most important predisposing factors. This is especially true for the vitamins of the B complex, and reference has been made to this when the following conditions were considered: beriberi (p. 114), pellagra

(p. 117) and nutritional amblyopia (p. 126). Alcoholism may precipitate deficiency by: (1) impaired appetite and reduced intake, (2) poor absorption, (3) reduced storage, and (4) increased requirements.

Zinc deficiency is especially likely to occur, as this element is part of several dehydrogenase enzymes including alcohol dehydrogenase. Night blindness in some alcoholic patients responds to zinc and not to vitamin A (p. 145).

Liver

Fatty infiltration. Alcoholics are prone to develop changes in the liver, ranging all the way from early fatty infiltration to severe cirrhosis with or without fatty changes. There has been considerable controversy as to whether alcohol by itself is toxic to the liver or acts by leading to nutritional disturbance which is ultimately responsible for the changes. It is now generally agreed that chronic excessive alcohol intake does damage the liver. In both experimental animals and man fatty infiltration and ultrastructural damage have been produced by the energetic substitution of alcohol for carbohydrate. These changes were evident within a week of starting alcohol administration and could not be prevented by increasing dietary protein, diminishing fat intake or by changing the type of fat.

Cirrhosis. Cirrhosis requires prolonged exposure to an injurious agent and is largely, if not entirely, irreversible. The incidence of cirrhosis of the liver in a country correlates fairly closely with the *per capita* consumption of alcohol but other factors such as viral hepatitis and the nutritional status complicate the picture (p. 180).

Other systems

Almost all parts of the body are affected but prominent among the changes are damage to the brain, heart, intestine, bone marrow, muscle and the gonads. High alcohol consumption during pregnancy may cause malformations in the infant. Although a number of studies have shown less CHD in moderate drinkers than non-drinkers, there is also evidence of high systolic and diastolic blood pressure.

36. CANCER

Relationship of diet to cancer formation

It has been suggested that up to 90 per cent of human cancers are associated with environmental factors. Dietary factors may have a direct impact on the occurrence of 30 to 40 per cent of cancers in men and 50 to 60 per cent in women in the western world and cause 50 per cent of cancer-related deaths. It is estimated that appropriate nutrition could reduce cancer deaths by an average of 35 per cent of the present 150 000 deaths per year. The wasting that accompanies the progress of cancer is partly due to anorexia but there is also increased metabolism, perhaps related to tumour growth. Carcinoma of the upper digestive tract impairs food intake.

The treatment of cancer often adversely affects nutritional status. Surgery of the alimentary tract may impair absorption of nutrients (p. 177). Cancer chemotherapy disturbs body metabolism and some drugs have a direct effect, for example methotrexate is a folic acid antagonist and 5-fluoracil damages the intestinal mucosa causing fat malabsorption. Radiotherapy causes destructive changes in tissues. Many cancer patients can only be prepared to withstand these forms of treatment by parenteral nutrition (p. 238).

Vitamin A deficiency has been associated with tumours of the gastro-intestinal tract, nasopharynx and lung. A high fat intake and obesity appear to relate to the incidence of carcinoma of the breast, colon and ovary. Many other relationships have been suggested (e.g. alcohol consumption and rectal cancer) but the evidence for all of these remains inconclusive at present.

The postulated mechanisms by which the food in our diet influences the development of cancer conceptually involve two distinct sequences: (1) the process of carcinogenic initiation — conversion of a normal cell to a neoplastic cell, followed by (2) promotion and progression. Dietary constituents, whether chemicals (e.g. nitrite, p. 22), nutrients, or xenobiotics (foreign compounds of no nutritional value requiring excretion by the body, e.g. aflatoxin p. 24) can promote or inhibit carcinogenic factors as outlined in the schema of Figure 20. Many chemicals known to produce cancer in experimental animals are introduced into the food chain from a variety of sources. Some well-documented food-borne carcinogens are shown in Table 49. In this regard, a distinction should be made between causes and mechanisms: a dietary cause of cancer is a food constituent which, when eaten, increases disease risk, while the mechanism is the means by which the cancer is engendered by the causative agent.

The induction of a cancer by a dietary constituent is a multistep process occurring during some period of time. Most of these substances need to be metabolically activated via a tissue-mediated chemical alteration before they

Table 49 Some food-borne carcinogens

Source	Example
Naturally occurring	Mycotoxins (e.g. aflatoxin), pyrrolizidine alkaloids
Contaminant 1. Introduced before processing 2. Introduced during processing	DDT, trichloroethylene, methylene chloride
Additive	Saccharin, nitrates and nitrites
Formed from food components 1. Formed during processing 2. Formed during preparation 3. Formed *in vivo*	Nitrosamines, aryldiazonium compounds Benzo(a)pyrene, heterocyclic amines Nitrosamides/nitrosamines

Reproduced with permission: Williams GM 1985 Food and cancer. Nutrition International 1: 49–59.

STAGE OF CARCINOGENIC ACTIVITY	INITIATION	PROMOTION	PROGRESSION
PROBABLE ACTION OF CARCINOGEN	Food-borne carcinogen → Electrophilic reactant or 'free-radical' → Binding of carcinogen to DNA/proteins → Alterations in DNA/proteins carcinogen-damaged cell	Expression → in altered cellular information → Growth of altered cells by proliferation promoter	Neoplasm → Metastasis
POSSIBLE SITES OF NUTRITIONAL INFLUENCE	• Detoxification of reactive carcinogenic compounds • Induction and inhibition of microsomal mixed-function oxidase enzyme systems • Interference with binding to macro-molecules • Modulation of DNA/protein damage repair	Induction & inhibition by: • Specific dietary lipid factors • Tumour growth factors • Inhibition of tumour promoting action	• Influence of diet on tumour behaviour e.g. lipids, proteins & hormones

Fig. 20 Aspects of the carcinogenic process that might be affected by nutrition. (Chen M, Meguid MM 1986 Postulated cancer prevention diets: a guide to food selection. Surgical Clinics of North America 6: 931–945).

can exert their carcinogenicity. This activation often requires multiple metabolic steps before resulting in a product which binds with DNA. After the requisite time, varying from months to years, the altered cell may express different growth properties due to new phenotypic characteristics. There may be altered cellular growth patterns which are either unregulated or are affected by unknown or poorly understood biochemical events. Also, the interactions of cells with a known carcinogen can be influenced by a variety of nutrients; i.e. types of diet may influence the occurrence, dosage and duration of exposure to carcinogens, and dietary constituents may regulate the activity of carcinogen-activating enzymes located in the endoplasmic reticulum of a cell.

The microsomal mixed-function oxidase enzyme systems (Figure 20) possess many of the enzymes capable of activating many carcinogens to their reactive form. This occurs by conversion of the often lipophilic carcinogen to a more hydrophilic compound, enabling it to enter the aqueous phase. Many drugs, including insecticides and xenobiotics, as well as dietary proteins and fats can induce the activition of this enzyme system. Conversely, the same enzyme systems can be inhibited by a variety of drugs, such as steroids.

The mixed-function oxidase system also contains enzymes which detoxify and inactivate ingested carcinogens — a process that leads to a decrease in carcinogenicity. Xenobiotics and dietary nutrients of both plant and animal origin can modify the effects of these enzymes by inducing the activity of these detoxifying systems, thereby directly participating in detoxification processes or inhibiting carcinogen-binding to critical cellular macromolecules.

A variety of cellular repair systems is available for repairing carcinogen-induced DNA damage and for excising DNA-carcinogen adducts. Dietary factors may play a role by either inhibiting the repair system, or by xenobiotic induction of repair system activity.

Several dietary factors, such as retinoids, carotenoids, vitamin A, selenium, different growth factors (protease inhibitors) and certain nutrient factors required by many cells inhibit experimental tumour promotion. Retinoids, synthetic compounds closely related to vitamin A, have been shown experimentally to suppress the development of precancerous changes in some epithelial tissues. In fully formed tumour, dietary lipids, proteins and hormones may affect growth by influencing tissue growth factors and hormones.

Relationship of malignant disease to nutrition

Protein-calorie malnutrition is a common problem in patients with cancer. Forty-five per cent of hospitalized cancer patients had lost 10 per cent or more of their body weight, and approximately 25 per cent lost more than 20 per cent of their body weight in some studies. Non-specific, tumour-related starvation is the primary cause of death in many cancer patients. Protein-calorie malnutrition is associated with a higher surgical risk.

The causes of this malnutrition in these patients are multiple; the common denominator is decreased nutrient intake. Other factors involve an altered nutrient requirement and the effects of anticancer therapy. These factors predispose the cancer patient to malnutrition, and indicate the need for nutritional support.

The marked anorexia and weight loss noted in cancer are so well recognized as to merit the term cancer cachexia. It bears no simple relationship to tumour burden, tumour cell type, or anatomic site of involvement, although it is seen most commonly in patients with dissemi-nated cancer or cancer of the gastrointestinal tract. Its aetiology remains incompletely understood. Figure 21 shows some of the possible factors that may lead to cachexia. It is probable that cachexia results from the interaction of a number of factors, including decreased food intake secondary to anorexia, decreased digestion and absorption, and increased nutrient needs due to the autonomous tumour metabolism.

Cachexia may be secondary to decreased intake resulting from the production by the tumour of peptides or other small molecular weight compounds which exert their effects on the central nervous system. Other factors include changes in taste perception, insulin sensitivity, as well as serum levels of lactate, fatty acids, and amino acids may be important in

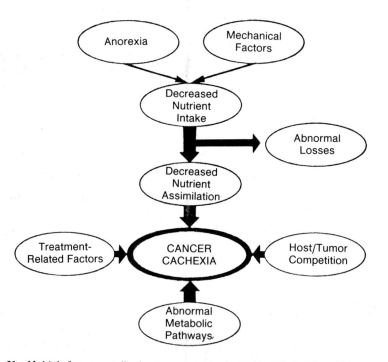

Fig. 21 Multiple factors contributing to cancer cachexia. (Buzby GP, Steinberg JJ 1981 Nutrition in cancer patients. Surgical Clinics of North America 61: 691–700).

regulating food intake. Depression and fear of cancer are still other factors, although they do not explain the anorexia and weight loss that often appear before diagnosis.

Weight loss also occurs in patients consuming adequate amounts of food, and weight loss in cancer patients has been said to be more rapid than that of simple starvation. These observations suggest that there may be alterations in overall metabolism, but particularly that of protein and fat metabolism.

Nutritional consequences of cancer treatment

Besides the metabolic effects of the disease itself, the cancer patient is predisposed to malnutrition as a result of therapy.

Chemotherapy. Chemotherapeutic agents affect the alimentary tract (Table 50). Most have in common the ability to produce nausea and vomiting. Nausea, vomiting, anorexia and altered taste perception not only result in decreased oral intake, but also lead to fluid and electrolyte imbalances and weight loss. A second feature of many of these drugs is the production of mucositis and stomatitis. The rapid turnover of cells in the gastrointestinal epithelium makes it particularly vulnerable to these agents. The resulting gastrointestinal changes lead to decreased oral intake. Decreased intestinal absorption may also occur.

Radiation therapy. The effects of radiation therapy which lead to nutritional alterations are related to the region irradiated (Table 51).

Surgery. The patient with cancer experiences the same metabolic response to surgery as do other patients. These include increased nitrogen losses and energy requirements. However, because cancer patients have frequently experienced significant weight loss prior to surgery, their ability to cope with these stresses is impaired.

The subsequent effects of cancer surgery on nutritional status are given in Table 52.

Benefits of nutrition support in patient receiving cancer treatment

Treatment of malnutrition generally results in improved physical strength, functional capacity and the subjective feeling of well-being. In addition, treatment can improve immune status and hypoalbuminaemia, contribute to a better surgical prognosis and increase the ability of the patient to tolerate radiation and chemotherapy.

37. DRUGS

The interrelationships of nutrition and drugs have received increasing attention as the metabolic consequences of drug treatment have been investigated and it has been better appreciated that many patients receiving drugs have nutritional disorders. There are three ways in which interaction

Table 50 Effects of cancer chemotherapeutic agents on the alimentary tract

Drug	Nausea	Vomiting	Anorexia	Mucositis	Intestinal Ulceration	Abdominal Pain	Diarrhoea	Constipation
Asparaginase	X	X	X					
BCNU	X	X	X					
Bleomycin				X				
Busulfan	X	X						
Cisplatinum	X	X	X					
Cyclophosphamide	X	X	X			X		
Cytarabine	X	X	X	X	X			
Dactinomycin	X	X	X	X		X	X	
Daunorubicin	X	X	X	X				
Doxorubicin	X	X	X					
Hydroxyurea	X	X		X			X	
Methotrexate	X		X	X	X	X	X	
Mithramycin	X	X	X		X			
Procarbazine	X		X					
Vinblastine	X	X						
Vincristine	X					X		X

Adapted from Shils ME 1980 Nutrition and neoplasia. In: Goodhart RS, Shils ME (eds) Modern nutrition in health and disease, 6th edn. Lea and Febiger, Philadelphia.

Table 51 Localized effects of radiotherapy leading to nutritional alterations

Region	Acute	Chronic
Central nervous system	Nausea	
Head and neck	Sore throat	Ulcer
	Dysphagia	Xerostomia
	Xerostomia	Dental caries
	Mucositis	Osteoradionecrosis
	Anorexia	Trismus
	Alteration in smell	Altered taste
	Loss of taste	
Thorax	Dysphagia	Fibrosis
		Stenosis
		Fistula
Abdomen-pelvis	Anorexia	Ulcer
	Nausea	Malabsorption
	Vomiting	Diarrhoea
	Diarrhoea	Chronic enteritis
	Acute enteritis	Chronic colitis
	Acute colitis	

Reproduced with permission from Donaldson SS, Lenon RA 1979 Alterations of nutritional status: Impact of chemotherapy and radiation therapy. Cancer 43:2036–2052.

Table 52 Potential nutritional sequelae of GI surgery for cancer

Radical resection of the oropharyngeal area	Impaired chewing and swallowing
Oesophagectomy and oesophageal reconstruction	Gastric stasis and hypochlorhydria secondary to vagotomy Diarrhoea and steatorrhoea
Gastrectomy	Dumping and malabsorption Achlorhydria and lack of intrinsic factor

Intestinal resection	Jejunum: decreased nutrient absorption
	Ileum: malabsorption of B_{12}, bile salts, and uric acid
	Diarrhoea
	Blind loop syndrome
	Massive bowel resection — severe malabsorption
	  Malnutrition
	  Metabolic acidosis
	Ileostomy and colostomy
	  Complications of salt and water balance

Pancreatectomy	Malabsorption Diabetes mellitus

Adapted from Shils ME 1980 Nutrition and neoplasia. In: Goodhart RS, Shils ME (eds) Modern nutrition in health and disease, 6th edn. Lea and Febiger, Philadelphia.

may take place: (1) effects of nutrition on drug metabolism, (2) effects of drugs on nutrient metabolism and (3) nutrients and the toxicity of drugs.

1. Protein-energy malnutrition (PEM), both in its endemic form in young children and as it may affect chronically ill patients of any age, may reduce the levels of enzymes including those involved in drug metabolism, and also of substrates derived from nutrients, used for the conjugation of drugs.

Malabsorption caused by this syndrome may impair the pharmacologic response of drugs. The clearance of a test dose of chloramphenicol has been shown to be delayed in children with PEM.

Mineral and vitamin deficiency may have similar effects. In animals zinc and magnesium deficiencies reduce lever levels of cytochrome P-450. Potassium deficiency induced by thiazide diuretics increases the risk of cardiac arrhythmias in patients receiving digitalis. Subclinical vitamin C deficiency, not uncommon in the elderly, may be a factor in the high incidence of adverse drug reactions in this age group.

2. There are many ways in which drugs affect the metabolism of nutrients and some are used with this effect in mind. Anorectic drugs such as fenfluramine are used to decrease appetite in the treatment of obesity (p. 153). Others, such as sulphonylureas, are used to stimulate appetite in prolonged convalescence or other causes or anorexia.

Carbohydrate metabolism is altered by drugs that cause either hyperglycaemia or hypoglycaemia. Those resulting in hyperglycaemia include thiazide diuretics, especially in those with impaired glucose tolerance as in diabetes mellitus. Corticosteroids, oral contraceptives, anticonvulsants such as dephenylhydantoin and nicotinic acid have had similar effects.

Hypoglycaemia may result from an overdose of sulphonylureas especially when they are given with other drugs that have a competitive effect. Ethanol may induce severe hypoglycaemia from inhibition of hepatic gluconeogenesis in acutely starved or chronically malnourished subjects.

A number of drugs may lower plasma lipids. Some cause a mild fat malabsorption (the antibiotics neomycin and kanamycin, p-amino-salicylic acid) or bind bile acids (cholestyramine resin, used in type II hyperlipidaemia, p. 190). D-Thyroxine lowers plasma cholesterol by increasing hepatic catabolism.

Clofibrate lowers plasma cholesterol, VLDL and triglyceride and is effective in the treatment of types IIb, III, IV and V hyperlipidaemias but its mechanism of action is uncertain. Nicotinic acid, but not nicotinamide, decreases tissue lipolysis.

Drugs which raise plasma lipids as a side effect of their use include oral contraceptives, large doses of adrenal corticosteroids, ethanol and growth hormone (triglycerides); and oral contraceptives, chlorpromazine, thiouracil and vitamin D (cholesterol). These adverse effects of oral contraceptives are of special concern in relation to their widespread use and the problem of coronary heart disease.

Nitrogen excretion in the urine is increased by costicosteroids, thyroid hormones and tetracyclines. Oral contraceptives and insulin decrease the circulating levels of some amino acids.

Mineral metabolism may be affected as in the potassium depletion induced by thiazide diuretics and sodium retention from corticosteroids and oral contraceptives. The enhancement or depression of iron absorption by various substances has been mentioned previously (p. 61). Impaired iodine uptake or release, leading to goitre, may be caused by sulphonylureas, phenylbutazone, cobalt and lithium. Oral contraceptives may lower zinc and increase copper in plasma. Prolonged use of adrenal steroids enhances osteoporosis and may lead to fractures in the elderly.

Vitamin status may be impaired in many ways by the use of drugs. Ethanol impairs the absorption of many vitamins including thiamin, folic acid and vitamin B_{12}. Isoniazid, used in the treatment of tuberculosis is a pyridoxine antagonist and may also cause pellagra as pyridoxine is required for the synthesis of niacin from tryptophan (p. 56). Pyridoxine has been shown to relieve the depression in women taking oestrogen-progestogen oral contraceptives. Those affected have been shown to have a defect in tryptophan metabolism, probably a result of induction of tryptophan pyrrolase, a rate-limiting enzyme on the pathway of tryptophan conversion to niacin, which would result in the use of pyridoxine in this pathway at the expense of the production of the neurotransmitter, 5-hydroxytryptamine.

Folic acid deficiency is common in patients receiving long-term anti-convulsant therapy (p. 125). Diphenylhydantoin has been most studied, but phenobarbital, primidone, phenothiazines and tricyclics have also been implicated. The mechanism is thought to be an effect on liver microsomal drug metabolizing enzymes which are known to require folate as cofactor, and also possibly on the synthesis of the enzymes themselves. Administration of folic acid appears to impair drug control of epilepsy but yeast tablet supplementation has been shown to improve folate status without causing any adverse effects.

Vitamin C status is impaired by tetracycline, oral contraceptives, cortico-steroids and high doses of aspirin. The antivitamin D action of anticonvul-sants has been mentioned elsewhere (p. 133).

3. Occasionally nutrients may counteract the harmful effects of toxic substances. Paracetamol is a safe analgesic in normal doses but attempted suicide by overdosage is frequent. The drug is excreted mainly as glucuronide and sulphate conjugates and the liver damage that results from overdosage is related to depletion of liver glutathione. Toxicity is increased by previous intake of phenobarbitol or protein deprivation and decreased by the sulphur donors cysteine and methionine, the latter being recommended in treatment.

Large intakes of vitamin C, 1 g or more per day, may increase the toxicity of mercury.

38. NUTRITIONAL DISORDERS AND THE LIFE-SPAN

THE FETUS
An infant may be born with low birth weight (2.5 kg) either because it is born earlier than normal, *preterm* or *premature*, or because it has not grown normally during a gestational period of normal duration, *'light'* or *'small for dates'* or *fetal malnutrition*. The generally accepted cut off point of 2.5 kg is an unsatisfactory compromise as many non-nutritional factors influence birth weight (p. 80).

The fetus is unable to regulate the fuel supply it receives from the mother, almost all in the form of glucose. In the overweight, glucose intolerant mother — a by no means infrequent occurrence in the west — the excess energy transferred to the fetus as a result of the hyperglycaemia can only be deposited as fat. In the third trimester fetal body adipose tissue may increase as much as 30-fold in what have hitherto been regarded as normal pregnancies.

THE NEONATE

Even more adipose tissue is laid down in the early months of postnatal life, under the influence of excessive energy feeding by the breast or the bottle, in western societies. In no other mammalian species does fat accumulation occur both pre- and postnatally. Healthy newborns in developing countries tend to be about 0.5 kg lighter and there is evidence to show that most of this is due to adipose tissue. Consequently the cut off point of low birth weight at 2.5 kg probably categorizes as low birth weight thousands of babies who only have less fat than the overfed western newborn. Confirmatory evidence for this view comes from the recognition in recent years that energy requirements for young infants have been overestimated and current weight standards are excessive and should be revised.

Preterm babies born before the 35th week are rarely able to suck or swallow effectively. Absorption, especially of fat, is limited and disorders in other systems such as the respiratory distress syndrome may preclude gastro-intestinal feeding and parenteral nutrition (p. 238) may have to be instituted. Nevertheless, once the initial feeding difficulties have been overcome these infants frequently catch up in growth and development, in contrast to those who are 'light for dates' who ofter suffer permanent physical and mental retardation.

About one-third to one-half of all low birth weight babies, the latter about 7 per cent of all births in Britain and as high as 35 per cent in India, are 'light for dates'. Congenital malformations, brain damage and hypoglycaemia are especially common in this group. The underlying causes of the fetal malnutrition that is reflected in low birth weight are multiple. The higher rates of low birth weight infants in developing countries are largely related to poor maternal nutrition. A high proportion of infants who receive this bad start in life go on to develop marasmus in infancy (p. 101). In technologically developed societies the not inconsiderable rates are related to placental defects and metabolic disorders of the fetus.

Children of low birth weight account for about 10 per cent of the child population and the impairment that may reveal itself at school age has been shown to relate more to attributes of the mother and family structure than to biological factors.

The proper nutrition of the low birth weight infant requires excellent nursing and close attention to feeding. Energy intake should be 110 to

130 kcal (0.46 to 0.54 MJ)/kg/day and water 150 to 200 ml/kg/day. There appears to be no advantage in increasing the energy density of formulae beyond the customary 67 kcal (0.28 MJ)/100 ml. Additional amino acids required by these infants are tyrosine and perhaps cystine. Mineral requirements are not increased but daily vitamin supplements are recommended. Those that feed or gain weight poorly may have to be fed by gastrostomy or parenterally but these should not be adopted routinely.

THE INFANT AND YOUNG CHILD

This age group is the most vulnerable of all to nutritional problems and much of Section II was devoted to these. Prominent among these are PEM (p. 100), various vitamin deficiencies (p. 109), iron deficiency (p. 141) and obesity (p. 147).

While poor growth is certainly the earliest manifestation of nutritional disorder to both mother and child is has many other causes. *Failure to thrive* may result from a disturbance of the mother-child relationship, as well as a variety of absorptive, metabolic, endocrine and other disorders which require investigation.

The displacement of traditional breast feeding by bottle feeding in developing countries has has especially disastrous consequences for child nutrition. Government policies of free milk distribution and the sometimes unscrupulous propaganda of baby milk companies have been partly responsible. The increasing tendency for young mothers to go out to work to supplement the meagre family income plays a part, but the added expense fritters much of this away. More important is the tendency to give very dilute formulae and the lack of care of the hygiene of the feeding bottle resulting in epidemics of fly-borne gastroenteritis especially in the hot months — 'summer diarrhoea'. Once this has occurred and the infant is vomiting and wasting the last straw to tip the balance into marasmus is often the ignorant advice of local lay and medical people alike to starve the child to stop the vomiting and diarrhoea (p. 278).

THE ADOLESCENT

This is a period of emotional and social as well as physical maturation. Especially related to this aspect are the occurrence of obesity (p. 141) and the opposite, but not unrelated, condition of anorexia nervosa (p. 213). Pregnancy brings its own nutritional stresses, but these are accentuated in the adolescent female (p. 254). The social circumstances are frequently adverse, to both mother and child, and it has been shown that the pregnant teenager usually has a food intake that does not differ from that of her non-pregnant peers. In general, the adolescent does not reach her full stature until four years after the onset of menstruation. Those who become pregnant within this period are especially at risk.

Anaemia is more frequent in adolescent girls than boys, largely related to menstruation in the former. Iron deficiency is the main cause but folic acid and vitamin B_{12} deficiencies also occur.

PREGNANCY AND LACTATION

Animal experiments have shown that deficiencies in the maternal diet have a profound effect on the size of litter, survival rates, size at birth, growth patterns and behaviour of the progeny. These results must not be applied to man without caution but they do suggest the importance of paying attention to the diet during pregnancy.

Birth weight of infants, neonatal mortality, maternal mortality and morbidity are influenced by the environment. It is very difficult to separate poor nutritional status from other factors such as low income, high parity, biological immaturity (under 17 years of age), short stature, low prepregnancy weight for height, low gain in weight during pregnancy, smoking, infections, chronic disease, complications of pregnancy and a history of unsuccessful pregnancies. Most of the factors tend to affect the same individuals.

The nutritional stress of pregnancy, often repeated at frequent intervals, in developing countries may precipitate such classical deficiency diseases as night blindness and xerosis conjuctivae due to vitamin A deficiency (p. 108), beriberi (p. 114), riboflavin deficiency (p. 119), and osteomalacia (p. 132). Much more widespread is anaemia due primarily to iron deficiency (p. 141) and to a lesser extent folate deficiency (p. 124). It is now believed that the usual diet in most countries cannot alone meet the increased needs for these nutrients in pregnancy.

Birth weight correlates with prepregnancy weight and total weight gain during pregnancy. A steady weight gain of 0·5 to 1·0 lb (0·23 to 0·46 kg) per week to a total of about 24 lb (11 kg) at term is recommended.

In adolescents, neonatal, postnatal and infant mortality rates are especially high. Pregnancy may have an adverse effect on the health and nutrition of the mother who is herself still immature. Intakes of iron, calcium, vitamin A and ascorbic acid tend to be particularly low and, on the other hand, obesity is not uncommon.

It has long been thought that nutrition is related to the occurrence and course of the *toxaemias of pregnancy*. Among these *pre-eclampsia* is usually defined as an acute hypertensive disorder appearing after about the 20th week of pregnancy and accompanied by oedema and/or proteinuria. *Eclampsia* is the end result of pre-eclampsia. The incidence of maternal mortality in toxaemia is inversely related to income. Contrary to popular belief energy restriction has not been demonstrated to be beneficial, the protein intake has not been shown to be related, and the practice of salt restriction and use of diuretics is not supported by scientific evidence.

Lactation increases nutritional requirements and the simplest evidence of an inadequate diet is loss of weight, and this may sometimes be masked by increase in body fluid. The volume and composition of milk tend to remain remarkably constant except in extreme deficiency, but this is probably only at the expense of maternal tissues and reserves when the diet is inadequate. Under these circumstances the deficiency states in pregnancy mentioned above all may be manifest also during lactation, especially if prolonged.

THE AGED

For a variety of reasons the aged may be especially vulnerable to developing nutritional deficiencies. Appetite is commonly poor, often because mastication is difficult from poor dentition or ill-fitting dentures. Malabsorption is not uncommon. Those immobilized or pyrexial for long periods suffer tissue breakdown. Ignorance of what constitutes a balanced diet, poverty, social isolation, mental disturbance and physical disabilities compound the problem.

Low levels of albumin, iron, folic acid, vitamin B_{12} and ascorbic acid in blood and biochemical evidence of low riboflavin, pyrodoxine and vitamin D status were much more frequent but did not necessarily correlate with clinical signs.

While, on the one hand, it is not possible to state with certainty that low biochemical levels are indicative of subclinical nutritional deficiency in the aged, on the other it must be recognized that they do form an especially vulnerable group, for reasons like those given above, and they should receive special attention.

Surveys of people over the age of 65 have shown a 1 to 2 per cent incidence of subnutrition with anaemia, osteomalacia and mild PEM being the most common forms.

MULTIPLE CHOICE QUESTIONS

Answer each question true *or* false

1. Food allergy:
   i) is more common than food intolerance
   ii) is associated with the production of IgE antibodies
   iii) can be caused by food additives
   iv) tends to lessen with advancing age
   v) is the most common form of allergy.

2. The following statements relate to total parenteral nutrition:
   i) The nitrogen: calorie ratio should be about 1:100
   ii) Fat emulsions may safely be given by peripheral vein
   iii) Selenium deficiency has been described in long-term parenteral nutrition
   iv) Urinary nitrogen excretion is a rough guide to protein requirement
   v) Energy needs are ideally met from dextrose (about 70 per cent) and fat (about 20 per cent).

3. Nutrient–drug interactions occur as follows:
   i) Potassium deficiency increases the risk of cardiac arrhythmias in patients receiving digitalis
   ii) Thiazide diuretics tend to induce hypoglycaemia
   iii) Thyroxine lowers plasma cholesterol by decreasing hepatic synthesis
   iv) Corticosteroids increase urinary nitrogen excretion
   v) Diphenylhydantoin induces folic acid deficiency.

4. In injury:
   i) release of catecholamines leads to inhibition of insulin and stimulation of corticosteroids
   ii) there is increased metabolic rate; about 100 per cent in multiple injuries
   iii) zinc assists in wound healing through formation of collagen cross-linkages
   iv) blood lactate is raised in the acute phase
   v) nitrogen balance usually becomes positive after about one week.

5. The following statements relate to nutrition and cancer:
   i) Dietary factors probably relate to 30 to 50 per cent of cancers in the western world
   ii) Nitrosamines have been shown to induce carcinoma in man
   iii) Cachexia is common in patients with disseminated cancer
   iv) The gastrointestinal mucosa is readily damaged by cancer chemotherapy
   v) Vitamin A deficiency has been associated with tumours of the lung and breast.

Explanation and answers on page 286.

FURTHER READING

31. Immunity and infection
Chandra R K, Newberne P M 1977 Nutrition immunity and infection. Plenum, New York
Selwyn P A 1986 AIDS: what is known. II Epidemiology. Hospital Practice 21: 127–164

32. Adverse reactions to food
Lessof M H (ed) 1983 Clinical reactions to food. Wiley, Chichester

33. Injury
Cuthbertson D P, Tilstone W J 1969 Metabolism during the post-injury period. Advances in Clinical Chemistry 12: 1
Fath J J, Meguid M M, Cerra F B 1985 The hormonal and metabolic response to surgery and stress. In: Practice of surgery, vol I. Harper & Row, Philadelphia, Ch 15A, p 1–26
Stoner H B, Frayn K N, Barton R N, Threlfall C J, Little R A 1979 The relationships between plasma substrates and hormones and the severity of injury in 277 recently injured patients. Clinical Science 56: 563–573

34. Elemental diets and parenteral nutrition
Fowell E, Lee H A, Dickerson J W T 1978 Intragastric tube feeds and elemental diets. In: Dickerson J W T, Lee H A (eds) Nutrition in the clinical management of disease. Arnold, London, p 332

Johnston I D A (ed) 1978 Advances in parenteral nutrition. MTP Press, Lancaster
Meguid M M, Aun F, Eldar S 1985 Nutrition in surgery. In: Goldsmith H S (eds) Practice of
surgery. Harper, & Row, Philadelphia

35. Alcoholism
Phillipson R V (ed) 1970 Modern trends in drug dependence and alcoholism. Butterworth,
London

36. Cancer
National Research Council, National Academy of Sciences 1982 Diet, nutrition and cancer.
National Academy Press, Washington, DC
Meguid M M, Dudrick S J (eds) 1966 Nutrition and cancer I. Surgical Clinics of
North America 66 (5) 869
Meguid M M, Dudrick S J (eds) 1966 Nutrition and cancer II. Surgical Clinics of
North America 66 (6) 1077
Williams G M 1985 Food and cancer. Nutrition International 1: 49–59

37. Drugs
Dickerson J W T 1978 The interrelationships of nutrition and drugs. In: Dickerson J W T,
Lee H A (eds) Nutrition in the clinical management of disease. Arnold, London, p 308
Roe D A 1986 Drugs and nutrition in the geriatric patient. Alan R Liss Inc, New York

38. Nutritional disorders and the life-span
Burman D 1982 Nutrition in systemic disease. In: McLaren D S, Burman D (eds) Textbook
of paediatric nutrition, 2nd edn. Churchill Livingstone, London
Exton-Smith A N 1978 Nutrition in the elderly. In: Dickerson J W T, Lee H A (eds)
Nutrition in the clinical management of disease. Arnold, London, p 72
Jacobson H N 1977 Nutrition. In: Philipp E E, Barnes J, Newton M (eds) Scientific
foundations of obstetrics and gynaecology, 2nd edn. Heinemann, London, p 511
McLaren D S 1987 A fresh look at perinatal growth and nutritional standards. World Review
of Nutrition and Dietetics 49: 87–120
Metcoff J 1982 Maternal nutrition and fetal growth. In: McLaren D S, Burman D (eds)
Textbook of paediatric nutrition, 2nd edn. Churchill Livingstone, London
Young E A (ed) 1986 Nutrition, aging and health. Alan R Liss Inc, New York

V

Food and nutrition in the community

'There are two sides to the life of every man: there is his individual existence which is free in proportion as his interests are abstract; and his elemental life as a unit in the human swarm, in which he must inevitably obey the laws laid down for him.'

L. N. TOLSTOY, *War and Peace*

39. INTRODUCTION

In recent years there has been a new emphasis placed upon the application of nutritional knowledge and expertise to the problems at the community level. This has come about largely as a result of a better understanding of the nature of the problems. They are now seen to be multifactorial in origin and incapable of solution by unilateral interventions as attempted in the past. It has also become appreciated by politicians and their advisers that good nutrition is not just a fortunate byproduct of development but is one of the necessary inputs to bring it about. Malnutrition in a population results in increased mortality, morbidity, diminished work efficiency and poor learning ability.

The Agent-Host-Environment concept should still provide a helpful approach to the problem as man in community is only individual man writ large. In Figure 22 the Host is now the *community;* local, national or world, and has to be considered both qualitatively *(nutritional status)* and quantitatively *(population)*. The food supply in its various aspects may be considered to be the quantitative aspect interacting with the community and within this is the qualitative aspect of *nutriment supply*. All of these are influenced by many factors inherent in society; such as *economics, technology, culture, education* and *hygiene*. It is they that are the ultimate determinants of nutrition. Those that seek to manipulate them rarely have the nutritional consequences of their actions in mind. It is therefore foolish of those who endeavour to bring about nutritional improvement to ignore them.

It should be clear from Figure 22 that a great variety of people are to a greater or lesser extent and directly or indirectly concerned with nutrition at the community level. Besides a variety of public health physicians, nurses, technicians, and other paramedical personnel they include administrators, politicians, economists, agriculturists, food technologists, educationalists,

258

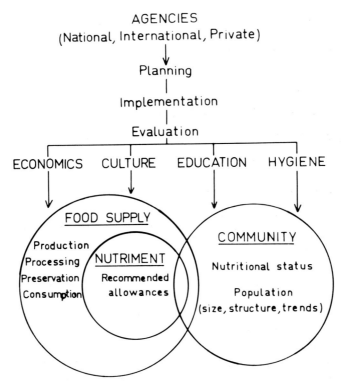

Fig. 22 The Agent-Host-Environment concept applied to nutrition in the community.

sociologists and others. From what has already been said it must be admitted that this gives a nutritionist's eyeview only; the vast majority of politicians and others do not recognize the need for their involvement.

What has been said applies equally to both developed and developing communities. Broadly speaking, the world can be divided into two unequal halves in relation to nutrition. While one half has never known hunger the other half has never known satiety. Throughout most of the developing world malnutrition mainly affects young children and to a lesser extent pregnant and lactating women. The forms taken by malnutrition and its underlying causes have been described previously (Section II). Among some, but by no means all, of these communities natural or man-made disasters may bring food shortages and famine. Increasingly in the towns and cities of the technologically developing countries, alongside the undernourished slum dwellers there are growing up affluent segments of society which are subject to the same lifestyle-related health problems as are the common lot in the west.

In the discussions that follow it will be necessary to draw distinctions between the widely contrasting conditions outlined above. However, in each set of circumstances similar principles apply for the improvement of nutrition and health, although the means to this end will differ.

40. WORLD FOOD SUPPLIES

When the problem of trying to meet the ever-increasing needs of the world's population for food is considered it is too often conceived of only in agricultural and economic terms. Measures aimed at growing more food and making it available at prices that all can afford are clearly of great importance. Ultimately, however, it is the quantity and quality of food that an individual actually consumes that determines his nutritional state.

Food supply

The relationship between food supply and population increase is not 1:1 but more like $4:2\frac{1}{2}$, i.e. a $2\frac{1}{2}$ per cent increase in population will necessitate a 4 per cent increase in food supply. This concept recognizes that there must be qualitative improvement among the poorest sections of populations. Secondly, relatively more people will be adults and children will tend to grow bigger.

There have been numerous technological developments in recent years that may potentially increase food supplies. Broadly speaking they are of four kinds:

1. Non-agricultural, such as food from petrol. This is not efficient and the nutrient mixture provided is not ideal.

2. Exploiting the ocean. There could be a three-fold increase but this would still meet only 10 per cent of the total need.

3. Food technology is the area where startling achievements are being attained but where at the same time many ill-conceived plans founder. Texturized protein, made from soya beans, provides a meat substitute nutritionally equivalent to hamburger, at about half the cost. In recent years it has been introduced in school and other mass feeding programmes and has met with general public acceptance. Fortification of foodstuffs with low-cost nutrients, especially vitamins and some elements, plays an important role in protecting vulnerable groups. In developing countries protein from leaves is being processed for human use. At present protein from single cell organisms is used in animal feeds but is not considered safe for human consumption.

4. Agricultural development. The expansion of subsistence farming has been the most important method of increasing food supplies up until the present time. Further extension is possible only to a limited extent. It is a very expensive method and generally speaking the available land is far away from the people to cultivate it, who are mainly in Asia.

During the past two decades startling results have been obtained by increasing the yield of certain cereal crops, notably maize, wheat and rice, by the use of fertilizers, ground water and improved protection, but most of all by the introduction of hybrid strains which have various characteristics favourable to high yield. These characteristics include high response to fertilizer, short growing season, lack of photosensitivity, resistance to disease, adaptability to flooding or to drought conditions, high nutritive quality and acceptable taste. This 'green revolution' has been very successful in those countries where climatic and political conditions are favourable. Despite the continued growth in population India has become an exporter of both wheat and rice. Rice is especially important. One-third of mankind depend on it for more than half their food and 90 per cent of low income people of the most densely populated regions rely on it. The green revolution can only be sustained if all the various necessary inputs are available together and can be purchased by the farmer. These inputs include such things as irrigation water, high-yielding seed, fertilizers, tools and machinery, transportation, plant protection, and storage. There is also a need for readily available credit at reasonable interest rates, and a whole fund of technical knowhow.

Food production

The annual production of food is about 1250 million tons. Technologically developed countries with only 25 per cent of the world's population consume 50 per cent of the food. Animals consume 25 per cent of all the grain; sufficient to feed the 1·3 billion people of China and India. It requires 20 lb of grain to produce each 1 lb of beef; 7 or 8 lb for 1 lb of pork and less per lb of chicken. In developed countries only 4 per cent of the population is employed in farming and superfarms in the USA, only 4 per cent of the total, produce 50 per cent of the food for that country and most of that for export. Most superfarms are but a small part of massive diversified companies. Under these conditions farming is very costly in money and energy; more than 1 kcal of energy is required to produce 1 kcal of food. Agribusiness is very flexible, responding rapidly to profit possibilities. Stocks built up in the 1960s rapidly disappeared when the four main grain-producing nations took one-third of the grain growing area out of production because of fall in prices.

In Asia 80 per cent, and in parts of Africa 95 per cent of the people live and work on the land, but land ownership is concentrated in the hands of the few. Of land greater than 100 hectares throughout the world only 2·5 per cent of the population own nearly 75 per cent of this land. In South America 17 per cent of land owners own 90 per cent of the land and many are absentee landlords and investment is low. Small farms have been shown to be more than 10 times as efficient as large in these circumstances. Cash crops mainly provide foreign exchange for the rich who monopolize the scarce imports of fertilizers and pesticides, and local employment is at the mercy of world prices. Even then much of the food is exported to developed countries and women and children suffer as a consequence.

Food production is not determined simply by an increase, or decrease, in total output from the present crops and livestock. Important adjustments occur as a result of changes in the contributions that make up the production. Livestock is a big adjuster. It is about seven times less efficient to feed people on livestock which has consumed crops than to feed them directly on those crops. In time of shortage livestock acts as a kind of shock-absorber. Most developing countries have little livestock and so no such provision to avert disaster.

Adjustment of food production is also brought about by changes in intensification of cropping systems. If population increases and the food supply is hard pressed the cropping system is intensified with greater production of those crops yielding more energy per acre, e.g. potatoes, rice, maize. Other important factors adjusting food production are the stocking of food on a short-term basis and trade which acts in the short and the long term.

Food distribution

The economist is concerned about maldistribution of food primarily at the international level. Because of the lack of purchasing power of the developing countries and the consequent failure under these circumstances of trade missions and promotional efforts Food Aid, especially from the United States (under Public Law 480), has appeared to some to be a solution. However, the snags have proved to be formidable, not least the cost to the donor countries and the depressing effect on food production by the recipient. Self-help with assistance is the present clarion call.

The efficiency of transport systems, both international and within a country, together with storage and preservation facilities, clearly form a vital link between the food produced and the food consumed. In some developing countries it has been estimated that as much as half the food produced is destroyed before it reaches the consumer. These matters have been touched on earlier (p. 19).

Food consumption

This may be assessed indirectly by the food balance sheet in which national data for total production of individual commodities are adjusted for imports and exports and for changes in stock to give estimates of gross food supplies. The estimates are rough; seasonal, regional and group differences are obscured. A carefully prepared food balance sheet can provide a government with valuable data regarding main food groups and energy and protein supplies.

Direct assessment involves household inquiries or measurement of the amount of food actually eaten by individuals. This method if properly applied collects more detailed information relating to rather limited groups. It supplements the information provided by the food balance sheet and is more appropriately considered in relation to nutritional status.

In Britain both these kinds of data have been collected regularly since 1940.

The first, known as CLE or consumption level estimates, corresponds roughly to the food available for human consumption. The second is derived from a National Food Survey (NFS) and represents food entering the family kitchen and does not include food eaten outside the home. Although the NFS is a valuable source of information concerning trends in food consumption its data have to be interpreted with caution as sizeable fractions of total food intake occur for most people outside the home.

In order to increase food intake there has to be overall economic growth. One of the major brakes preventing increased food consumption by very poor families is their low purchasing power. As high a proportion as 70 per cent of any increase in family spending in developing countries goes on food, while the figure is only 10 per cent in developed countries. Thus the problem is not a technological one, as had been assumed for years, but economic.

Nutriment supply

This is the qualitative aspect of food supply, i.e. a concern for ensuring the consumption of sufficient food to meet, but not exceed, energy and nitrogen requirements and an adequacy of the various nutrients.

In general, affluent societies consume more than is good for them of total energy, saturated fat, refined carbohydrate and more protein than they need. There are encouraging signs that governments are increasingly concerned to advise people to eat prudently (see p. 280)

The mass of people in developing countries are undernourished to some degree by western standards. There has long been a tendency to assume that deficiency of protein in the diet of young children is largely responsible and terms such as the 'protein gap' and 'protein crisis' have been freely used. While this is no doubt true for the 100 million or so of the world's people subsisting on poor quality staples, it is not true for the majority of cereal-eating peoples (p. 11). Several studies in different countries show that total energy is the limiting factor (see p. 100) in relation to the pre-school child. However, the question still needs to be asked, 'why is the total food intake suboptimal?'. In the young child, poverty, ignorance and infections are largely responsible and these cannot be overcome merely by producing more or even better food.

41. POPULATION AND FOOD

It will take twice as much food by A.D. 2000 to feed twice as many people no better than the people of the 1960s were fed. To feed the world's population at the end of the century (probably well over 6000 million as 5 billion was passed in mid-1987) adequately will require very much more.

Population studies conducted by the United Nations show that the projected growth is more than twice as great for the less-developed regions (average rate 2·4 per cent) as for the more-developed regions (1·0 per cent). In addition the less-developed regions carry a very heavy load of youth dependency. In 1960, 40 per cent of the total population of these regions was under 15 years of age.

Population growth has important repercussions on economic development. A typical situation in developing countries is a rise in total income of 4 per cent which, with 2.4 per cent population growth, lifts *per capita* income by only 1.6 per cent, requiring 43 years to double. With widespread unemployment and underemployment only slower rates of population growth will help economic growth.

The need for population policies by the governments of developing countries has been forced on them by unprecedentedly high rates of population growth in recent years resulting from efficient control of disease coupled with high fertility of traditional peasant societies. About 75 per cent of all people in such regions live in countries whose governments formally favour reduction of birth rates as national policy. Population growth approaching zero at the present time has resulted largely from individual choice in many western countries and as a result of government policy only in a few small developing countries. China, with its draconian policy of one child per family, has put a brake on population growth at about 1 billion. For the remaining three-quarters of the world's population rapid growth will inevitably continue unchecked until at least the end of the century and control will eventually come through either development or catastrophe.

Of major importance is the distribution of wealth within a country. Between 1965 and 1972 the gross national product (GNP) in Brazil increased by 5·6 per cent and the population only by 2·9 per cent. The GNP went up by only 2 per cent in the USA and Britain and yet there is widespread malnutrition in Brazil.

Population density does not correlate with food supply. A World Bank study in Asian showed that there were more hectares per person in the four worst-fed countries: India (0·30), Pakistan (0·40), Bangladesh (0·16) and Indonesia (0·15); than in the four best-fed countries: China (0·13), South Korea (0·07), Vietnam (0·10) and Taiwan (0·06).

A study made by the Population Council in 1972 showed that 31 developing countries, with 75 per cent of the population of all developing countries, had public birth control policies. Twenty eight others, with a further 13 per cent of the population, suggested family planning in some form. Most of these programmes have failed to reach their objectives; mainly because of the lack of social and economic reform, together with a reduction in infant mortality and the continuing preference for male children.

Population control is one thing, and family planning is another. The former is the concern of nations and works only one way, towards limitation. Family planning deals with: (1) having children if this is difficult, (2) limiting the size of the family (3) spacing the children that are born. Motivation is most important and the improved chances of survival of children and their better education can be strong motives for limiting their number. Numerous studies show that spacing of children has a favourable effect on their survival. While much effort is being spent on developing better contraceptive devices than the pill or the loop, not enough attention is being paid to influencing motivation. It has been calculated that prolonged breast feeding has a more significant contraceptive effect than all the artificial means put together in the third world (p. 82).

The world food supply is increasingly being determined by climate and politics. When the previous edition was written most western countries had very little food in reserve. Now the situation has dramatically changed; at the end of 1987 the barns, granaries and cold stores are bulging with more unwanted food than the world has ever previously seen. The EEC food 'mountains' and drink 'lakes' are notorious and only now are policies beginning to be agreed to set matters right. It is an additional folly that technological developments continue to make productivity ever more efficient under these circumstances.

In the third world many poor countries penalize their farmers by denying them a proper price for their produce; these governments prefer to subsidize the urban masses' food, among whom discontent is likely to breed revolution. Fundamental also to food and famine in developing countries is land impoverishment and erosion, consequent upon rapid increase in human and animal populations.

42. NUTRITIONAL ASSESSMENT AND SURVEILLANCE

Hitherto methodology has not developed sufficiently to make possible the assessment of the nutritional status of a community in quantitative terms. Part of the probem lies in the fact that we cannot define good, or normal, nutrition. Deviations from the normal form a gradual spectrum of change and a dividing line between normal and abnormal can only be drawn arbitrarily. Two questions require answers: (1) Where will the line be drawn between the 'normal' and 'subnormal' (and in some cases the 'supranormal')? (2) What proportion of 'abnormal' findings in a population will it be necessary to have in order to warrant some action?

In recent years attention has been given to the need for the surveillance of the nutritional status of populations in relation to activities in the fields of food, agriculture and health. A surveillance system is designed to provide the continuous collection of data as an integral part of the formulation and execution of policies in these areas. A methodology of nutritional surveillance has been outlined by a Joint FAO/UNICEF/WHO Expert Committee (see Further Reading).

The kinds of information needed for the assessment of nutritional status of a community are shown in Table 53. Some are more directly of medical concern and these will be dealt with here.

Table 53 Information needed for assessment of nutritional status

Source of information	Nature of information obtained	Nutritional implications
1. Agricutural data Food balance sheets	Gross estimates of agricultural production Agricultural methods Soil fertility Predominance of cash crops Overproduction of staples Food imports and exports	Approximate availability of food supplies to a population
2. Socio-economic data Information on marketing, distribution and storage	Purchasing power Distribution and storage of foodstuffs	Unequal distribution of available foods between the socioeconomic groups in the community and within the family
3. Food consumption patterns Cultural-anthropological data	Lack of knowledge, erroneous beliefs and prejudices, indifference	
4. Dietary surveys	Food consumption	Low, excessive or unbalanced nutrient intake
5. Special studies on foods	Biological value of diets Presence of interfering factors (e.g. goitrogens) Effects of food processing	Special problems related to nutrient utilization
6. Vital and health statistics	Morbidity and mortality data	Extent of risk to community Identification of high-risk groups
7. Anthropometric studies	Physical development	Effect of nutrition on physical development
8. Clinical nutritional surveys	Physical signs	Deviation from health due to malnutrition
9. Biochemical studies	Levels of nutrients, metabolites and other components of body tissues and fluids	Nutrient supplies in the body Impairment of biochemical function
10. Additional medical information	Prevalent disease patterns, including infections and infestations	Interrelationships of state of nutrition and disease

(WHO 1963 Technical report series 258.)

VITAL STATISTICS

The type of data that may be considered to be in some way public health indicators of malnutrition are morbidity rates for certain diseases (such as tuberculosis), mortality rates in the perinatal and early childhood periods, maternal mortality, and life expectancy figures. Such data are often not available or, if available, often unreliable. The method of collection of data will clearly be important, e.g. although the number of deaths recorded may be quite reliable this will not be true of the causes of death of those not seen by a physician and those not autopsied.

Nutrition is only one of many factors influencing morbidity and mortality statistics. Actuarial tables of life insurance companies have for long indicated that there is a direct correlation between overweight (not necessarily obesity) and life expectation. The use of vital statistics as an indicator of malnutrition has been virtually confined to the preschool child period when malnutrition (mostly PEM p. 100) is commonest.

Age-specific mortality rates

Infant mortality rate. This has long been used as an indicator of the health of a community. It is much higher in developing than in industralized countries. The difference is greater if the perinatal period (first month) is excluded as malnutrition plays little part at this time, but data according to special age periods like this are normally not kept. The contrast will be especially great in those places where rapid social change is taking place. As we have seen (p. 102), urbanizing influences tend to favour the occurrence of marasmus, mainly a disease of the first 12 months of life. In the relatively few parts of the world where kwashiorkor predominates, the peak age incidence of PEM falls later than the first year. The future trend is for marasmus to replace kwashiorkor. Consequently marasmus may be expected to play an important part in infant mortality in those places where economic growth does not keep up with social change.

Mortality rate, 1 to 4 years. This rate has been suggested as a public health index of malnutrition, as it is in this, the preschool period, that much of the stress from maternal deprivation, malnutrition and infection falls. This rate may be even 30 to 50 times higher in some developing countries than it is in Europe or North America. The influence of malnutrition on this rate will be greatest in those places where kwashiorkor, rather than marasmus, predominates.

Second year mortality rate. This is a more recent refinement of the 1 to 4 year rate by those who contend, and rightly, that most of the high level of the latter rate in developing countries can be attributed to the contribution made by the second year. Many of the late cases of marasmus and of kwashiorkor can be expected during this year.

These rates should not not be regarded as a 'public health index of malnutrition'. They can show what the chances of survival of a child are, but in order to know what is causing the poor survival detailed information on disease is necessary.

Cause-specific morbidity and mortality

At the clinical level it is possible through special surveys, outpatient clinics and hospitals to record the prevalence of (1) malnutrition in its various forms, and (2) nutrition-related diseases, especially 'gastroenteritis', measles and pertussis. This approach has often been the basis for practical measures to be taken. In its simplest terms this may not amount to more than a competent expert visiting an area for a few days, discussing the problem with government health officials and examining patients in hospitals and clinics. It is then possible to report whether or not a serious problem exists, although the causes and the remedies may not at that stage be evident.

Cause-of-death records are not to be relied upon to indicate specific death rates due to malnutrition, even where official records are reasonably accurate. There is universal reluctance to have the primary cause of death recorded as 'malnutrition' because of the social and ethical implications of such a diagnosis. Kwashiorkor with its florid clinical picture is much more often recorded than marasmus, which is less spectacular and is usually masked by the frequently accompanying 'gastroenteritis'.

CLINICAL SIGNS

A careful and complete physical examination remains one of the cornerstones of clinical medicine, despite the proliferation of laboratory tests in recent years. In the field attention has to be confined to a few externally visible areas such as limited parts of the skin, mouth, hair and eyes. In any population, however, instances of frank nutritional disease giving rise to symptoms and signs of alarming degree will be very few indeed. Almost all the signs observed in a nutrition survey are entirely trivial.

Furthermore, being confined to the surface of the body, factors such as dirt, smoke, cold, heat and infections of the surfaces play a major part in actually causing the lesions, or at least in modifying them. A related problem is the lack of specificity of the signs in nutrition surveys. Some, such as scars of the cornea and rhagades of the angles of the mouth, are stigmas of former conditions. It is very difficult in retrospect to know how such lesions were caused in the first place. Other signs are symptomless, usually of a very chronic nature, showing only a minimal deviation from the normal appearance of the tissue which they affect. None of these signs can be attributed with certainty to a single nutrient deficiency. Furthermore, many non-nutritional factors also have to be included in the differential diagnosis.

The amount of disagreement among observers as to the decision concerning whether a sign is present or absent and, if present, as to the degree of presence, is very great and inversely proportional to the magnitude of the lesions. Observers tend to 'overdiagnose' to begin with and then become accustomed to the presence of what they considered deviations from normal.

Abnormal appearances in the covering tissues of the body imply structural and histological alterations. Before this can happen there must be depletion of what stores the body has and a 'biochemical lesion' in the tissue. Thus at best these signs are indicative of a rather advanced stage of deficiency.

Signs used in nutrition surveys

A WHO Expert Committee on Medical Assessment of Nutritional Status (1963) classified such signs as: those (1) not related to nutrition; (2) that need further investigation, and (3) known to be of value. The first group consists of various appearances which have clearly no relation to nutrition, e.g. alopecia, pyorrhoea, and some others which were at one time thought to be related, e.g. pinguecula, pterygium. In the second group are many signs for which there is still no good evidence for a nutritional aetiology, they include malar pigmentation, geographic tongue and changes in blood pressure. The third group includes the signs shown in Table 54. These signs have been described in Section II on undernutrition in relation to one or other of the nutritional deficiency states. Under field conditions, however, few examples of such signs will be encountered in even the most undernourished community. Rather will the signs observed in the field be very mild, easy to overlook and regarded by some as normal, or easy to mistake for other lesions. Apart from mottled enamel of the teeth and thyroid enlargement these signs are either clearly recognizable only in advanced deficiency, or else are non-specific.

ANTHROPOMETRY

Poor nutrition is only one, although perhaps the most important, of the adverse factors leading to stunted growth and retarded development. Especially in childhood, in developing regions of the world infections are so closely bound up with poor diet that their respective effects on growth cannot be separated. The evidence from controlled experiments for the influence nutrition has on the growth of animals is conclusive, but for man it is circumstantial only. Even so the secular trend of increase in height observed over many decades in schoolchildren in some western countries, which recently appears to have reached a maximum, and studies in special groups, such as the increase in size of Japanese observed first in those who migrated to the USA and then more recently in indigenous Japanese, provide evidence that changes in the way of life, of which nutrition is probably the most important, do affect growth and development of whole populations.

Field anthropometry usually has to be undertaken with a limited number of relatively simple methods, with due care paid to the technique used in performing the test and the interpretation of the results. The apparent simplicity of the tests, such as measuring weight and length, should not allow these tasks to be delegated to an inexperienced person. Instruments used must be accurate, in good working order, adjusted for use, procedures have to be standardized, and lack of co-operation in subjects, especially important in young children, has to be overcome.

Somatic measurements of various kinds are especially important in assessing growth in childhood. The results obtained, whether in an individual or a population, have to be compared with some standard. Standards for some

Table 54 Signs known to be of value in nutrition surveys and their interpretation
Kanawati AA 1976 In: McLaren DS (ed) Nutrition in the community. John Wiley and Sons, Chichester)

Signs	Associated disorder or nutrient
Hair	
Lack of lustre	Protein energy malnutrition
Thinness and sparseness*	Protein energy malnutrition
Straightness	Protein energy malnutrition
Dyspigmentation*	Protein energy malnutrition
Flag sign	Protein energy malnutrition
Easy pluckability*	Protein energy malnutrition
Face	
Nasolabial dyssebacea	Riboflavin
Moon-face	Kwashiorkor
Eyes	
Pale conjunctiva*	Anaemia (iron etc.)
Bitot's spot*	Vitamin A
Conjunctival xerosis*	Vitamin A
Corneal xerosis	Vitamin A
Keratomalacia*	Vitamin A
Angular palpebritis	Riboflavin, pyridoxine
Lips	
Angular stomatitis*	Riboflavin
Angular scars	Riboflavin
Cheilosis*	Riboflavin
Tongue	
Scarlet and raw tongue*	Nicotinic acid
Magenta tongue	Riboflavin
Teeth	
Mottled enamel*	Fluorosis
Gums	
Spongy bleeding gums*	Ascorbic acid
Glands	
Thyroid enlargement*	Iodine
Parotid enlargement	Starvation
Skin	
Xerosis	Vitamin A
Perifollicular hyperkeratosis*	Vitamin A
Petechiae	Ascorbic acid
Pellagrous dermatosis*	Nicotinic acid
Flaky paint dermatosis*	Kwashiorkor
Scrotal and vulval dermatosis	Riboflavin
Nails	
Koilonychia	Iron
Subcutaneous tissue	
Oedema*	Kwashiorkor
Fat decreased	Starvation, marasmus,
Fat increased	Obesity

* Suggested for use in rapid survey.

Signs	Associated disorder or nutrient
Muscular and skeletal systems	
Muscle wasting*	Starvation, marasmus, kwashiorkor
Craniotabes	Vitamin D
Frontal and parietal bossing	Vitamin D
Epiphyseal enlargement*	Vitamin D
Beading of ribs	Vitamin D
Persistently open anterior fontanelle*	Vitamin D
Knock-knees or bow legs*	Vitamin D
Thoracic rosary	Vitamin D, ascorbic acid
Musculoskeletal haemorrhages	Ascorbic acid
Internal systems	
(a) Gastrointestinal	
Hepatomegaly*	Kwashiorkor
(b) Nervous	
Psychomotor changes	Kwashiorkor
Mental confusion	Thiamin, nicotinic acid
Sensory loss	Thiamin, nicotinic acid
Motor weakness	Thiamin, nicotinic acid
Loss of position sense	Thiamin, nicotinic acid
Loss of vibration	Thiamin
Loss of ankle and knee jerks	Thiamin
Calf tenderness	Thiamin
(c) Cardiac	
Cardiac enlargement	Thiamin
Tachycardia	Thiamin

* Suggested for use in rapid survey.

commonly used measurements, such as weight, height and head circumference, are available from North America and Europe. These were obtained by measuring a statistically satisfactory sample of what were considered to be healthy, well-fed subjects of known age. Longitudinal data are used for children. Percentile charts have been constructed for weight and height separately and several versions are in general use to follow the growth of individual children or plot cross-sectional data of a population.

Considerable attention is being paid in various countries at the present time to the development of local standards. This is a major undertaking but, wherever suitable subjects have been available, the results have been found to be closely comparable to those developed earlier in the west. One of the most serious difficulties in most developing countries is to know the exact age of children. If registration is not in force or not strictly adhered to, it is possible sometimes to date the birth approximately by the use of a calendar made up of local events, such as religious holidays or special happenings such as earthquakes. Comparison of certain measurements may be made to get round the problem of unknown age: head circumference/mid-arm circumference is an example.

Somatic measurements

The following require a minimum of simple equipment and may each contribute particular information: (a) weight (body mass), (b) length (overall size), (c) head circumference (possible relationship to mental development), (d) mid-arm circumference; variations being due mainly to changes in muscle mass (protein) and fat (energy). Chest circumference is also of value, especially in relation to head circumference, when the exact age of a child is not known. Weight-for-length and weight-for-head-circumference may also be used in the same way.

Reliance should not be placed on any single measurement for the evaluation of the growth of a child. Weight, the measurement most commonly used in clinics, is subject to quite gross errors when made routinely by harassed personnel. Furthermore, quite considerable body compositional variation occurs in healthy young children of the same age. Increase in body water, not evident clinically as oedema, may be marked by an apparently satisfactory rise in body weight. If a strong measuring board is used for height and a flexible steel tape measure for the circumferences of head, chest and arm, reproducible results may be obtained indefinitely by unskilled personnel with the minimum of supervision. Increase in weight, in the absence of normal increase in the skeletal measurements, will draw attention to failure to thrive, probably of nutritional origin. Further disadvantages are the inappropriate nature of western standards for developing countries and in the case of the weight alone the incorrect assumption that all children of a given age should ideally have the same weight, and its inability to distinguish between past and present effects of malnutrition.

As a consequence weight/length/age is being used increasingly. This is based on the not unreasonable assumption that at any given age all children should ideally have a certain mass (weight)/size (length) irrespective of actual weight or length. Figure 23 shows how any child or group of children can have their nutritional status assessed in this way. Those who show considerable stunting (90 per cent or less of length for age) and a normal weight/length/age value are classed as nutritional dwarfs as a result of malnutrition in the past but no longer active in the present.

The anthropometric approach is only capable of identifying what one might call 'thriving', especially in the growing child. Many factors may result in 'failure to thrive' in the individual but, if a considerable proportion of the children of a community are considered not to be thriving, then the main reason will be undernutrition.

For adults ideal weight for height in relation to body frame (large, medium or small) in the form of tables based on life insurance company data are in general use. Here the problem is usually one of overweight and this is usually considered to exist when the actual weight is more than 10 per cent above the ideal, and obesity to be present when the figure is more than 20 per cent above the ideal. The visual assessment of frame is recognized to be inaccurate and

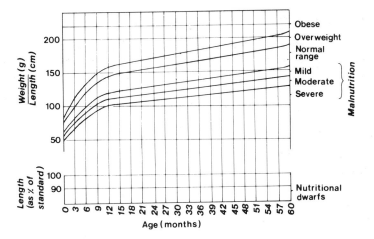

Fig. 23 Chart for the assessment of nutritional status (McLaren D S, Read W W C 1975 Lancet 219).

measurements of the frame are being introduced. Skinfold measurements are used for the same purpose.

LABORATORY TESTS

Field conditions impose various limitations on the kinds of tests. Subjects who voluntarily participate in a survey cannot be subjected to tests that might carry some risks which can legitimately be taken in patients seeking investigation and treatment of disease. Sampling has to be confined virtually to blood and urine. The range of values found in healthy individuals is very wide. Consequently individual values are meaningless and the results for the sample of a population have to be considered with regard to the proportion of the population with values lying within certain ranges. Besides deficient intake, abnormal values may be caused by malabsorption, failure in transport, or destruction or excretion of a particular constituent. The conditions of collection of the sample (e.g. time of day, relation to meals), of storage, preparation for estimation and technique of estimation all introduce probabilities of variation in results obtained, even for the same individual at the same time. The error is likely to be greater the smaller the amount of material available and the lower the concentration of the constituent in the sample. Duplicate estimations are often not carried out because of lack of material, sometimes conditioned by the desire to do a whole battery of tests on a single sample.

A list of currently advocated tests applicable in nutrition surveys is shown in Table 55. This is quite comprehensive and relatively few surveys will be able to have all these tests performed. Those requiring sampling after dosing (load tests) or timed urine specimens are difficult to carry out under the exigencies

Table 55 Laboratory tests for nutrients and metabolites

Nutrient	Most sensitive	Less sensitive	Least sensitive
Protein	plasma amino acids, transferrin, prealbumin urine 3-methyl histidine	serum albumin, urine hydroxyproline, urea/creatinine	total serum protein
Lipids	serum high density lipoproteins	serum cholesterol, triglycerides	
Vitamin A		serum vitamin A, retinol-binding protein	
Vitamin D	serum $25(OH)D_3,1,25\ (OH)_2D_3$	serum alkaline phosphatase	serum calcium and phosphorus
Vitamin E	serum tocopherol	H_2O_2 erythrocyte fragility	
Vitamin K	prothrombin time (PT)	bleeding and coagulation times	
Vitamin C	whole blood ascorbic acid	serum ascorbic acid	
Thiamin	erythrocyte transketolase and TPP effect	urine thiamin	blood pyruvate
Riboflavin	erythrocyte glutathione reductase	urine riboflavin	
Nicotinic Acid		urine N_1 methyl nicotinamide and its pyridone	
Folic acid	erythrocyte folate	serum folate	bone marrow film, thin blood film
Vitamin B_6		tryptophan load test and urine xanthurenic acid, plasma and urine pyridoxine	erythrocyte glutamic pyruvate and oxaloacetic transaminase
Vitamin B_{12}	serum vitamin B_{12}, thymidylate synthetase	urine methylmalonic acid	bone marrow film, thin blood film
Iron	serum ferritin, iron in bone marrow	serum iron saturation transferrin	blood film
Iodine	T_3, T_4	serum protein-bound iodine	urine iodine
Zinc	serum zinc	hair zinc	
Selenium	erythrocyte glutathione peroxidase	serum selenium	

of field conditions. Even the collection of 'spot' urine samples in the field poses problems, especially from uncooperative young children.

Recently hair root morphology has been shown to be an aid in differentiating the severer degrees of PEM. Trace element status is now considered not to be accurately reflected by concentration in hair.

DIETARY EVALUATION

Dietary evaluation consists of an assessment of food consumption in relation to nutrient and energy requirements. This may be done at different levels: worldwide (FAO Indicative Food Plan), national, community, special group (young children, pregnant women).

At the international and national level three sets of data need to be known: (1) food balance data, i.e. figures for production, import and export of various foods; (2) age and sex structure of the population; and (3) the nutritional requirements of the population in terms of its structure.

At the community level items (2) and (3) still apply but item (1) can be replaced by a more accurate assessment of actual intake by direct measurement. This usually consists of some form of household food-consumption survey. There are three steps in such a survey:

1. Assessment of food consumption, e.g. by recording quantities of food eaten during a set period, say 7 days; by weighing and measuring foods in the raw state and perhaps cooked portions.

2. Calculation of nutritive value of food. Food composition tables, preferably local if available, are used to calculate nutritive value. Chemical analyses of foods may be made for special purposes and if laboratory facilities are available. Food composition should be calculated *per capita* per day and the composition of the family taken into account. Cooked servings have to be weighed if distribution within the family is to be gauged.

3. Comparison with nutritional requirements. Recommended allowances, taking into account such factors as sex, age, weight, and physiological state, have been worked out for a number of technologically developed countries and by FAO/WHO with the developing regions especially in mind.

Although dietary surveys are difficult to carry out, are time-consuming, and need well-trained personnel, and although results are difficult to interpret and are subject to numerous errors, they have the distinct advantage that the results form the very basis for practical measures to improve the nutrient intake, including nutrition education.

Interpreting the results

It was earlier suggested that there was a need for some criteria, however arbitrary, in order to form a basis for interpretation of the results obtained by the methods just described and to serve as the basis for recommendations for action. Each of the five types of data has to be interpreted separately but it is advantageous if all or several of the methods have been used in one survey so that comparisons may be made. In Table 56 an attempt is made to lay down some guide lines. A positive result in a majority of these criteria could be taken as an indication for the need for action.

The further question remains: 'Having decided to take action, what form should the action take?' It is hoped that some clues to the answer will be found in the pages of this book.

Table 57 gives a very rough indication of the magnitude of food and nutritional problems on the world scale.

43. MEASURES TO COMBAT MALNUTRITION

Improving nutritive quality

Measures are likely to be most effective if applied to staple foods. Programmes are expensive and have to be carefully controlled. Before they are embarked upon due consideration must be given to whether they will achieve their objective and benefit a considerable proportion of the needy population.

Nutritive quality may be improved in several kinds of ways. Selective breeding, notably of wheat, rice and maize can induce a higher protein content although the amino acid pattern and the physical properties of the protein complex are not necessarily improved at the same time. The enhancement of other qualities, especially yield, may conflict.

The nutritive value of cereals is preserved by processing; notably parboiling and home pounding of rice (p. 19).

Table 56 Suggested criteria for recommending control measures against childhood malnutrition

1. Vital statistics	
infant mortality	> 50/1000 live births
1–4 years mortality	> 10/1000 population of same age
2. Clinical signs	
Frank marasmus, kwashiorkor, xerophthalmia	> 1/100 0–5 years inpatients
Oedema, dermatosis of kwashiorkor	> 5/1000 affected individuals 0 — 5 years field survey
3. Anthropometry	
Weight/length/age	> 20/100 below normal range McLaren and Read 1975
4. Laboratory tests	> 15/100 'low' ICNND standard or >5/100 'deficient' ICNND standards
5. Dietary evalution	> 20/100 below 75 per cent of FAO/WHO recommended allowances

The nutritive value of a processed food may be increased by *enrichment* (restored to what it had been in the raw product), or by *fortification* (increasing nutritive value above that of the raw product).

Thiamin to white rice and several B vitamins and iron to wheat are added for fortification. Lysine fortification of wheat, aimed at combating protein-energy malnutrition, has been abandoned as inappropriate (p.000). Other fortification measures in common use are vitamins A and D to margarine and non-fat dried milk (the latter being an especially important measure where latent vitamin A deficiency accompanies protein-energy malnutrition), iodate to common salt and fluoride to water.

Special groups

Preschool children and to a less extent, pregnant and lactating women, have special nutritional requirements. Partly because of the physiological stress to which they are subject, but also because of ignorance, susceptibility to disease, or taboos they are prone to receive an inadequate diet. School children and workers may have their performance improved considerably by the provision of meals at work.

The measures that need to be taken will be determined by the causes and the nature of the problem. Particularly in the case of preschool child malnutrition it is now recognized that the causes are multifactorial and complex and the problem in most instances concerns inadequate intake to meet energy requirements and not a specific deficiency of protein. Much effort has been misspent on protein rich food mixtures aimed at combating a mythical protein crisis (see Further Reading).

Nutrition education

This can have the effect of making more efficient use of money when it is scarce and also helping to prevent its waste when more abundant. Especially in urbanizing situations many non-food items attract available money and among foods those with prestige associations are preferred. Furthermore, living conditions in towns and cities for the poor are overcrowded and insanitary. The brunt is especially borne by the young child for whom the protection afforded by breast feeding during the first 6 months or more together with supplementary feeding after the first few months is frequently never provided under these circumstances or withdrawn prematurely when the mother goes out to work, becomes pregnant again or is unable to produce enough milk (p. 102). Maternal and child health centres are ideally placed to educate mothers in child feeding practices and in some countries where protein-energy malnutrition is rife special mothercraft centres or nutritional rehabilitation centres have been set up for this purpose. Considerable success, with a modest outlay, has been achieved in rural areas of several countries where through the work of such centres frank malnutrition of the kwashiorkor type in young children has been virtually abolished. However, in rapidly urbanizing communities where the more intractable factors such as overcrowding, bad sanitation and poverty are causal, similar success has not been reported to date and seems unlikely in the absence of total social uplift.

The malnutrition-infection complex

It has been estimated that about 20 million children die annually as a consequence of malnutrition and infection. Almost all are in the third world and 80 per cent are under the age of 2 years. About a quarter of these deaths are due to acute diarrhoeal diseases for which there is no vaccine at present. Immunization is available for six other major childhood infections: measles, diphtheria, pertussis, tetanus, poliomyelitis and tuberculosis and encouraging results of its Expanded Immunization Programme (EPI) have been reported recently by WHO. UNICEF has developed a four-fold strategy towards the control of the complex called GOBI (Growth monitoring, Oral rehydration, Breast feeding, and Immunization).

Health for all by the year 2000

This is the slogan adopted by WHO in its campaign to combat worldwide health problems through primary health care. Improved nutrition, especially of the young child and its mother, is an integral part of this programme. There are some signs that a number of countries in the third world are making considerable progress towards the goal and these can be followed in the annual reports of the Director General of UNICEF *The State of the World's Children*. On the other hand misgivings have been expressed about the enormity of the task and the nature of the approach. References in Further Reading explore these issues fully.

Food and nutrition in a disaster

Disaster, whether due to 'natural' causes such as drought, flood or earthquake; or man-made as a consequence of war and civil strife, results alike through displacement from home and disruption of life, in privation that includes malnutrition and starvation. While a total lack of food can be withstood much longer than exposure to extreme cold and heat or lack of water, it has a bad influence on morale. Consequently some form of nourishment should be provided for victims as soon as possible but the provision of a full diet is not as urgent as some other considerations. Deaths from epidemic diseases far outnumber those from starvation although the latter contributes to the former by decreasing resistance. There have been recent reports from Africa that refeeding of starving people in camps may be associated with the outbreak of malaria and the activation of chronic diseases such as brucellosis and tuberculosis. It has been suggested that improved iron

Table 57 Hunger and malnutrition

Disorder	Nutritional factor(s) involved	Precipitating factors	Major features	Vulnerable groups	Geographic distribution	Numbers affected (v.approx.) at any time
Hunger	All, especially energy sources	Food shortage, poverty	Impaired physical, mental performance	All	Lowest socio-economic group developing countries	1000 million
Protein-energy malnutrition	Protein, energy mainly	Early weaning, gastroenteritis, measles, etc	Retarded physical, mental development, marasmus, kwashiorkor	Infants and preschool children	Marasmus mainly urbanizing developing countries, kwashiorkor mainly Africa	Mild 500 m moderate 100 m severe 10 m
Xerophthalmia	Vitamin A	Rice staple, measles, early weaning	Night blindness, xerosis, keratomalacia, morbidity, mortality	Young children	S & E Asia, parts of M. East, Africa, L.America	250 000 blind/year 10 million Xerosis
Rickets, Osteomalacia	Vitamin D	Unfortified milk, sunlight lack, drugs	Skeletal deformities	Infants, pregnant, aged	Urbanizing developing countries, Asian immigrants to U K	Thousands
Beriberi	Thiamin	Non-parboiled rice, alcoholism	Heart failure, nerve and brain damage	Mainly adults	Parts of Asia, cities of Europe, N.America	Thousands
Pellagra	Niacin	Maize (as porridge)	dermatosis, diarrhoea, dementia	Mainly adults	Parts of Africa M. East, C.India	Uncommon
Scurvy	Vitamin C	Lack of fruit, excess cooking	Haemorrhages, impaired wound healing	Infants, aged	Mainly desert areas	Rare
Iron deficiency	Iron	Prematurity, milk diet, menstruation	Anaemia	Infants, child-bearing period	World wide	100s of millions
Goitre	Iodine	Leached soil, ? goitrogens	Thyroid enlargement, cretinism, deaf mutism	Females	Hill areas of Asia, M. East, L. America	100 million

status might be partly responsible (p.000).

If the food available is not especially deficient in certain nutrients a balanced inanition will be produced by diminished food intake with progressive emaciation as the only obvious clinical sign. Specific deficiency diseases are only likely to become evident if the basic diet is that of an area where these deficiencies have been occurring among the poorest sections of the population in normal times (e.g. total inanition in prisoners of war in Europe, vitamin deficiencies in prisoners of war in Asia, and kwashiorkor in the Nigerian civil war).

Recent experience in Africa shows that early warning systems fail when governments suppress the facts and that voluntary bodies are often more sensitive and effective in reacting to emergencies than governmental agencies. However, as situations become stabilized and become chronic, long-term solutions require continuing local commitment and massive outside support. Despite the unfortunate wealth of experience available now in famine relief and rehabilitation, it is distressing to find that outbreaks of frank deficiency disease, such as nutritional blindness due to vitamin A deficiency, constantly recur as they have in Ethiopia and Sudan recently.

44. FOOD AND NUTRITION POLICY AND PLANNING

It might well be argued that policy making and planning should precede all other considerations in relation to nutrition and the community. In the best of all possible worlds this would indeed be so, but in the world as it is, with nutrition and health — especially of the underprivileged — given very low priority and with the existing paucity of data and lack of control of many determining factors, this holistic approach is unrealistic. A practical balance has to be struck between the enthusiastic, ivory tower day dreaming of planners and the fragmented, sporadic piecemeal interventions of those running the services at the grassroots.

Nutrition, like any subject of academic and practical concern, has gone through phases of waxing and waning enthusiasm for some new emphasis. This is not only natural but has usually proved to be beneficial as sound contributions to knowledge provide a firmer basis for practical solutions to the problems. The effects of malnutrition on the developing nervous system and on the immune response are but two recent examples. Important contributions are to be made to nutritional science by research in other related disciplines. However, when activism has outstripped or ignored nutritional knowledge, as in the ill-fated protein-rich food mixture and amino acid fortification programmes to combat childhood malnutrition, lamentable setbacks occur. The recent interest of economists and planners in the problems of food and nutrition can only be welcomed, but this must be tempered with full acknowledgment of the state of knowledge and a realistic approach to the possibilities for change.

Within the confines of existing realities a positive contribution can result from the application to food and nutrition problems of the recognized steps in any planning sequence. These consist of: (1) definition of the problem, (2) causal analysis, (3) statement of broad objectives, (4) comparison of alternative measures, (5) decision making, (6) implementation of plan and (7) evaluation.

The demise of multisectoral nutrition planning occurred in developing countries over the short period of about a decade from its rise in the early 1970s. The reasons for failure probably lie in such things as an overemphasis on policy itself, its divorce from operational responsibility, the divorce of nutrition from other activities, and an insensitivity to the recipients as people and to the political issues. Lessons should have been learned from these ill-conceived and poorly executed experiences that may permit greater success with intrasectoral activities that are now receiving emphasis, in which nutrition is being treated as an integral part of agricultural development and of primary health care.

Although western governments and agencies have become heavily involved in nutrition planning for developing countries there is only one western country that has so far put its own national nutrition policy into effect; this is Norway about a decade ago. There are special reasons why it could happen in this small country and is unlikely to take place elsewhere (see Further Reading). It is doubtful, too, whether it can ever be proved satisfactorily to have been directly responsible for any improvement in health; there are too many other unknown and uncontrollable variables. Further-more, it is questionable whether enough is known about the role of diet in disease for sweeping statements to be made concerning desirable eating for the majority of the healthy population. For example, it has been estimated that as much as 80 per cent of the variance is unaccounted for by the known risk factors in the aetiology of coronary heart disease. Then again, there is very little agreement among the experts as to what recommendations to make to the public. Moreover there is inevitably strong pressure brought to bear by any threatened segment of the powerful food industry and of the agricultural lobby when dietary modification is proposed at an official level.

In 1977 Dietary Goals for the United States were promulgated; the six main goals being:

1. Increase carbohydrate (as complex carbohydrate) to 55 to 60 per cent of the energy intake.

2. Reduce overall fat consumption from present 40 per cent to 30 per cent of energy intake.

3. Reduce saturated fat to 10 per cent of dietary intake and balance with 10 per cent non-saturated and 10 per cent polyunsaturated fats (all as percentage total energy).

4. Reduce dietary cholesterol to 300 mg per day.

5. Reduce refined sugar consumption to 15 per cent of dietary energy.

6. Reduce salt consumption to approximately 3 g per day.

This approach is still largely directed to the nutritionists rather than the public as it is framed in terms of nutrients and not items of food. In Britain

Table 58 Facets of malnutrition — infection interrelationships

	Effects	Remarks
Malnutrition	Impaired cell-mediated immunity (CMI)	Especially kwashiorkor; vitamin A deficiency
	Impaired humoral immunity	Less than CMI
	Damage to epithelial barriers to infection	Especially vitamin A deficiency
	Damage to intestinal mucosa, also microbial contamination of small intestine	Causing malabsorption
Infections	Anorexia	Causing diminished intake
	Pyrexia	Increasing requirements
	Malabsorption	Due to damage especially by enteroinvasive bacteria and enteroviruses
	Increased secretion	
	Protein-losing enteropathy	

this further step has been taken, albeit at an unofficial level, by a prescription for a better British diet (see Further Reading). It is based on economic as well as nutritional considerations and recommends that trends over the next decade or so should proceed long the following lines (it may be added that such trends are indeed taking place, although there is no indication yet one way or the other as to what the consequences may be):

Decreased consumption: Fats and oils, sugar, meat — all by 15 per cent
Alcohol by 25 per cent

Increased consumption: Potatoes, other vegetables, fruit — all by 15 per cent
Grain products by 20 per cent

No change: dairy products (excluding butter), fish, eggs, pulses (and nuts).

It has often been claimed that dietary changes have been largely responsible for the marked reduction in deaths from coronary heart disease over the past 20 years in the United States. However, there are a number of facts against this interpretation (p. 207).

At the end of 1987 in the UK affairs in this area are in a most unsatisfactory state. In summary, the NACNE (National Advisory Committee on Nutrition Education) report which appeared in 1983 failed to gain government approval as a result of pressure that was brought to bear. It was followed in 1984 by a COMA (Committee on Medical Aspects of Food Policy) report on diet and cardiovascular disease in which its principal recommendation concerning fat intake differed from that in the NACNE report and that of WHO. Although many nutritionists are disappointed that these attempts to implement some kind of nutrition policy have foundered, others are relieved, believing that the moves were premature in our present state of considerable ignorance.

MULTIPLE CHOICE QUESTIONS

Answer each question true *or* false.

1. In connection with world food supplies:
   i) a 5 per cent increase in population necessitates an 8 per cent increase in food supply
   ii) bringing more land under cultivation is the main method to feed more people in the future
   iii) 90 per cent of low income people in the most densely populated places have rice as staple
   iv) technologically developed countries have 10 per cent of the world's population and consume 30 per cent of the food
   v) the major constraint on increased food consumption of low income families is their low purchasing power.

2. Concerning population and food:
   i) the projected population growth rate is twice as high in less developed regions compared with more developed regions
   ii) population density tends to correlate with food supply
   iii) prolonged breast feeding has a greater contraceptive effect than all artificial measures
   iv) population control and family planning are synonymous
   v) GNP gives an indication of distribution of wealth in a country.

3. Concerning nutritional assessment in a community:
   i) infant mortality is considerably influenced by the occurrence of marasmus
   ii) cause of death records reflect quite well death rates due to malnutrition
   iii) stunting is reflected by height/age
   iv) scarlet raw tongue often indicates niacin deficiency
   v) glutathione peroxidase activity measures riboflavin status.

4. Concerning measures to combat malnutrition:
   i) lysine fortification of wheat is currently used to combat PEM
   ii) about 20 million children die annually from malnutrition-infection complex
   iii) contraception is part of the GOBI program of UNICEF
   iv) diarrhoeal diseases are covered by UNICEF's immunization programe
   v) refeeding of starving populations may lead to outbreaks of infection.

5. Food and nutrition policy and planning:
   i) of a holistic type is no longer advocated
   ii) has been adopted by only one government, that of the USA
   iii) rests on a sound footing of scientific knowledge

iv) in the US Dietary Goals of 1977 included restriction of overall fat consumption to 30 per cent of total energy

v) generally states that the average intake of a community in the west of salt should be lowered and that of fibre increased.

Explanation and answers on page 286.

FURTHER READING

39. Introduction
Berg A 1973 The nutrition factor: its role in national development. Brookings Institute, Washington DC
George S 1976 How the other half dies: the real reasons for world hunger. Penguin, Harmondsworth
McLaren D S (ed) 1983 Nutrition in the community 2nd edn. Wiley, Chichester

40. World food supplies
Jennings P R 1974 Rice breeding and world food production. Science 186: 1085
Pirie N W 1969 Food resources, convential and novel. Penguin, Harmondsworth
Scientific American 1976 Food and Agriculture 235: no 3

41. Population and food
Food and Agriculture Organization 1983 World system of information and rapid alert on food and agriculture. FAO, Rome
Scientific American 1974 The human population 231: no 3

42. Nutritional assessment and surveillance
Habicht J-P, Mason J 1983 Nutritional surveillance. In McLaren D S (ed) Nutrition in the community, 2nd edn. Wiley, Chichester
Joint FAO/UNICEF/WHO Expert Committee 1976 Methodology of nutritional surveillance. WHO Technical Report Series no 593. WHO, Geneva
Sauberlich H E, Dowdy R P, Skala J H 1977 Laboratory tests for the assessment of nutritional status, 2nd edn. CRC Press, Cleveland
United States Department of Health, Education and Welfare 1972 Ten-State Nutrition Survey 1968-70, NEW Publication no (HSM) 72-8134. HEW, Washington DC

43. Measures to combat malnutrition
Bryant J 1969 Health and the developing world. Cornell University Press, Ithaca
Chen L C 1986 Primary health care in developing countries: overcoming operational, technical, and social barriers. Lancet ii: 1260-1265
Gracey M (ed) 1986 Diarrhoeal disease and malnutrition: a clinical update. Churchill Livingstone, Edinburgh
Kielmann A A, Taylor C E, Parker R L 1978 The Narangwal nutrition study: a summary review. American Journal of Clinical Nutrition 31, 2040-2052
Latham M C 1982 Control of malnutrition In: McLaren D S, Burman D (eds) Textbook of paediatric nutrition, 2nd edn. Churchill Livingstone, London, p 364
Navarro V 1986 A critique of the ideological and political positions of the Willy Brandt Report and the WHO Alma Ata Declaration. In: Crisis, health and medicine. Tavistock, New York
Williams C D, Jelliffe D B 1972 Mother and child health: delivering the services. Oxford University Press, Oxford

44. Food and nutrition planning
Berg A, Scrimshaw NS, Call D L (eds) 1973 Nutrition, national development and planning. MIT Press, Cambridge, Mass
deVille de Goyer C, Seaman J, Geiger U 1978 The management of nutritional emergencies in large populations. WHO, Geneva

Field J O 1977 The soft underbelly of applied knowledge: conceptual and operational problems in nutrition planning. Food Policy 2: 228

Food and Agriculture Organization 1969 Manual on food and nutrition policy. FAO Nutritional Series, no 22. FAO, Rome

McLaren D S 1974 The great protein fiasco. Lancet 2: 93

McLaren D S 1977 Nutrition planning: the poverty of holism. Nature 267: 742

McLaren D S 1978 Nutrition planning day dreams at the United Nations. American Journal of Clinical Nutrition 31: 1295

National Advisory Committee on Nutritional Education 1983 Proposals for nutritional guidelines for health education in Britain. Health Education Council, London

Townsend P, Davidson N (eds) 1982 Inequalities in health. Penguin, London

ANSWERS TO MULTIPLE CHOICE QUESTIONS

It is customary when marking MCQs to give one mark for a correct answer, to deduct one mark for an incorrect answer, and to give no mark for a question not attempted.

It is often considered that with this system of marking a total mark of 50 out of 100 (or a similar proportion) is a pass mark.

The questions given here are in no way intended to be comprehensive, but rather to serve as an indication as to how other suitable questions might be formulated.

Answers

Section I

1. F, F, F, T, F
2. T, T, F, T, F
3. T, F, T, T, F
4. T, F, T, F, F
5. F, T, F, F, F

Section II

1. F, T, F, F, T
2. T, T, F, F, T
3. F, F, T, T, T
4. F, T, T, T, F
5. T, F, T, T, F

Section III

1. F, F, T, F, F
2. F, T, F, T, F
3. F, T, T, T, F
4. F, T, T, F, T
5. T, F, T, F, T

Section IV

1. F, T, T, T, F
2. F, T, T, T, T
3. T, F, F, T, T
4. T, F, F, T, T
5. T, F, T, T, F

Section V

1. T, F, T, F, T
2. T, F, T, F, F
3. T, F, T, T, F
4. F, T, F, F, T
5. T, F, F, T, T

Index